D1378011

HORMONE THERAPY
IN BREAST AND PROSTATE CANCER

CANCER DRUG DISCOVERY AND DEVELOPMENT

Beverly A. Teicher, *Series Editor*

HORMONE THERAPY IN BREAST AND PROSTATE CANCER

Edited by

V. CRAIG JORDAN

Robert H. Lurie Comprehensive Cancer Center, Northwestern University, Chicago, IL

and

BARRINGTON J. A. FURR

AstraZeneca Pharmaceuticals, Macclesfield, UK

Foreword by ELWOOD V. JENSEN

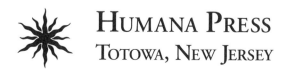

HUMANA PRESS
TOTOWA, NEW JERSEY

Due diligence has been taken by the publishers, editors, and authors of this book to assure the accuracy of the information published and to describe generally accepted practices. The contributors herein have carefully checked to ensure that the drug selections and dosages set forth in this text are accurate and in accord with the standards accepted at the time of publication. Notwithstanding, as new research, changes in government regulations, and knowledge from clinical experience relating to drug therapy and drug reactions constantly occurs, the reader is advised to check the product information provided by the manufacturer of each drug for any change in dosages or for additional warnings and contraindications. This is of utmost importance when the recommended drug herein is a new or infrequently used drug. It is the responsibility of the treating physician to determine dosages and treatment strategies for individual patients. Further it is the responsibility of the health care provider to ascertain the Food and Drug Administration status of each drug or device used in their clinical practice. The publisher, editors, and authors are not responsible for errors or omissions or for any consequences from the application of the information presented in this book and make no warranty, express or implied, with respect to the contents in this publication.

This publication is printed on acid-free paper. ∞
ANSI Z39.48-1984 (American National Standards Institute) Permanence of Paper for Printed Library Materials.

Cover Design by: Patricia F. Cleary.

Production Editor: Mark J. Breaugh.

Photocopy Authorization Policy:
Authorization to photocopy items for internal or personal use, or the internal or personal use of specific clients, is granted by Humana Press Inc., provided that the base fee of US $10.00 per copy, plus US $00.25 per page, is paid directly to the Copyright Clearance Center at 222 Rosewood Drive, Danvers, MA 01923. For those organizations that have been granted a photocopy license from the CCC, a separate system of payment has been arranged and is acceptable to Humana Press Inc. The fee code for users of the Transactional Reporting Service is: [0-89603-673-1/02 $10.00 + $00.25].

Printed in the United States of America. 10 9 8 7 6 5 4 3 2 1

Library of Congress Cataloging-in-Publication Data

Hormone therapy in breast and prostate cancer / edited by V. Craig Jordan and
Barrington J. A. Furr.
     p. ; cm.
  Includes bibliographical references and index.
  ISBN 0-89603-673-1 (alk. paper)
    1. Breast--Cancer--Hormone therapy. 2. Prostate--Cancer--Hormone therapy. 3.
Estrogen--Antagonists--therapeutic use. 4. Antiandrogens--therapeutic use. I. Jordan,
V. Craig (Virgil Craig) II. Furr, B. J. A.
    [DNLM: 1. Breast Neoplasms--drug therapy. 2. Prostatic Neoplasms--drug therapy. 3.
Androgen Antagonists--therapeutic use. 4. Antineoplastic Agents, Hormonal--therapeutic
use. 5. Selective Estrogen Receptor Modulators--therapeutic use. 6.
Tamoxifen--therapeutic use. WP 870 E557 2001]
RC280.B8 E523 2001
616.99'449061--dc21

WP
870
E557
2002

FOREWORD

It has been said that the control of disease has three goals, which, in increasing order of attraction are palliation, cure, and prevention. For most types of disseminated cancer, medical science has achieved only the first of these objectives, while for some malignancies the side effects of the therapeutic agents employed rival the disease itself in precluding a desirable quality of life. In contrast, those cancers of the breast and prostate that retain the hormone dependency of the tissue of origin, and thus are sensitive to endocrine manipulation, offer a more favorable situation for control. *Hormone Therapy in Breast and Prostate Cancer* takes the reader on a fascinating scientific journey that illustrates how the combination of clinical and basic investigations has realized the first two objectives for both of these prevalent malignancies and, with breast cancer, the promise of being close to the third goal.

Our endocrinological tour begins with the surgeons, who, more than a century ago, with remarkable insight at a time when estrogenic hormones were still unknown, excised the ovaries of premenopausal women with advanced breast cancer, causing tumor regression in some patients. Forty-five years later, after animal experiments had established that the growth of the prostate gland depends on androgenic hormone produced by the testes, it was shown that removal of these organs leads to striking remissions in most men with disseminated prostate cancer. Subsequently, it was found that some, but not all, postmenopausal women with metastatic breast cancer respond favorably to excision of either the pituitary or adrenal glands. For those patients with tumors of the hormone-dependent type, the remissions obtained by endocrine ablation were superior to those provided by cytotoxic chemotherapy, and, during the 1950s and 1960s, surgical removal of the sex hormone-producing organs became the standard therapeutic approach for treating advanced breast and prostatic neoplasia.

Despite the benefit derived from endocrine ablation in many patients with hitherto untreatable disease, these procedures are not perfect. Although most prostatic cancers respond to castration, only one-third of all breast cancer patients have tumors that are hormone-dependent. Thus, most patients with mammary cancer were being subjected to a non-reversible surgical procedure that did not help them. Moreover, those undergoing adrenalectomy or hypophysectomy required the continual administration of glucocorticoids for their maintenance.

As described in the chapters that follow, a combination of research in chemistry, biochemistry, physiology, and pharmacology has provided alternative approaches to the therapy of breast and prostate cancer that have eliminated most of the disadvantages associated with surgical removal of the hormone factories. Elucidation of the pathways of estrogen and androgen biosynthesis led to the discovery of compounds that block their production, and identification of substances from the pituitary that control the factories has permitted the development of antagonists of their action. The demonstration that estrogens, and later androgens, exert their stimulatory effects in combination with specific receptor proteins explained the ability of certain compounds to block hormone action at the target cell level and offered a rational means for finding improved antagonists that compete with the hormone for binding to the receptor. Finally, analysis of the estrogen receptor content of excised tumor specimens permitted the identification of those breast cancers that will not respond to either endocrine ablation

v

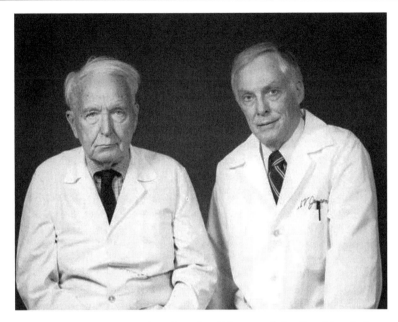

Nobel Laureate Dr. Charles Huggins, founding Director of the Ben May Laboratory for Cancer Research (left), and Dr. Elwood Jensen, his successor (right).

or antiestrogen therapy, thus excluding the majority of patients from therapeutic procedures that will not help them.

Not only have antiestrogens replaced surgical ablation as first-line treatment for advanced breast cancer, as well as for adjuvant therapy at the time of mastectomy, but recent clinical trials indicate that certain of these agents, such as tamoxifen, that are tolerated on prolonged administration can prevent the occurrence of breast cancer, at least in high-risk individuals. Thus, for this malignancy, one seems close to achieving the third and most elusive goal of cancer control, that of prevention.

When one surveys the development of tamoxifen and related antiestrogens as therapeutic and, possibly, preventive agents for breast cancer, one is impressed by the insight, fortitude, and persistence of the scientist whom we all recognize as the father of the clinical utility of tamoxifen. This was all the more remarkable given the disastrous experience of others with the side effects of certain earlier antiestrogens. To illustrate the progress that has been made over the past thirty years, it may be appropriate to dedicate the following thought to Craig Jordan:

> "A lady with growth neoplastic
> Thought ablation was just a bit drastic.
> She preferred that her ill
> Could be cured with a pill,
> Which today is no longer fantastic."

Elwood V. Jensen
Professor Emeritus
University of Chicago

PREFACE

There is enormous public interest in the successful use of endocrine therapy for the treatment of cancer. Newspapers and magazines daily extol the virtues of one product versus another. Tamoxifen is a household name and millions of people are now taking hormone antagonists in one form or another. This is the reason for writing this book.

We have lived through a revolution of translational research that, we believe, can be used as a model for future progress. The principle was simple—find a target in the cancer cell and attack a critical pathway for growth. But at the start, there was no guarantee of success. History is lived forward, but written in retrospect. We know the end before we describe the beginning and so we can never really recapture what it was like.

Thirty years ago, when we were starting our careers in endocrinology and pharmacology, the treatment of breast and prostate cancer was very different from what it is today. Patients were treated in the later stages of the disease based on clinical observations and experience accumulated over three generations. Strategies were not mechanism-based, although translational research had been important in defining the role of the ovaries and the testes in the growth of breast and prostate cancer, respectively.

In the case of breast cancer, radical mastectomy was the standard of care, with radiation therapy available to control recurrences. Advanced breast cancer was showing encouraging responses to combination chemotherapy, which led to the widespread belief among the medical community (that is still held by many today) that the appropriate cocktail of new and powerful chemotherapies would be found that would cure cancer. Adjuvant chemotherapy was not an option because the concept of destroying the last micrometastasis after "curative" surgery had not yet evolved into the lexicon of clinical trials. Although hormonal therapy had fewer side effects than any of the chemotherapies, the clinical studies in the 1950s and 1960s had proven, to the satisfaction of nearly everyone, that endocrine therapy was not a useful path for clinical investigation. High dose estrogen or androgen therapy showed advantages for about a year in one third of postmenopausal women with metastatic disease. Diethylstilbestrol produced higher response rates in prostate cancer, but most patients relapsed and many had serious cardiovascular complications caused by the therapy. The medical and scientific community concluded that hormonal approaches could not provide any long-term benefits for patients. Rather than adding high doses of hormones, the other strategy was endocrine ablation to remove the ovaries, adrenal glands, or the pituitary gland. These approaches could be life-threatening and, more often than not, did not produce any beneficial response for the patient. Clearly, a test was needed to predict who to treat successfully, thereby avoiding unnecessary surgery.

The treatment of prostate cancer was also empiric. Although Professor Charles Huggins had received the Nobel Prize in 1966 for his contributions to the endocrine control of prostate cancer, it is fair to say that basic research on prostate cancer was at least a decade behind breast cancer research at this time. Nevertheless, the seeds for success had been sown that would develop into a molecular approach to drug treatment in the 1970s.

Elwood Jensen synthesized the first high specific activity tritiated estradiol and showed that it was localized and retained in the estrogen target tissues of immature rats. Jensen proposed the existence of an estrogen receptor (ER) that modulated estrogen action within different target cells. He thus established the molecular foundation for steroid endocrinology. But perhaps of greater importance, he also translated this knowledge to propose that the ER assay would predict the response of breast cancer patients to endocrine ablation. However, the concept that the presence of ER would predict endocrine responsiveness only became widely accepted following an NCI conference in Bethesda in 1974. Jensen had solved the important issue of targeting ablative therapy to those who were most likely to respond but perhaps more important, in our view, he identified a target for rational drug discovery. Unfortunately, in 1970, there was little or no enthusiasm for drug development in this area.

The first nonsteroidal antiestrogen was discovered serendipitously in the 1950s by Leonard Lerner and associates at the William S. Merrill Company, Cincinnati, but the analogs were not developed for cancer therapy because of toxicological concerns. One compound, clomiphene, was developed to induce ovulation in subfertile women, but the original enthusiasm that nonsteroidal antiestrogens would be effective "morning after" contraceptives had waned by the late 1960s. No one was suggesting research in antiestrogens as the way to a successful career. However, Arthur Walpole and Dora Richardson working at the laboratories of ICI Pharmaceuticals (now AstraZeneca) in Alderley Park, Cheshire, discovered a novel series of triphenylethylenes with reduced toxicity. In the patents, it was recognized that the drugs had the potential to regulate the reproductive cycle and to treat hormone-dependent cancers. The latter application alone, if it were achieved, would be a major advance as there would now be little need for ablative surgery. Walpole was the head of the Fertility Control Program at ICI Pharmaceuticals throughout the 1960s and his work provided the basis for the development of tamoxifen for the induction of ovulation and for the treatment of advanced breast cancer in the 1970s. Unfortunately, Walpole died in July 1977 and never saw the full application of the results of his discoveries. He was an outstanding individual who was responsible not only for antiestrogens but also for the investigation of drugs that regulated gonadotrophin release. His contributions were essential to the progress we see today in the endocrine treatment of both breast and prostate cancer.

We are, therefore, both beneficiaries of Walpole's legacy. Walpole played an important role in our careers by encouraging us to develop our own ideas. One of us (VCJ) experienced Walpole "the PhD thesis examiner" in 1972 for a study

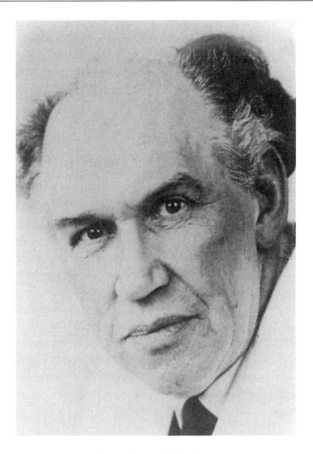

Dr. Arthur L. Walpole

of the structure activity relationships of nonsteroidal antiestrogens at Leeds University. Walpole subsequently approved the resources to conduct the first laboratory studies of tamoxifen (then ICI 46,474) as a treatment and preventative for breast cancer in laboratory animals. These studies by VCJ were conducted at the Worcester Foundation between 1972 and 1974 so the results could be used to support clinical trials in the United States. Also, with the help of Elwood Jensen, then Director of the Ben May Laboratories at the University of Chicago, studies showed that tamoxifen blocked estradiol binding to human ER. Walpole subsequently strongly supported a Joint Research Scheme between Leeds University (VCJ) and ICI Pharmaceuticals (1975–1979). The results of this collaboration identified the potential of antiestrogens with high affinity for ER and the relationship between duration of tamoxifen treatment and the effectiveness of the antitumor actions. This was a key discovery for the future clinical application of tamoxifen as an adjuvant therapy.

One of us (BJAF) was recruited to ICI Pharmaceuticals in 1972 by Arthur Walpole to work in the Reproductive Endocrinology Group. His leadership and encouragement led to the discovery, with Dr. Anand Dutta, of the LHRH agonist, Zoladex, and its depot formulation with Dr. Frank Hutchinson. Although Walpole also supported strongly the antiandrogen project that led to the discovery of what is currently the leading antiandrogen, Casodex, sadly he did not live to see this triumph either.

Today, tamoxifen has reached it full potential as an endocrine agent used to treat all stages of breast cancer. Millions of women with breast cancer have benefited from the use of tamoxifen. Long-term adjuvant tamoxifen therapy is proven to save lives, and it can be estimated that 400,000 women are alive today because of this appropriate treatment strategy. The recognition that tamoxifen was becoming a "treatment of choice" encouraged the subsequent development of selective aromatase inhibitors and pure antiestrogens and pioneered the development of a whole new drug class: the selective estrogen receptor modulators (SERMs) to treat osteoporosis and to test in the prevention of coronary heart disease and breast cancer.

The lessons learned with tamoxifen were applied to prostate cancer with the development of nonsteroidal antiandrogens and luteinizing hormone releasing hormone (LHRH) superagonists to interrupt gonadotrophin release. These latter agents are used to treat both breast and prostate cancer.

The chapters in *Hormone Therapy in Breast and Prostate Cancer* describe the laboratory and clinical development of concepts that are now successfully applied for the treatment of breast and prostate cancer. We are pleased to thank our friends and colleagues who have contributed to the chapters and created a balance of history, laboratory discovery, and clinical practice. Our book is offered as a foundation and guide to progress for researchers and clinicians alike.

The clinical progress during the past three decades would not have happened but for the conceptual shift in reasoning that occurred in the early 1970s. The central role of steroid receptors in our story was the direct result of Elwood Jensen's seminal studies in translational research. We are honored that Professor Jensen generously agreed to write the Foreword for our book.

V. Craig Jordan
Barrington J. A. Furr

CONTENTS

Contributors

ROGER W. BLAMEY • *Professorial Unit of Surgery, Nottingham City Hospital, Nottingham, UK*

JASON S. CARROLL • *Cancer Research Program, Garvan Institute of Medical Research, St. Vincent's Hospital, Darlinghurst, Australia*

MITCHELL DOWSETT • *Academic Department of Biochemistry, Royal Marsden Hospital, London, UK*

YVONNE P. DRAGAN • *School of Public Health, Ohio State University, Columbus, OH*

MICHAEL DUKES • *Academic Department of Biochemistry, Royal Marsden Hospital, London, UK*

GALE M. ENGLAND • *Northwestern University Medical Program, Chicago, IL*

ROBIN FUCHS-YOUNG • *Department of Carcinogenesis, The University of Texas M.D. Anderson Cancer Center, Science Park Research Division, Smithville, TX*

JUNICHI FUKUCHI • *The Ben May Institute for Cancer Research and the Department of Biochemistry and Molecular Biology, University of Chicago, Chicago, IL*

BARRINGTON J. A. FURR • *AstraZeneca Pharmaceuticals, Mereside, Alderley Park, Macclesfield, Cheshire, UK*

PAUL E. GOSS • *The Toronto Hospital-General Division, Toronto, ON, Canada*

WILLIAM J. GRADISHAR • *The Robert H. Lurie Comprehensive Cancer Center, Division of Hematology/Oncology, Department of Medicine, Northwestern University Medical Program, Chicago, IL*

V. CRAIG JORDAN • *Northwestern University Medical Program, Chicago, IL*

AMIR V. KAISARY • *The Royal Free Hospital NHS Trust and School of Medicine, London, UK*

YUNG-HSI KAO • *The Ben May Institute for Cancer Research and the Department of Biochemistry and Molecular Biology, University of Chicago, Chicago, IL*

GEERT J. C. M. KOLVENBAG • *AstraZeneca Pharmaceuticals, Wilmington, DE*

ANAIT S. LEVENSON • *Northwestern University Medical Program, Chicago, IL*

SHUTSUNG LIAO • *The Ben May Institute for Cancer Research and the Department of Biochemistry and Molecular Biology, University of Chicago, Chicago, IL*

MONICA MORROW • *Lynn Sage Breast Cancer Research Program, Northwestern University Medical School, Chicago, IL*

HENRY D. MUENZNER • *Northwestern University Medical Program, Chicago, IL*

ELIZABETH A. MUSGROVE • *Cancer Research Program, Garvan Institute of Medical Research, St. Vincent's Hospital, Darlinghurst, Australia*

RUTH M. O'REGAN • *The Robert H. Lurie Comprehensive Cancer Center, Division of Hematology/Oncology, Department of Medicine, Northwestern University Medical Program, Chicago, IL*

DAVID H. PHILLIPS • *Institute of Cancer Research, Haddow Laboratories, Sutton, Surrey, UK*

HENRY C. PITOT • *Departments of Oncology and of Pathology and Laboratory Medicine, McArdle Laboratory for Cancer Research, University of Wisconsin Medical School, Madison, WI*

OWEN W. J. PRALL • *Cancer Research Program, Garvan Institute of Medical Research, St. Vincent's Hospital, Darlinghurst, Australia*

ALBERT RADLMAIER • *Clinical Development Oncology, Schering AG, Berlin, Germany*

CAROLINE C. REID • *The Toronto Hospital-General Division, Toronto, ON, Canada*

EILEEN M. ROGAN • *Cancer Research Program, Garvan Institute of Medical Research, St. Vincent's Hospital, Darlinghurst, Australia*

FRITZ H. SCHRÖDER • *Department of Urology, Erasmus University and Academic Hospital Rotterdam, Rotterdam, The Netherlands*

K. SHENTON • *Academic Department of Biochemistry, Royal Marsden Hospital, London, UK*

ROBERT L. SUTHERLAND • *Cancer Research Program, Garvan Institute of Medical Research, St. Vincent's Hospital, Darlinghurst, Australia*

HIROYUKI TAKEI • *Second Department of Surgery, Gunma University School of Medicine, Maebashi, Japan*

A. E. WAKELING • *AstraZeneca Pharmaceuticals, Mereside, Alderley Park, Macclesfield, Cheshire, UK*

COLIN K. W. WATTS • *Cancer Research Program, Garvan Institute of Medical Research, St. Vincent's Hospital, Darlinghurst, Australia*

NICHOLAS R. C. WILCKEN • *Cancer Research Program, Garvan Institute of Medical Research, St. Vincent's Hospital, Darlinghurst, Australia*

KATHY A. YAO • *Northwestern University Medical Program, Chicago, IL*

1

An Introduction to the
Regulation of Sex Steroids
for the Treatment of Cancer

V. Craig Jordan and Barrington J.A. Furr

CONTENTS

1. INTRODUCTION

The reduction of circulating steroid hormones or the blockade of steroid action in cancer tissue are primary goals in the current strategy of breast- and prostate-cancer treatment. Antiestrogens, antiandrogens, aromatase inhibitors, and highly potent luteinizing hormone-releasing hormone (LH-RH) agonists (used to desensitize the pituitary gland and perform a "medical hypophysec-tomy") are all drugs that have been proven to be valuable cancer treatments over the past two decades. However, the knowledge that there is a link between sex steroids and growth of some breast and prostate tumors has taken a century to piece together.

In 1896, George Beatson [1] reported that some premenopausal women with inoperable advanced breast cancer could benefit from the removal of the ovaries. Beatson based his strategy on the knowledge that the histology of mammary tissue could be affected in rabbits or farm animals by spaying. One could argue that these data, from a single physician, were the first successful attempt to conduct translational research in breast cancer. In a similar vein, Stanley Boyd at the Charing Cross Hospital could be said to have performed the first "clinical trials overview" of the effect of oophorectomy to treat advanced breast cancer in premenopausal women. Boyd collected information on 54

From: *Hormone Therapy in Breast and Prostate Cancer*
Edited by: V. C. Jordan and B. J. A. Furr © Humana Press Inc., Totowa, NJ

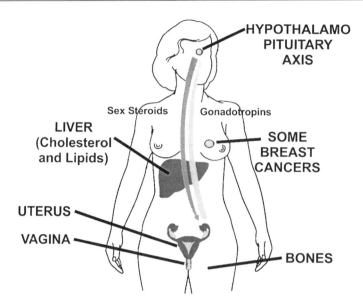

Fig. 1. Estrogen-target tissues around a women's body. The appreciation of the regulation of menstrual cycle and the mechanism of estrogen action has been key to the use of nonsteroidal antiestrogens in the treatment and prevention of breast cancer.

patients who had undergone oophorectomy and found that about 30% had an objective response to the procedure *(2)*. This important result has defined the response rate of advanced breast cancer to any good single agent endocrine therapy since that time. The identification of individual tumors that were more likely to respond to endocrine therapy did not become a clinical reality until the 1970s. In the late 1950s, Jensen discovered the estrogen receptor (ER) *(3)* and proposed a predictive test for hormone-responsive breast cancer based on the identification of ER in tumors *(4)* (Fig. 1). However, if the receptor is the target for antihormonal therapy, the evolving understanding of hormone synthesis and action has also played a pivotal role in current treatment.

The discovery of an estrogenic principle in the follicular fluid of pig ovaries by Allen and Doisy in 1923 *(5)* was a major breakthrough that proved to be invaluable in all future research endeavors in the area. Allen and Doisy established a vaginal-cornification assay in ovariectomized mice to identify estrogenic compounds *(5)* and Doisy subsequently crystallized the first steroid hormone estrone in 1929 *(6)*.

Historically, the vaginal cornification assay was important to identify synthetic estrogens during the 1930s *(7–9)* and was used to demonstrate the potency of the synthetic nonsteroidal estrogen diethylstilbestrol (DES) by Sir Charles Dodds *(10)*. High doses of DES were subsequently used for the successful treatment of both prostate *(11)* and breast cancer *(12)*. This work was pioneering because the reported success of pharmacological doses of a synthetic estrogen heralded the era of chemotherapy for cancer. The mechanism of action of DES in suppressing growth of prostate cancer was clear: it prevented secretion of luteinizing hormone from the pituitary gland, which consequently led to a fall in androgen secretion from the testes. In essence, this produced the first medical castration. Although the actual mechanism of action of high-dose estrogen is obscure in the case of breast-cancer treatment, the therapeutic approach proposed by Professor Paul Erhlich at the turn of the century that a drug could be synthesized to produce selective toxicity on bacteria *(13)*, now became a reality for cancer. However, a full understanding of steroidogenesis and the control of the reproductive system was necessary before a logical strategy of targeted drug development could be fully implemented.

The discovery that the pulsatile release of a small peptide, known as LH-RH, regulates the secretion of luteinizing and follicle-stimulating hormones (FSH) was initially viewed therapeutically as a way to induce ovulation in infertile women and stimulate spermatogenesis and androgen production in infertile men *(14)*. However, the finding that the pituitary gland becomes rapidly desensitized by prolonged stimulation with LH-RH raised the possibility that contraceptive agents could be developed *(14)*. Sustained release preparations of highly potent LH-RH agonist analogs effectively produce a medical oophorectomy and stop ovarian-estrogen synthesis in women and testicular-androgen synthesis in men *(15)*. The application of sustained release preparations used to treat premenopausal breast cancer and prostate cancer is now known to be an effective therapy, thereby avoiding surgical procedures and endocrine ablation *(16,17)*.

Breast-cancer incidence increases with age, but the same proportion of postmenopausal women respond to endocrine therapy as premenopausal women. The ovaries are the primary site for estrogen synthesis but significant levels of estrogen are produced by postmenopausal women. The adrenal glands are an important site for steroidogenesis. Huggins and Bergenstal *(18)* found that adrenalectomy, with maintenance of patients on cortisone acetate, could cause some regression of late advanced breast and prostate cancer. Hypophysectomy *(19,20)* was also effective but morbidity was high and patients again had to be maintained on corticoids. In fact, high doses of corticoids alone were also able to control adrenal steroidogenesis. However, the finding that the steroid androstenedione was converted to estrone *(21,22)* in postmenopausal women and that there was significant local production of estrogens by aromatization in breast cancers *(23,24)*, provided a rationale to explain the efficacy of inhibitors of aromatization as therapeutic agents in breast cancer *(25–27)*.

If estrogen and androgen are essential to cause the growth of breast and prostate cancer, then antagonist drugs that block hormone action would be valuable therapeutic agents. The discovery of antiestrogens built on the extensive knowledge that nonsteroidal estrogens could be identified rationally *(7–9)*. Lerner and coworkers *(28)* reported the first nonsteroidal antiestrogen, MER25 in 1958. This simple triphenylethanol had only antiestrogenic actions and no other hormonal or antihormonal properties. However, MER25 was too toxic for clinical use and analogues of the estrogen triphenylethylene were investigated. Harper and Walpole *(29)* reported that ICI 46,474 (tamoxifen) was a potent antiestrogen in the rat and this was pursued as a treatment for advanced breast cancer *(30)*. Today, tamoxifen is the endocrine treatment of choice for all stages of breast cancer and the first drug to be approved (in the United States) for the reduction of the incidence of breast cancer in high-risk women *(31,32)*.

The world-wide success of tamoxifen encouraged a close examination of the mechanism of action. The discovery of the ER by Jensen *(3)* and the proposal to use the ER assay to identify women who were more likely to respond to a hormonal treatment played a fundamental conceptual role in the use of tamoxifen to treat breast cancer. It is now known that tamoxifen is more likely to enhance the survival of women with ER-positive tumors *(31)* and prevents the development of ER-positive breast cancer *(32)*. However, the discovery of selective ER modulation with tamoxifen and keoxifene (now called raloxifene) in the laboratory *(33,34)* and the demonstration that tamoxifen and raloxifene have estrogen-like effects on bone *(35)* but antiestrogenic effect on the breast has opened the door to new opportunities for the discovery of novel compounds to treat a number of diseases associated with the menopause such as osteoporosis, coronary heart disease, and breast and endometrial cancers *(34–37)*.

New knowledge about estrogen action has been advanced by the sequencing and cloning of the ER *(38–39)* and the discovery of a new ER *(40)* that modulates estrogen action in different tissues around the body of both males and females. The classical ER is referred to as ERα and the new receptor is ERβ (Fig. 2). What is particularly interesting is the fact that ERβ was discovered by examining a cDNA library from rat prostate and that it appears to act antagonistically to the classical ERα. The tools of molecular biology have demonstrated that the endocrinology of the different sexes can be interrelated at the subcellular level.

Considerable effort is now focused on attempts to improve further response rates and duration of remission in breast cancer by other endocrine maneuvres. Depot administration of the LH-RH agonist, Zoladex, was shown to be as effective as combination cytotoxic chemotherapy in premenopausal women with ER-positive breast cancer and was much better tolerated in the ZEBRA trial *(41,42)*. Combination of LH-RH agonists with tamoxifen gives greater efficacy in pre-peri-menopausal breast-cancer patients than either agent alone *(43–45)*.

The newer aromatase inhibitors have been shown to be at least equivalent to tamoxifen, the gold standard in postmenopausal women with advanced

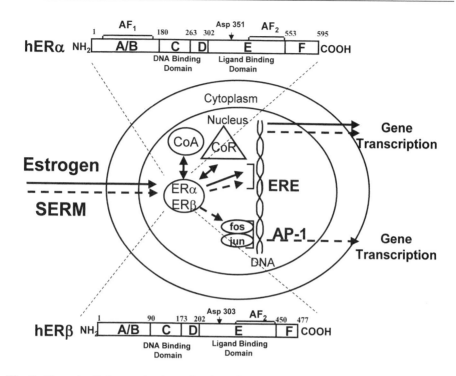

Fig. 2. The subcellular mechanism of action of estrogen in a target issue, i.e., ER-positive breast cancer. Estrogen action is regulated by two estrogen receptors: the classical ER now referred to as ERα and the newly described estrogen receptor ERβ. Once estrogen binds to the receptor, the complex changes shape and dimerizes before binding to estrogen response elements (EREs) in the promoter region of an estrogen-responsive gene. Gene translation occurs by the binding of coactivator (CoA) molecules to the ER complex that contribute to the transcription complex. RNA polymerase and DNA unwinding enzymes are recruited to ensure gene transcription. Antiestrogen ER complexes could incorporate novel corepressor (CoR) molecules to block gene transcription.

breast cancer *(46)* and trials are now in progress to delineate their role in adjuvant therapy. Building on the observations made by Harris and colleagues *(47)* over a decade ago, that epidermal growth factor (EGF) receptor content of breast tumors was inversely correlated with ER and response to contemporary endocrine therapy was poorest in tumors with high EGF content, new trials are evaluating EGF receptor tyrosine kinase inhibitors as endocrine therapy in breast cancer: promising preliminary results have been reported *(48)*. Thus, it seems likely that we are again on the threshold of significant improvements in therapy for breast cancer but careful and logical clinical trials supported by strong preclinical studies are necessary to realise this exciting potential.

Preclinical and clinical research in prostate cancer reflects the advances made in breast cancer, although progress has lagged behind until recently. Professor Charles Huggins, the Nobel Laureate, was the first to reason that castration would improve the prognosis of prostate cancer by androgen withdrawal *(11)*. Antiandrogens that block the binding of dihydrotestoserone to the androgen receptor (AR) in the prostate, and thereby prevent androgen stimulation of prostate-cancer growth have now been discovered and developed clinically.

Cyproterone acetate was the first clinically effective antiandrogen produced by Neumann and colleagues at Schering AG *(49)*. It proved effective in prostate cancer, but had a range of steroid-related side effects including liver toxicity. It was also a potent progestin and suppressed libido. The subsequent discovery of a nonsteroidal antiandrogen, flutamide by Neri and associates at Schering-Plough *(50)* was a major step forward because this was a pure antiandrogen that had negligible effects on libido: it still had some hepatoxicity and caused diarrhea in some patients, but due to its short half-life had to be given three times a day. The discovery and development of the pure nonsteroidal antiandrogens, nilutamide *(51)* and Casodex *(52)*, allowed once-daily dosing to be introduced. Casodex has now become established as the antiandrogen of choice based on its proven efficacy and its superior tolerance and half-life. Casodex (150 mg) monotherapy is as effective as castration in Mo prostate-cancer patients but without the psychological morbidity *(53)*. Recent results show that Casodex monotherapy is also effective in men with early prostate cancer *(54)*. This is consistent with preclinical data showing that early endocrine intervention is superior to delayed treatment *(55)* and with the results of an Medical Research Council clinical trial where castration given early was better than delayed treatment *(56)*.

Combination therapy of LH-RH agonists with pure antiandrogens was heralded as a major breakthrough in improving response in patients with prostate cancer *(57)*. Extensive trials with a range of LH-RH agonists and antiandrogens have given variable results and a single large trial of surgical castration alone vs combination with antiandrogen *(58)* failed to show any difference between the treatment arms. Meta-analysis of a majority of the trial data *(59)* has shown a small but significant advantage for combination therapy. It is possible also that there is a greater benefit for some subgroups than others. In the overview of these trials, it certainly appeared that pure nonsteroidal antiandrogens were more likely to be beneficial than cyproterone acetate.

Potent inhibitors of a 5α-reductase, like finasteride, have been shown to reduce markedly production of the potent androgen, 5α-dihydrotestosterone, but this is accompanied by increased concentrations of testosterone *(60)*. Since testosterone can also bind to the androgen receptor and effect cellular proliferation, this may explain why results with finasteride in treatment of prostate cancer have been disappointing *(61)*.

Just as with breast cancer, there are several new endocrine approaches being evaluated in prostate cancer. LH-RH antagonists *(62)* are being used and appear to give comparable results to surgical castration and LH-RH agonists. Claims that they have longer-term clinical advantages, particularly as a result of lack of a transient initial rise in testosterone frequently seen with LH-RH agonists, have yet to be substantiated in randomized clinical trials. LH-RH antagonists appear to have an acceptable safety profile and histamine-releasing effects have been eliminated in the newer agents, but clinical experience, at present, is far more limited than with LH-RH agonists.

EGF receptors have also been found in prostate cancer (63) and EGF has been shown to induce cellular proliferation (64). Potent inhibitors of EGF receptor tyrosine kinase have, therefore, also been used to inhibit prostate-cancer growth in early clinical trials (65).

The pace of research in prostate cancer is accelerating and we can expect significant further advances in the next few years, both in new treatment options and effective therapies in early disease and premalignant conditions such as prostate intraepithelial neoplasa.

2. STRATEGIES FOR THE ENDOCRINE TREATMENT OF CANCER

This volume describes the enormous advances that have been made in the treatment of breast and prostate cancer by the rational application of endocrine pharmacology. Thirty years ago, novel endocrine therapy for breast and prostate cancer was not viewed clinically as a priority for investigation. This perspective has changed and hundreds of thousands of patients are alive today because of improvements in endocrine therapy. The story traces the collaboration between the laboratory and clinic to provide safe and effective medicines to aid patients with cancer. Indeed, the effectiveness of endocrine therapy has resulted in the testing of the worth of tamoxifen as a chemopreventive in well women (32) and its approval as the first preventive for any form of cancer.

The description of the target site specificity of steroid hormones and the regulation of steroidogenesis through the hypothalamic-pituitary axis have been fundamental to the current strategies that can rationally regulate the flow of steroids to a tumor site.

We believe it is appropriate to summarize the principal therapeutic strategies that have proved, through clinical trials, to be successful approaches to control tumor growth.

Most of the work was originally focused on postmenopausal patients with metastatic breast cancer (Fig. 3). Antiestrogens bind specifically to the ER in the breast tumor so the action of the group was a direct application of the emerging knowledge of estrogen actions in its target tissue during the 1960s (3). In contrast, aminoglutethimide restricted the availability of circulating estrogen in postmenopausal women. Aminogluthethimide blocks the biosynthesis of steroids in

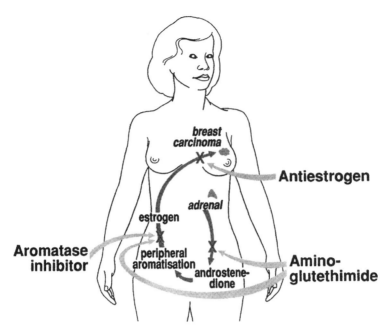

Fig. 3. The evolution of strategies for endocrine treatment of advanced breast cancer in postmenopausal patients. Antiestrogens block estrogen action in the tumor. Amino-glutethimide blocks steroidogenesis in the adrenal glands and the conversion of androstenedione by aromatase enzymes in peripheral body fat. Aromatase inhibitors are available that block the enzyme specifically.

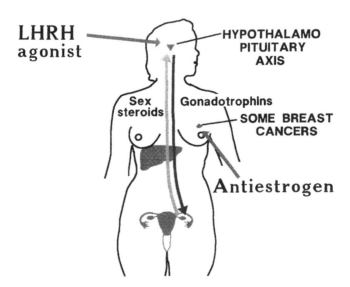

Fig. 4. Premenopausal women with advanced breast cancer can be successfully treated with either LH-RH agonists (that cause a chemical oophorectomy by blocking gonadotrophin release) or tamoxifen a nonsteroidal antiestrogen. The combination is proving to be a valuable new treatment strategy.

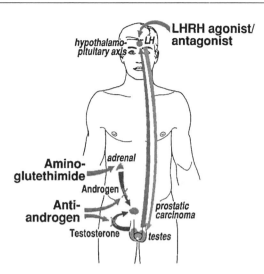

Fig. 5. Prostate cancer can be treated with LH-RH agonists/antagonists to prevent androgen synthesis in the testis by blocking gonadotrophin release. Antiandrogens block the direct effects of androgens in the prostate cancer. Aminogluthethimide blocks adrenal steroidogenesis but is rarely used since the development of effective specific nonsteroidal antiandrogens.

the adrenal glands and blocks the conversion of androstendione to estrone by aromatase enzymes in the peripheral body fat. Although the approach of using aminogluthethimide was clinically successful, the incidence of side effects focused efforts on designing more specific agents. The result is a variety of aromatase inhibitors that are specific for the enzyme at peripheral sites.

The antiestrogen tamoxifen has been proven to be effective in premenopausal patients (Fig. 4) despite increases in circulating estrogen *(66,67)* caused by interruption of the hypothalamic-pituitary axis feedback system. The sensitivity of the hypothalamic-pituitary axis to falling estrogen levels from the ovary causes a reflex rise in gonadotrophins. Aromatase inhibitors are not used in premenopausal women because the powerful action of gonadotrophins can reverse ovarian aromatase blockade. Another strategy, that is proving to be successful in pre- and peri-menopausal women, is the use of sustained release preparations of LH-RH to cause desensitization of the pituitary gland. As a result, the reduction in gonadotrophins causes a medical oophorectomy. A combination of a sustained release preparation of an LH-RH agonist and an antiestrogen will effectively decrease further the availability of estrogen to the tumor as will combination of LH-RH agonist and aromatase inhibitor.

Similar treatment strategies are used in men to control the growth of androgen responsive prostate cancer (Fig. 5). LH-RH agonists/antagonists reduce androgen availability by preventing gonadotrophin release from the pituitary gland and nonsteroidal antiandrogens specifically block androgen action in the tumor by binding to the androgen receptor.

Overall, this volume describes the evolution of these treatment strategies. This is a rapidly evolving story so we have chosen to contribute an updated chapter at the end of the book.

REFERENCES

1. Beatson GT. On the treatment of inoperable cases of carcinoma of the mamma: suggestions for a new method of treatment with illustrative cases. *Lancet* 1896; 2:104–107.
2. Boyd S. On oophorectomy in cancer of the breast. *BMJ* 1900; ii:1161–1167.
3. Jensen EV, Jacobson HI. Basic guides to the mechanism of estrogen action. *Recent Prog Horm Res* 1962; 18:387–414.
4. Jensen EV, Block GE, Smith S, Kyser K, DeSombre ER. Estrogen receptors and breast cancer response to adrenalectomy. *Natl Cancer Inst Monogr* 1971; 34:55–70.
5. Allen E, Doisy EA. An ovarian hormone: Preliminary report on its localization, extraction and partial purification and action in test animals. *JAMA* 1923; 81:819–821.
6. Doisy EA, Veler CD, Thayer S. Folliculin from urine of pregnant women. *Am J Physiol* 1929; 90:329–330.
7. Dodds EC, Lawson W. Synthetic oestrogenic agents without the phenanthrene nucleus. *Nature* 1936; 137:996.
8. Cook JW, Dodds EC, Hewett CL. A synthetic oestrus-exciting compound. *Nature* 1933; 131:56–57.
9. Robson JM, Schonberg A. Oestrous reactions, including mating, produced by triphenylethylene. *Nature* 1937; 140:196.
10. Dodds EC, Lawson W, Noble RL. Biological effects of the synthetic oestrogenic substance 4:4′-dihydroxy-alpha:beta-diethylstilbene. *Lancet* 1938; 1:1389–1391.
11. Huggins C, Hodges CV. Studies on prostatic cancer 1. The effect of castration, of estrogen and of androgen injection on serum phosphatases in metastatic carcinoma. *Cancer Res* 1941; 1:293–297.
12. Haddow A, Watkinson JM, Paterson E. Influence of synthetic oestrogens upon advanced malignant disease. *BMJ* 1944; 2:393–398.
13. Baumler E. Paul Ehrlich, Scientist for Life. Holmes & Meier, New York, 1984, p 288.
14. Dutta AS, Furr BJA. Luteinizing hormone releasing hormone (LHRH) analogues. *Ann Rep Med Chem* 1985; 20:203–214.
15. Furr BJA, Milsted RAV. LHRH analogues in cancer treatment, in *Endocrine Management of Cancer 2. Contemporary therapy.* Stoll BA, ed. Karger, Basel, 1988, pp 16–29.
16. Blamey RW. The introduction of the LHRH agonist, goserelin (Zoladex), into clinical practice. *Endocr Rel Cancer* 1997; 4:229–232.
17. Kaisary AV, Tyrell CJ, Peeling WB, Griffiths K. Comparaison of LHRH analogue (Zoladex) with orchidectomy in patients with metastatic prostatic carcinoma. *Br J Urol* 1991; 67:502–508.
18. Huggins C, Bergenstal DM. Inhibition of human mammary and prostatic cancers by adrenalectomy. *Cancer Res* 1952; 12:134–141.
19. Luft R, Olivercrona H, Sjogren B. Hypofysektomi pa manniska. *Nordisk Medicin* 1952; 47:351–354.
20. Pearson OJ, Ray BS, Harrold CC, West CD, Li MC, Maclean JP. Hypophysectomy in treatment of advanced cancer. *JAMA* 1956; 161:17–21.
21. Longcope C. Metabolic clearance and blood production rates of estrogens in postmenopausal women. *Am J Obstet Gynecol* 1971; 111:778–781.

22. Hemsell DL, Grodin JM, Brenner PF, Siiteri PK, MacDonald PC. Plasma precursors of estrogen. II. Correlation of the extent of conversion of plasma androstenedione to estrone with age. *J Clin Endocrinol Metab* 1974; 38:476–479.
23. O'Neill JS, Miller WR. Aromatase activity in breast adipose tissue from women with benign and malignant breast diseases. *Br J Cancer* 1987; 56:601–604.
24. Miller WR, Forrest APM. Oestradiol synthesis by a human breast carcinoma. *Lancet* 1974; 2:866–868.
25. Griffiths CT, Hall TC, Saba Z, Barlow JJ, Nevinny HB. Preliminary trial of aminoglutethimide in breast cancer. *Cancer* 1973; 32:31–37.
26. Cash R, Brough AJ, Cohen MNP, Satoh PS. Aminoglutethimide (Elipten-Ciba) as an inhibitor of adrenal steroidogenesis: Mechanism of action and therapeutic trial. *J Clin Endocrinol Metab* 1967; 27:1239–1248.
27. Santen RJ, Lipton A, Kendall J. Successful medical adrenalectomy with aminoglutethimide. *JAMA* 1974; 230:1661–1665.
28. Lerner LJ, Holthaus JF, Thompson CR. A non-steroidal estrogen antagonist 1-(p-2-diethylaminoethoxyphenyl)-1-phenyl-2-p-methoxyphenylethanol. *Endocrinology* 1958; 63:295–318.
29. Harper ML, Walpole AL. A new derivative of triphenylethylene: effect on implantation and mode of action in rats. *J Reprod Fertil* 1967; 13:101–119.
30. Cole MP, Jones CT, Todd ID. A new anti-oestrogenic agent in late breast cancer. An early clinical appraisal of ICI 46474. *Br J Cancer* 1971; 25:270–275.
31. EBCTCG. Tamoxifen for early breast cancer: an overview of the randomised trials. *Lancet* 1998; 351:1451–1467.
32. Fisher B, Costantino JP, Wickerham DL, et al. Tamoxifen for prevention of breast cancer: report of the National Surgical Adjuvant Breast and Bowel Project P-1 Study. *J Natl Cancer Inst* 1998; 90:1371–1388.
33. Jordan VC. Designer estrogens. *Sci Am* 1998; 279:60–67.
34. Levenson AS, Jordan VC. Selective oestrogen receptor modulation: molecular pharmacology for the millennium. *Eur J Cancer* 1999; 35:1628–1639.
35. Jordan VC, Phelps E, Lindgren JU. Effects of anti-estrogens on bone in castrated and intact female rats. *Breast Cancer Res Treat* 1987; 10:31–35.
36. Gottardis MM, Jordan VC. Antitumour actions of keoxifene and tamoxifen in the N-nitrosomethylurea-induced rat mammary carcinoma model. *Cancer Res* 1987; 47:4020–4024.
37. Lerner LJ, Jordan VC. Development of antiestrogens and their use in breast cancer: eighth Cain memorial award lecture. *Cancer Res* 1990; 50:4177–4189.
38. Green S, Walter P, Kumar V, et al. Human oestrogen receptor cDNA: sequence, expression and homology to v-erb-A. *Nature* 1986; 320:134–139.
39. Greene GL, Gilna P, Waterfield M, Baker A, Hort Y, Shine J. Sequence and expression of human estrogen receptor complementary DNA. *Science* 1986; 231:1150–1154.
40. Kuiper GG, Enmark E, Pelto-Huikko M, Nilsson S, Gustafsson JA. Cloning of a novel receptor expressed in rat prostate and ovary. *Proc Natl Acad Sci USA* 1996; 93:5925–5930.
41. Kaufman M. Zoladex (Goserelin) Vs CMF as adjuvant therapy in pre/perimenopausal, node positive, early breast cancer: preliminary efficacy results from the ZEBRA study. *Breast* 2001; 10 (Suppl 1):S30.
42. Jonat W. Zoladex versus CMF adjuvant therapy in pre/perimenopausal breast cancer: tolerability comparisons. *Proc ASCO* 2000; 19:87a.
43. Jonat W, Kaufmann M, Blamey RW, et al. A randomised study to compare the effect of the luteinising hormone releasing hormone (LHRH) analogue goserelin with or without tamoxifen in pre and perimenopausal patients with advanced breast cancer. *Eur J Cancer* 1995; 31A:137–142.
44. Klein JGM, Beex L, Mauriac L, et al. Combined treatment with the LHRH agonist buserelin (LHRH-A) and tamoxifen (TAM) vs single treatment with each drug alone in pre-

menopausal metastatic breast cancer. Final results of EORTC study 10881. *Ann Oncol* 1998; 9 (Suppl 4):11.

45. Klijn JGM, Blamey RW, Boccardo F, et al. A new standard treatment for advanced pre-menopausal breast cancer: a meta-analysis of the Combined Hormonal Agents Trialists' Group (CHAT). *Eur J Cancer* 1998; 34 (Suppl 5):S90.

46. Nabholtz JM, Buzdar A, Pollak et al. Anastrozole is superior to tamoxifen as first-line therapy for advanced breast cancer in postmenopausal women: Results of a North American multicenter randomized trial. *J Clin Oncol* 2000; 18:3758–3767.

47. Harris AL. EGF receptor as a target for therapy and interactions with angiogenesis, in *EGF Receptors in Tumour Growth and Progression* (Lichtner RB, Harkins RN, eds). Ernst Schering Foundation Workshop 19, Springer Verlag, Berlin, 1997, pp 3–17.

48. Ciardiello F, Caputo R, Bianco R, et al. Antitumor effect and potentiation of cytotoxic drugs activity in human cancer cells by ZD-1839 (Iressa), an epidermal growth factor receptor-selective tyrosine kinase inhibitor. *Clin Cancer Res* 2000; 6:2053–2063.

49. Neumann F Pharmacology and clinical uses of cyproterone acetate, in *Pharmacology and Clinical Uses of Inhibitors of Hormone Secretion and Action* (Furr BJA, Wakeling AE, eds). Bailliere-Tindall, London 1987, pp 132–159.

50. Neri RO. Clinical Utility of flutamide. *J Drug Dev* 1987; 1 (Suppl):5–9.

51. Ojasoo J. Nilutamide. *Drugs of the future* 1987; 12:763–770.

52. Kolvenbag G, Furr B. Bicalutamide development: from theory to therapy. *Cancer J* 1997; 3:192–203.

53. Iverson P, Tyrell CJ, Anderson JB. Comparison of Casodex (bicalutamide) 150mg monotherapy with castration in previously untreated non-metastatic prostate cancer: mature survival results. *Eur Urol* 2000; 37 (Suppl):128.

54. Wirth M, Tyrrell C, Wallace M, et al. Bicalutamide ('Casodex') 150mg as immediate therapy in patients with localized or locally advanced prostate cancer significantly reduces the risk of disease progression.

55. Furr BJA. Treatment of hormone-responsive rat mammary and prostate tumours with Zoladex depot, in *Hormonal Manipulation of Cancer: Peptides, Growth Factors and New (anti) Steroidal Agents* (Klijn, JGM, Paridaens R, Foekens JA eds). Raven Press, New York, 1987, pp 213–223.

56. MRC Prostate Cancer Working Party Investigators Group. Immediate versus deferred treatment for advanced prostatic cancer: initial results of the Medical Research Council trial. *Br J Urol* 1997; 79:235–246.

57. Labrie F, Dupont A, Belanger A. Complete androgen blockade for the treatment of prostate cancer, in *Important Advances in Oncology* (De Vita VT, Hellman S, Rosenberg SA, eds). Lippincott, Philadelphia, 1985, pp 193–217.

58. Eisenberger MA, Blumenstein BA, Crawford et al. Bilaterial orchiectomy with or without flutamide for metastatic prostate cancer. *New Engl J Med* 1998; 339:1036–1042.

59. Prostate Cancer Trialists' Collaborative Group. Maximum androgen blockade in advanced prostate cancer: an overview of the randomised trials. *Lancet* 2000; 355:1491–1498.

60. Span PN, Voller MCW, Smals AGH, et al. Selectivity of finasteride as an in vivo inhibitor of 5α reductase isozyme enzymatic activity in the human prostate. *J Urol* 1999; 161:332–337.

61. Ornstein DK, Rao GS, Johnson B, et al. Combined finasteride and flutamide therapy in men with advanced prostate cancer. *Urology* 1996; 48:901–905.

62. Garnick MB, Tomera K, Campion M, Kuca B. Abarelix-depot (A-D), a sustained-release (SR) formulation of a potent GnRH pure antagonist in patients with prostate cancer: Phase II clinical results and endocrine comparison with superagonists Lupron and Zoladex. *J Urol* 1996; 161(Suppl):340, Abs 1312.

63. Djakiew D. Dysregulated expression of growth factors and their receptors in the development of prostate cancer. *Prostate* 2000; 42:150–160.

64. Parczyk K, Schneider MR. The future of antihormone therapy: innovations based on an established principle. *J Cancer Res Clin Oncol* 1996; 122:383–396.

65. Barton J, Blackledge G, Wakeling A. Growth factors and their receptors: new targets for prostate cancer therapy. In press.

66. Jordan VC, Fritz NF, Tormey DC. Endocrine effects of adjuvant chemotherapy and long-term tamoxifen administration on node-positive patients with breast cancer. *Cancer Res* 1987; 47:624–630.

67. Jordan VC, Fritz NF, Langan-Fahey S, Thompson M, Tormey DC. Alteration of endocrine parameters in premenopausal women with breast cancer during long-term adjuvant therapy with tamoxifen as the single agent. *J Natl Cancer Inst* 1991; 83:1488–1491.

I PRECLINICAL ANTIESTROGENS

2 Antiestrogens and the Cell Cycle

*Colin K. W. Watts, Owen W.J. Prall,
Jason S. Carroll, Nicholas R.C. Wilcken,
Eileen M. Rogan, Elizabeth A. Musgrove,
and Robert L. Sutherland*

Contents

1. INTRODUCTION

Recognition of the involvement of estrogen in the growth of breast cancer stemmed from observations made a century ago, when it was shown that ovariectomy in cases of pre-menopausal breast cancer could lead to tumor regression *(1)*. Subsequent research in experimental models of carcinogen-induced mammary cancer revealed that estrogen was essential for both the initiation and progression of the disease. These observations, together with the demonstration that some breast tumors had a specific binding protein for estrogen, the estrogen receptor (ER), and that ER status was correlated with response to endocrine therapy, provided the rationale for the introduction of the antiestrogen tamoxifen in the treatment of breast cancer *(2)*. Tamoxifen is currently the

From: *Hormone Therapy in Breast and Prostate Cancer*
Edited by: V. C. Jordan and B. J. A. Furr © Humana Press Inc., Totowa, NJ

treatment of choice for hormone-dependent breast cancer both in advanced disease and as an adjuvant to surgery in early breast cancer. Recent overviews of the outcome of randomized clinical trials of adjuvant tamoxifen therapy demonstrate significant reductions in risk of recurrence, increased overall survival, and reduced incidence of contralateral breast cancer *(3,4)*. In addition to tamoxifen and other nonsteroidal antiestrogens, steroidal antiestrogens have been described *(5,6)* that generally exhibit pure antagonist activity, in contrast to the partial antagonist properties of tamoxifen. Such compounds are potentially more potent therapeutically than tamoxifen and early experience in the clinic shows efficacy in cases where tumors are resistant to tamoxifen. Thus antiestrogens of various structural classes with differing tissue-specific estrogen agonist/antagonist properties have an established and expanding role in the treatment of breast cancer. The accepted basis of their clinical efficacy in breast cancer is inhibition of estrogen-induced mitogenesis but the molecular basis of this action has not been fully elucidated. This chapter summarizes research from this laboratory aimed at understanding the mechanistic basis for estrogen/antiestrogen control of breast cancer cell-cycle progression.

2. EFFECTS OF ANTIESTROGENS
ON CELL-CYCLE PROGRESSION
2.1 Cell-Cycle Effects In Vitro

Initial insights into mechanisms of antiestrogen action as growth inhibitory agents came from studies on the effects of antiestrogens on breast cancer cell proliferation in vitro. Early experiments showed that the relative cell number and rate of thymidine incorporation into DNA of ER-positive (but not ER-negative) breast cancer cells were markedly reduced by antiestrogen treatment *(7,8)*. These compounds are predominantly cytostatic rather than cytotoxic in vitro and this is associated with arrest of cells in the G_1 phase of the cell cycle, with a resulting decrease in the relative proportion of cells synthesising DNA (S phase, Fig. 1A) *(9–13)*. A typical response to antiestrogens of all structural classes is shown in Fig. 1B where MCF-7 breast-cancer cells growing exponentially in 5% fetal calf serum (FCS) with a doubling time of 28 h are treated with the steroidal pure antiestrogen ICI 182780. Little change is apparent over the first 8 h of exposure, but the proportion of cells in S phase then falls continuously to reach a minimum by 24 h. These decreases are mirrored by increases in the proportion of cells in G_1 phase. Experiments with cells synchronized by mitotic selection demonstrate that only those cells in early-to-mid G_1 phase are susceptible to growth arrest *(9,11)*. Cells in plateau phase, where the proportion of proliferating cells is reduced, are relatively insensitive, suggesting that only actively cycling cells are sensitive to antiestrogen *(13,14)*. Compatible with an antiestrogen-mediated, reversible inhibition of cell-cycle progression

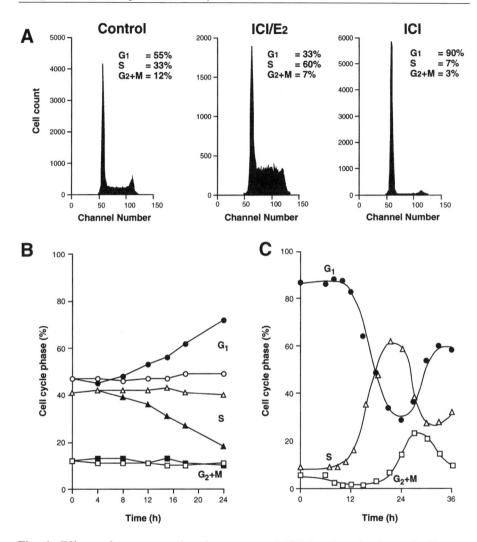

Fig. 1. Effects of estrogen and antiestrogen on MCF-7 cell-cycle phase distribution. MCF-7 cells were growth-arrested for up to 48 h with 10 nM ICI 182780 and then treated with 100 nM estradiol or vehicle (ethanol). Harvested cells were stained for DNA content and the proportion of cells in G_1, S and G_2 + M phases of the cell cycle determined. **(A)** Representative DNA histograms for untreated, exponentially growing cells (Exp), cells treated with ICI 182780 (ICI) for 59 h and cells treated with ICI 182780 for 48 h and then rescued by estradiol for 21 h (ICI +E2). **(B)** Antiestrogen inhibition. Cells were treated with 10 nM ICI 182780 (solid symbols) or with 0.1% ethanol vehicle (open symbols) between 0–24 h. G_1 (J, E); S (H, C); and G_2 + M (B, G) phase. From ref. *(62)*. **(C)** Estrogen rescue. After 48 h of ICI 182780 cells were treated with estradiol. At intervals thereafter, cells were harvested and the proportion of cells in G_1 (J), S (C), and G_2 + M (G) phases determined. From ref. *(17)*.

in G_0/G_1 phase are data demonstrating semi-synchronous progression into S phase following estrogen "rescue" of antiestrogen-treated cells (Fig. 1A, 1C). This phenomenon was first noted by Lippman and Bolan (7) and has recently been exploited by us and others to gain new insights into estrogen control of cell-cycle progression (15–17).

These data provide strong evidence that antiestrogens inhibit breast cancer cell proliferation in culture by inhibiting cell-cycle progression in early to mid G_1 phase. The exact state at which they are arrested, i.e., in G_0 or G_1, has yet to be defined but this does not involve permanent exit from the cell cycle as estrogen (but not several growth factors, e.g. insulin-like growth factor [IGF]-1, epidermal growth factor [EGF] and heregulin) can re-initiate cell cycle progression.

Because the response to antiestrogens can be modulated by interactions with steroids and growth factors, such as those present in FCS (see ref. 18 and references therein) we have also defined the growth-regulatory actions of antiestrogens in estrogen-free, serum-free medium (19–21). Under these culture conditions the proliferation of MCF-7 and T-47D cells was markedly inhibited by nonsteroidal or steroidal antiestrogens, both being essentially cytostatic after 24 h exposure. The concentration-dependence of growth inhibition of these antiestrogens appears to be little affected by the absence of serum and estrogens. As in serum-containing medium, the changes in cell-cycle phase distribution that accompanied growth inhibition were similar for both classes of antiestrogens with the proportion of cells in S phase falling rapidly after 9 h to reach a minimum within 24 h. Other studies have also shown that antiestrogens are able to inhibit proliferation under steroid-depleted conditions (10,22–26) and that antiestrogens inhibit cells stimulated to proliferate by insulin (10,26), IGF-I (10), EGF (26), or transforming growth factor (TGF-α) (10). The diversity of mitogenic stimuli inhibited by antiestrogen treatment suggests that the molecular targets of inhibition are common to estrogen- and growth factor-activated pathways.

Although the mechanisms by which antiestrogens inhibit growth factor-induced proliferation in the apparent absence of estrogen are unknown, several potential mechanisms for antiestrogen inhibition of gene expression have been suggested that might operate under such conditions (27–29). These include: inhibition of the function of unoccupied ER bound to DNA; DNA binding of antiestrogen-ER complexes to estrogen-response elements resulting in transcriptional interference of basal expression or expression driven by other promoter elements; and inhibition of AP-1 activity, possibly resulting from protein-protein interactions between the antiestrogen-ER complex and Fos/Jun.

2.2 Cell-Cycle Effects In Vivo

Although growth inhibition by antiestrogens in vitro is primarily due to cell-cycle arrest in G_0/G_1 phase, data obtained from breast cancer cell lines grown as solid tumors in nude mice are less clear-cut. Antiestrogen inhibition of tumor growth in vivo has been reported to result primarily from cell loss that is not cell-cycle-phase specific *(30)*. To further address this issue we examined the effects of tamoxifen on the growth and cell cycle-phase distribution of MCF-7 cells grown as tumors in nude mice *(19)*. Under conditions of estradiol (E_2) stimulation tumors grew rapidly. This estrogen-stimulated growth was almost completely abolished by the simultaneous administration of tamoxifen (Fig. 2A). However, at longer tamoxifen treatment times, slow tumor growth became apparent, consistent with results seen in other studies in which large MCF-7 tumors eventually re-grew in the presence of tamoxifen *(31,32)*. Flow cytometric analysis showed control tumors had an S phase fraction of more than 20%, consistent with their rapid growth rate (Fig. 2B). While the differences in cell cycle-phase distribution were not as large as those observed in vitro, tamoxifen treatment resulted in significant decreases in the proportion of cells in S phase with a corresponding increase in cells in G_1 phase (Fig. 2C). These data clearly demonstrate that cell cycle phase-specific cytostatic effects of tamoxifen can occur both in vitro and in vivo but do not rule out other concurrent mechanisms of growth inhibition in vivo. Although we saw no evidence for tumor regression on tamoxifen treatment in agreement with others *(31,32)*, Brünner et al. *(30)* found tamoxifen led to growth inhibition and shrinkage of MCF-7 tumors in nude mice and concluded its effects in vivo were not mediated through a G_1 phase block but rather through non-cell cycle-phase-specific cell loss. If tamoxifen has this activity, it may be equivalent to estrogen withdrawal, which has also been shown to result in apoptosis and tumor regression of E_2-stimulated MCF-7 tumors *(33)*. There is some direct evidence for apoptotic effects of antiestrogens in xenograft models *(34,35)* and in primary breast cancer *(36)*. However, it should also be noted that the extent of tumor shrinkage induced by tamoxifen treatment in another study *(32)* was no different from placebo controls suggesting tamoxifen has no cytotoxic effect *per se*. Thus the relative contributions of decreased cell proliferation and increased cell death to the antitumor activity of antioestrogens in vivo is a major unanswered question.

3. MOLECULAR MECHANISMS OF ANTIESTROGEN INHIBITION OF CELL-CYCLE PROGRESSION

Despite current knowledge of the effects of antiestrogens at the whole-cell level, a precise understanding of the molecular events underlying estrogen and antiestrogen action is not yet available, particularly with regard to effects on cell proliferation. The effects of antiestrogens at submicromolar concentrations can generally be reversed by the simultaneous or subsequent addition of estrogen *(8,12,13,37)*. Antiestrogen action is therefore believed to be medi-

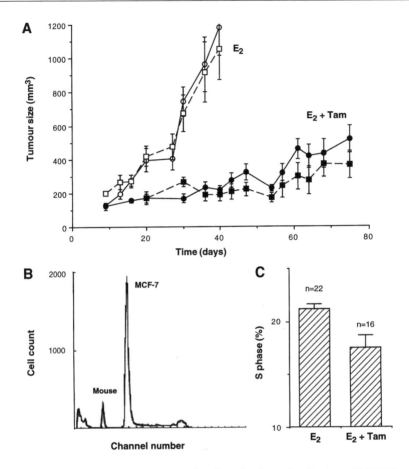

Fig. 2. Effects of tamoxifen on growth and cell-cycle phase distribution of MCF-7 tumors in nude mice. Nude mice bearing MCF-7 tumors were treated twice weekly with either estradiol or estradiol plus tamoxifen dissolved in peanut oil to a final dose of 20 (squares) or 50 (circles) mg/wk estradiol and 200 mg/wk tamoxifen. Tumor volumes were measured at intervals (Fig. **2A**). At the conclusion of the experiment, tumors were harvested for DNA analysis. Figure **2B** shows a representative DNA histogram of an estradiol treated tumor, where 'Mouse' indicates cells originating from the host animal. Figure **2C** shows pooled results for the S-phase content of estradiol-treated tumors (both doses) and estradiol plus tamoxifen-treated tumors. From ref. *(19).*

ated primarily through competitive binding to the ER, with direct effects on the transactivation of estrogen-responsive genes, which in turn can subsequently alter the expression and activity of numerous additional gene products. The identity of the set of such genes specifically involved in antiestrogen control of cell-cycle progression has yet to be fully defined, although the action of antiestrogens to arrest cells at a point within the G_0/G_1 phase of the breast-cancer-cell-cycle focuses the search for antiestrogen target genes on those with known activities in controlling progression through G_1 phase. Restriction of antiestrogen sensitivity to cells in early to mid G_1 phase further defines the potential genes that are the initial targets of antiestrogen action. To date most attention has been focused on the cyclin-dependent kinases (CDKs), their inhibitors and substrates, and the proto-oncogene c-*myc*.

3.1. Control of Cell-Cycle Progression

Progress through the cell cycle is governed by the sequential activation of a family of CDKs with the consequent phosphorylation of specific substrates to allow progression through checkpoints in the cell cycle. Since normal physiological regulation of cell-cycle progression by extracellular stimuli, including growth factors and steroid hormones *(38–40)*, is mediated during G_1 phase *(41)*, the major interactions controlling G_1 progression are a central focus and these are illustrated in Fig. 3. Key substrates of the CDKs with G_1-phase specific actions (i.e., Cdk2, Cdk4, and Cdk6) include the retinoblastoma gene product, pRB, and the related pocket protein p107, although it is likely that other important substrates remain to be identified *(38)*. The consequence of inactivation of the pRB protein by phosphorylation is the release of a number of bound and functionally inactive factors including the E2F family of transcription factors *(42–45)*. Upon release from pRB complexes, these transcription factors activate transcription of genes whose products are required for S-phase progression *(42–45)*. CDK activity is subject to multiple levels of regulation. Since CDKs are inactive in the absence of cyclin binding, cyclin abundance is a major determinant of cyclin-CDK activity *(46)*. Each cyclin is thus typically present for only a restricted portion of the cell cycle, and cyclin induction is an integral part of mitogenic signaling. Alteration of cyclin abundance is sufficient to alter the rate of cell-cycle progression since overexpression of the principal G_1 cyclins, cyclins D1-3 or E, accelerates cells through G_1 and conversely, inhibition of their function by antibody microinjection prevents entry into S phase *(38,39,41)*. An essential role for cyclin D1 in normal mammary-gland development and breast cancer is indicated by the absence of lobular-alveolar compartments in transgenic mice with disruption of the cyclin D1 gene *(47,48)*, and evidence that cyclin D1 overexpression is an early *(49)* and common *(50)* event in human breast cancer.

CDK activity is also regulated by a network of kinases and phosphatases so that cyclin binding is sufficient only for partial activation *(46,51)*. Phosphorylation by the CDK-activating kinase (CAK) on a conserved threonine residue is necessary for full activity *(46,51)*. However, even in the presence of phosphorylation at this residue and cyclin binding, CDKs can be inhibited by phosphorylation of N-terminal threonine and tyrosine residues within the catalytic cleft *(51)*. The dual specificity Cdc25 phosphatases activate CDKs by dephosphorylating these inhibitory residues *(51)*.

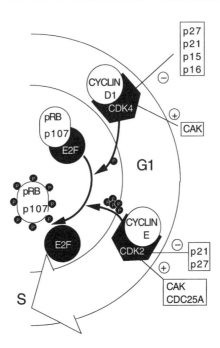

Fig. 3. Cell-cycle regulation during G_1 phase. Progress from G_1 into S phase is regulated by the actions of the molecular pathways illustrated schematically. The major G_1 cyclin complexes in breast-cancer cells, cyclin D1-Cdk4, and cyclin E-Cdk2 are illustrated. The activity of these complexes is regulated at several levels including cyclin abundance, consequent assembly of the cyclin/CDK complex, and activation by both kinases (CAK) and phosphatases (CDC25). Once active the CDKs phosphorylate substrates including pRB and the related "pocket protein," p107, leading to the release of molecules including the transcription factor E2F and consequent transcription of genes necessary for entry into S phase. The CDK inhibitors p21 and p27 not only interfere with the phosphorylation steps leading to the activation of the CDK but inhibit active CDK complexes. While the p16 CDK inhibitor may also inhibit holoenzyme complexes, a major function is to inhibit the assembly of cyclin D1-Cdk4 complexes. Redrawn from ref. *(92)*.

A further level of control results from the actions of two families of specific CDK inhibitory proteins (CDKIs). One family, of which the prototypic member is p16^{INK4}, specifically targets the kinases which associate with the D-type cyclins, Cdk4 and Cdk6. The inhibitory activity of this family appears to result largely from competition with the cyclin for CDK binding although there is also evidence that p16 family members bind to and inhibit cyclin D-Cdk4 and cyclin D-Cdk6 complexes *(52,53)*. The other family, of which p21 (WAF1, Cip1, sdi1) and p27 (Kip1) are the best-studied, interact with cyclin/CDK complexes containing Cdk2 as well as Cdk4 and Cdk6. Recent structural studies of p27 bound to cyclin A-Cdk2 indicate that p27 interacts with both cyclin A and Cdk2, occluding the catalytic cleft of Cdk2, causing multiple structural changes within the complex *(54)*. Despite these multiple modes of inhibition of CDK activity, cyclin/CDK complexes containing p21 or p27 can retain activity in in vitro kinase assays *(55–57)*. More recent data indicate that p21 and p27 as well as a related inhibitor, p57[Kip2], stabilize cyclin D-Cdk4 and cyclin D-Cdk6 complexes in vitro *(55)*. Thus low stoichiometry p21 binding promotes assembly of active complexes while at higher stoichiometry kinase activity is inhibited *(55)*. Consequently, these molecules appear to have functions in addition to CDK inhibition, perhaps as adaptors which not only promote assembly of the cyclin-CDK complexes but also target these complexes to specific intracellular compartments or substrates.

In addition to the G_1 cyclins, the proto-oncogene product c-Myc is one of only a limited number of proteins that are known to be rate-limiting for progression through G_1 phase *(58)*. c-Myc-induced stimulation of DNA synthesis is preceded by modulation of the expression or activation of cyclins, CDKs, and CDK inhibitors, although it appears that there are differences in the specific responses to c-Myc activation, perhaps related to cell type or the presence of functional pRB *(58)*. While some data suggest close links between c-Myc and cyclin D1, other data argue that they may be involved in alternative pathways for progression through G_1 phase *(58)*. There is, however, increasing evidence of a role for c-Myc in the activation of cyclin E-Cdk2 *(59–61)*. This activation appears to be indirect, rather than by direct transcriptional regulation of components of the cyclin-CDK complex.

The complexity of control of cyclin-CDK activity provides multiple targets through which physiological regulators of cell proliferation might mediate their effects. However, only a restricted range of these potential targets appear to be utilized. Thus, regulation of cyclin or CDK inhibitor expression is a frequent response to mitogens including steroid hormones, peptide-growth factors and cytokines, and to growth arrest following induction of differentiation or treatment with inhibitory factors, e.g., TGF-β *(38–40)*. In contrast, regulation of the expression or activity of the kinases and phosphatases controlling CDK phosphorylation and hence activation appears to be rare. Consequently, examination of the effects of antiestrogens and estrogens on cell-cycle regulatory molecules has focused on regulation of c-Myc, cyclins/CDKs, and CDK inhibitors.

4. EFFECTS OF ANTIESTROGENS ON CELL-CYCLE REGULATORY MOLECULES

4.1. Antiestrogen Increases Hypophosphorylated Retinoblastoma Protein

Because of the central role of pRB as a regulator of cell-cycle progression in late G_1 phase, we examined whether pRB phosphorylation is altered by antiestrogen treatment, in particular whether this occurs at times compatible with a

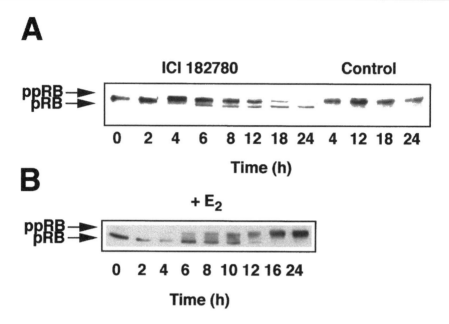

Fig. 4. Effects of estrogen and antiestrogen on phosphorylation of the RB protein. (**A**) Whole-cell lysates from MCF-7 cells treated with 10 nM ICI 182780 or with 0.1% ethanol vehicle (control) were Western blotted with an anti-RB antibody. The upper band, ppRB, represents the hyperphosphorylated form of RB and the lower band, pRB, the hypophosphorylated form. From ref *(62).* (**B**) Antiestrogen-treated MCF-7 cells were rescued with estradiol as described in Fig. 1. At intervals thereafter, whole-cell lysates were prepared and Western blotted for pRB as above. From ref. *(17).*

role for pRB in mediating the cell-cycle effects of antiestrogens, and whether changes in phosphorylation are consistent with antiestrogen regulation of G_1 cyclin/CDK activities *(62,63).* Western blotting of MCF-7 cell lysates from untreated exponentially growing control cells demonstrated that almost all pRB exists in the more highly phosphorylated, slowly migrating form (Fig. 4A). Treatment with ICI 182780 resulted in a time-dependent decrease in pRB phosphorylation, with a corresponding increase in the growth-inhibitory, hypophosphorylated form of pRB from 4–6 h *(62).* These early changes in pRB phosphorylation preceded decreases in % S phase cells by several hours, indicating that they are likely to be a cause, rather than a consequence, of antiestrogen-induced inhibition of cell-cycle progression. At 12 h both forms of pRB were still present but at 18 h and 24 h additional hypophosphorylation and a decrease in total pRB protein were observed, such that little or none of the hyperphosphorylated pRB remained. These later changes in phosphorylation occur when major effects on inhibition of entry into S phase are already apparent. Similar results were seen in another ER-positive breast-cancer cell line, T-47D *(63)*, and with both steroidal and nonsteroidal antiestrogens. Thus given the known function of pRB in controlling progression through G_1 to S phase, early decreases in the degree of pRB phosphorylation may be central to the inhibition of entry into S phase that is the ultimate consequence of anti-estrogen action.

Further support for this conclusion is provided by experiments where cells growth arrested with ICI 182780 for 48 h were "rescued" by addition of E_2 *(16,17)*. This resulted in the synchronous entry of cells into S phase commencing at 12 h, the proportion of cells in S phase reaching a maximum of 60% at 21–24 h (Fig. 1C). After 48 h of ICI 182780 pretreatment, almost all pRB is hypophosphorylated (time 0, Fig. 4B). Following estradiol treatment an increase in more slowly migrating, phosphorylated forms of pRB is first apparent at 6 h. The proportion of phosphorylated pRB increases at subsequent time points such that after 12 h, when cells commence their synchronous entry into S phase, little or no hypophosphorylated pRB remains. Similar results are obtained in estrogen rescue of tamoxifen arrested MCF-7 cells *(15)*. Estrogen treatment also increased the total cellular concentration of pRB (Fig. 4B). These observations, then, are essentially the reverse of those seen when cells are treated with antiestrogen supporting a central role for pRB in mediating the opposing effects of estrogens and antiestrogens on G_1 to S-phase progression in target cells.

Recently we have shown that ICI 182780 not only influences the phosphorylation state of pRB, but also results in hypophosphorylation of p107 and p130 (two related pRB family members) *(63a)*. p107 total protein levels also decrease, but p130 levels accumulate, which is characteristic of growth arrest. Coupled with this, we have detected the association of p130 with its preferred transcription factor (E2F4), suggesting that antiestrogens arrest cells in quiescence (G_0 phase) as opposed to the G_1 phase.

4.2. Antiestrogen Inhibition of Cdk4 and Cdk2 Activities

While the mechanisms responsible for the antiestrogen regulation of pRB phosphorylation have yet to be fully defined, reductions in CDK activity are the most likely explanation, although an alternative explanation that requires further investigation is the possible action of protein phosphatases suggested to control pRB reactivation *(44)*. To investigate which of the CDKs that act during G_1 phase might be responsible, cyclin D1-associated kinase activity (principally Cdk4 activity in MCF-7 cells [*(64)*]) following ICI 182780 treatment was measured in immunoprecipitates of cyclin D1. Kinase activity towards a recombinant, truncated pRB substrate fell by 40% at 12 h and by 80% at 24 h (Fig. 5A), indicating that initial alterations in kinase activity precede the cell-cycle effects of antiestrogens: only small effects on inhibition of entry of cells

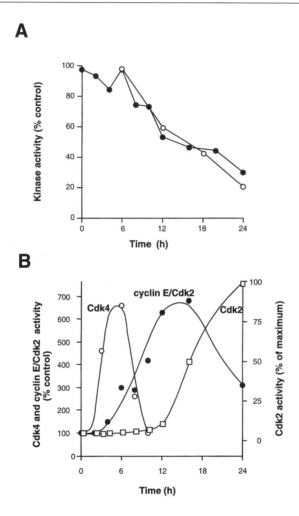

Fig. 5. Effect of estrogen and antiestrogen on cyclin D1- and cyclin E-associated kinase activities. (**A**) Immunoprecipitates were prepared from whole-cell lysates of MCF-7 cells treated with 10 nM ICI 182780 using anti-cyclin E or -cyclin D1 antibodies. Cyclin D1-associated Cdk4 activity (○) was determined using recombinant pRB(379–928) as a substrate. Cyclin E-associated Cdk2 activity (●) was assayed using a histone H1 substrate. From ref. *(62)* and unpublished data. (**B**) MCF-7 cells were rescued with estradiol as described in Fig. 1. At intervals thereafter, whole-cell lysates were prepared, immunoprecipitated with antibodies to either Cdk4, cyclin E, or Cdk2, and kinase activity determined. Cdk4 activity (○), cyclin E/Cdk2 activity (●) and total Cdk2 activity (□). From ref. *(17)*.

into S phase were apparent at 12 h (Fig. 1B). This inhibition is rapidly, though transiently reversed in the estrogen-rescue model, where Cdk4 activity (determined in Cdk4 immunoprecipitates) was elevated several fold by 3 h after estradiol treatment, maximally elevated at 6 h, and thereafter declined (Fig. 5B). Given that the cyclin D1/Cdk4 complex is active in mid-G_1 phase *(65)*, a decrease in cyclin D1/Cdk4 activity is consistent with involvement of this complex in mediating the early- to mid-G_1 phase point of action of antiestrogens on pRB phosphorylation.

Cdk2 is the second major CDK acting in the G_1 phase and its total cellular activity, as measured in Cdk2-immunoprecipitates, appeared to be unaffected by antiestrogen treatment between 2 and 6 h but decreased starting at 8 h *(62,63)*. This profound inhibition of Cdk2 activity might result in pRB hypophosphorylation at late times and contribute to the sustained antiestrogen blockade of cell-cycle progression. However, cyclin A/Cdk2 is the predominant form of this complex and when the subcomponent of Cdk2 associated with cyclin E was examined, a more complex picture emerged as significant decreases in kinase activity were seen prior to 12 h (Fig. 5A). This inhibition increased to 24 h and beyond and suggests that inhibition of cyclin E/Cdk2 complexes contributes to the early effects of antiestrogens on pRB phosphorylation.

Like antiestrogens, estradiol had little effect on total Cdk2 activity prior to changes in S phase and pRB phosphorylation *(17)* (Fig. 5B). After antiestrogen pretreatment, cyclin E-associated kinase activity is low and estradiol restores this activity by threefold at 6 h (Fig. 5B), coinciding with the time when both the increase in Cdk4 activity and the shift in pRB phosphorylation are first apparent. The substantial and early changes in both Cdk4 activity and cyclin E-associated kinase activity between 4 and 6 h indicate that both kinases were likely to contribute to the initial changes in pRB phosphorylation following estradiol treatment. These results suggest that estrogens and antiestrogens have early specific effects on the activities of both cyclin D1/Cdk4 and cyclin E/Cdk2, which in turn are responsible for the observed changes in pRB phosphorylation associated with their opposing effects on G_1 to S-phase progression.

4.3. Mechanisms of Antiestrogen Regulation of G_1 Phase CDK Activity

CDKs are regulated at multiple levels, each of which, potentially, could be influenced by antiestrogens to inhibit kinase activity. Protein levels of Cdk4, Cdk2, and their partners cyclin D3 and cyclin E are unaltered by antiestrogen treatment over 12 h *(62,63)*. Consistent with their known expression in late G_1/S and S phase, respectively, cyclin D3 and cyclin A protein levels declined significantly at late times probably as a consequence of the decreasing S-phase population. The latter decrease probably results in the observed decreases in total Cdk2 activity. In contrast, decreases in cyclin D1 mRNA expression are

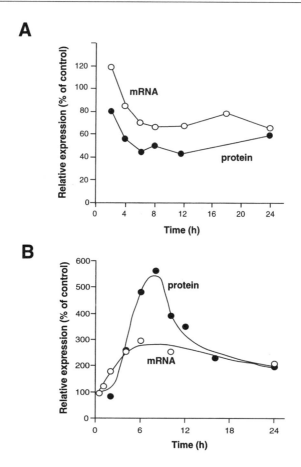

Fig. 6. Effects of estrogen and antiestrogen on cyclin D1 mRNA and protein levels. **(A)** MCF-7 cells were treated with 10 nM ICI 182780 and harvested at intervals thereafter for RNA extraction or preparation of whole-cell lysates. Northern blots were probed for cyclin D1, and mRNA levels were determined by phosphorimager analysis and expressed relative to the ethanol controls. Western blots were probed with an antibody to cyclin D1 and protein levels were determined by phosphorimager analysis and are expressed relative to the ethanol controls. From ref. *(62)*. **(B)** MCF-7 cells were rescued with estradiol as described in Fig. 1 and harvested and analyzed for cyclin D1 mRNA and protein expression as described earlier. From ref. *(17)*.

detected 2–4 h after a variety of antiestrogen treatments, with maximal decreases of approx 50% occurring by 6 h (Fig. 6A), before any major changes in the proportion of cells in S phase *(19,21,62,63)*. Cyclin D1 protein also falls to a minimum level of 50% or less at 6 h (Fig. 6A) in MCF-7 cells and ER-positive MDA-MB-134 cells, a change of similar magnitude to decreases in % S phase, but occuring several hours earlier. Although mRNA levels fall significantly, no detectable changes in cyclin D1 levels were observed in T-47D cells treated with ICI 164384, perhaps because of Western-blot-sensitivity limitations (63). Close correspondence between the timing of the disappearance of mRNA and protein is in agreement with the known short half-life of cyclin D1 protein in the MCF-7 cell line (less than 1 h) and other cell types (66).

In confirmation of a specific antiestrogen effect on cyclin D1 expression, early and pronounced changes in mRNA and protein expression are also seen in response to estradiol prior to any change in % S phase (15,17,67,68) (Fig. 6B). Although cyclin D1 levels are rapidly altered by antiestrogens and estradiol, it remains to be determined whether these are directly transcriptionally mediated effects or require prior activity of other gene products. Experiments with actinomycin D suggest that the effects of estrogen on cyclin D1 mRNA levels are transcriptionally mediated but the ability of cycloheximide to abolish mRNA induction shows that this is not a direct effect on the cyclin D1 gene and implies a requirement for *de novo* synthesis of intermediary proteins, which mediate either cyclin D1 gene transcription or mRNA stabilization (17). Studies on the cyclin D1 gene promoter have identified several regulatory regions including an AP-1 site (69) providing a link between estrogen-induced AP-1 activity (27) and cyclin D1 induction. A more recent study confirms that this AP-1 site is within the promoter region responsible for estrogen regulation of this gene (67).

Several studies provide evidence for a pivotal role of cyclin D1 in G_1 progression in breast-cancer cells. Ectopic expression of cyclin D1 is sufficient and rate-limiting for G_1-S phase progression in pRB-positive breast cancer cells, and results in increases in cyclin D1-Cdk4 and Cdk2 kinase activities (16,70–72). Furthermore, microinjection of either cyclin D1 antibodies or recombinant dominant negative Cdk4 or p16[INK4] (protein or cDNA) prevents estradiol-induced G_1-S phase progression in MCF-7 cells (73). Therefore it is possible that the inhibition of cell-cycle progression following antiestrogen treatment may be a consequence of reduced cyclin D1 expression. To examine this further, we generated stable transfectants of T-47D and MCF-7 cells that contained cyclin D1 cDNA downstream of a metal-responsive metallothionein promoter. Cells were treated with the steroidal antiestrogens ICI 164384 or ICI 182780 or the nonsteroidal antiestrogens tamoxifen and 4-hydroxytamoxifen, arresting cells in G_1 phase as described earlier. Subsequent treatment with Zn-induced cyclin D1 protein expression and this was accompanied by cyclin D1-Cdk4 complex formation, activation of cyclin D1-Cdk4 and cyclin E-Cdk2 activities, pRB phosphorylation, and entry into S phase (Fig. 7). Treatment of control cell lines with Zn was without significant effect. Therefore expression of cyclin D1 alone was sufficient to overcome antiestrogen-induced G_1 arrest, suggesting a role for cyclin D1 in antiestrogen arrest. However, a critical role

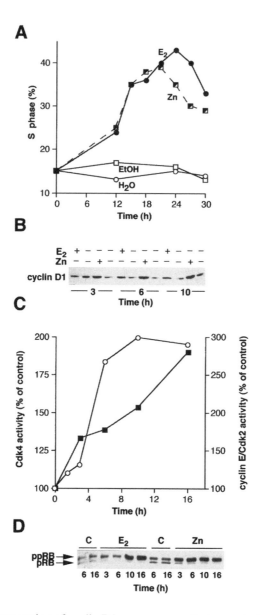

Fig. 7. Inducible expression of cyclin D1 can reverse antiestrogen-induced growth arrest. **(A)** An MCF-7 cell line stably transfected with the Zn-inducible pΔMT vector containing cyclin D1 cDNA was growth-arrested for 48 h with 10 nM of the antiestrogen ICI 182780. Cells were treated at time 0 with either 50 μ*M* Zn (▨), vehicle (H₂O, ○), 100 nM estradiol (E₂) (●), or vehicle (EtOH). At intervals thereafter, the proportion of cells in S phase was determined by flow cytometry. **(B)** Whole-cell lysates were prepared at intervals following treatment (shown in hours) and immunoblotted with antibodies against cyclin D1. **(C)** Zinc-treated whole-cell lysates were prepared and assessed for Cdk4 (■) and cyclin E/Cdk2 (○) activity as described in Fig. 5. Autoradiographs were quantitated by densitometry and expressed relative to time-matched controls. **(D)** Cell lysates from the same experiment were immunoblotted with a pRB antibody. From ref. *(16)*.

of cyclin D1 in estrogen-dependent proliferation in other target tissues is less certain since mice carrying null mutations of both cyclin D1 alleles exhibit mammary-gland ductal development and pregnancy-related uterine hyperplasia, known classical estrogen-mediated biological responses *(47,48)*.

4.4. Antiestrogen Effects on the CDK Inhibitors p21[WAF1/CIP1] and p27[KIP1]

Although decreases in Cdk2 and cyclin D1-associated kinase activities are predicted in response to antiestrogen treatment as the consequence of corresponding changes in the levels of cyclin D1 and cyclin A proteins, cyclin levels only fall by approx 50% *(62)*. This suggests that antiestrogen action necessitates the activation of additional factors that are responsible for the quantitatively greater inhibition of kinase activities, particularly beyond 12 h. We have therefore examined whether antiestrogens might regulate the levels of expression of the specific inhibitors of CDK activity, p21[WAF1/CIP1] and p27[KIP1]. In MCF-7 cells, Western-blot analysis of p21 expression shows little or no change in the first 12 h and an approximate threefold induction by ICI 182780 at 18–24 h *(62)*, coinciding with the timing of inhibition of total Cdk2 activity but later than the first changes in inhibition of cyclin D1-associated pRB kinase and cyclin E/Cdk2 histone H1 kinase activity (Fig. 5A). Similarly, p27 protein levels increased approx 50% by 12 h and attained an approximate threefold maximal increase between 18 and 24 h. Neither inhibitor is markedly altered prior to changes in % S phase indicating that the late changes are more likely a consequence, than a cause, of inhibition of cell-cycle progression. p27[KIP1] could play a role in the decrease in Cdk4 activity over this period. Similarly, increased expression of p21[WAF1/CIP1], also an inhibitor of both Cdk4 and Cdk2 *(74,75)*, may well contribute to inactivation of Cdk4 at these times but neither is likely to be responsible for the earlier inhibition of Cdk4 or cyclin E/Cdk2. The dramatic downregulation of total Cdk2 activity at 18–24 h that occurs without corresponding large decreases in cyclin E or cyclin A levels also suggests the possible inhibitory action of p21 and p27. It will be interesting to determine whether raised levels of these CDKIs contribute to continued growth arrest by antiestrogens upon longer term treatment by maintaining pRB hypophosphorylation.

Further investigation into the inhibition of cyclin D1/Cdk4 and cyclin E/Cdk2 at early timepoints has revealed that the loss of cyclin D1-containing complexes as the result of repressed cyclin D1 transcription resulted in release of free p21 and p27, which was subsequently recruited by and inhibited cyclin E/Cdk2. This shift in inhibitors between cyclin D1/Cdk4 and cyclin E/Cdk2 occurred prior to the increase in total protein levels of p21 and p27, and highlights the general importance to cell-cycle control of redistribution of CDKIs between different cyclin/CDK complexes.

4.5. CDK Complex Formation in Antiestrogen and Estrogen Action

The full interpretation of the previous results will depend on analysis of the components that make up antiestrogen-inhibited cyclin D1/Cdk4 and cyclin E/Cdk2 complexes. Such studies are underway but clues to the possible mode of antiestrogen action come from our most recent studies on the activation of these complexes in the estrogen-rescue model. It is necessary to bear in mind, however, that antiestrogens may not simply act in a way that is the mirror image of estrogen action. The most likely explanation for Cdk4 activation following estrogen rescue is that it is the direct consequence of increased cyclin D1/Cdk4 complex formation resulting from estrogen-induced expression of cyclin D1 protein, a conclusion reached by several recent studies *(15,67,68)*. This is illustrated in Fig. 8A, which shows the alterations in composition of immunoprecipitated cyclin D1 complexes in MCF-7 cells treated with estradiol. This is also a property shared with a number of other mitogens. In T-47D breast cancer-cells progestins, IGF-1, insulin, serum, and bFGF induce cyclin D1 mRNA, protein, and cyclin D1/CDK complex formation (*see* ref. *21* and unpublished observations) as do many other mitogens in a variety of other cell types *(66,76)*. However, the presence of elevated levels of cyclin D1 is not always sufficient for increased kinase activity in quiescent cells stimulated by growth factors, leading to the postulation that an "assembly factor" governs formation of active complexes *(65);* other authors have suggested that this factor might be p21 *(55,57)*. The increased relative content of p21 in cyclin D1/CDK complexes concurrent with increased activity of the complexes following estrogen rescue (Fig. 8A) is consistent with this possibility. At present the mechanism that allows enrichment of p21 in the cyclin D1/Cdk4 complex is unknown.

As noted earlier (Fig. 5B), estrogen rescue also results in activation of cyclin E-associated Cdk2 at early time points, i.e., 4–6 h *(16,17)*. In contrast to the action of most other mitogens, where activation of cyclin E/Cdk2 occurs through increases in total or Cdk2-associated cyclin E *(77,78)*, we detected no change in either cyclin E mRNA or protein or Cdk2 protein at early times. Furthermore, examination of cyclin E complexes immunoprecipitated from lysates from estrogen-treated cells revealed that the levels of cyclin E, Cdk2, p21, and p27 remained unchanged in cyclin E complexes until 10 h after estradiol treatment *(17)*. While activation of cyclin E/Cdk2 at 16 h was likely to involve loss of p21 and p27 from the complex due to a decline in their total intracellular levels *(17)*, these experiments did not identify a mechanism for the activation of cyclin E/Cdk2 prior to 16 h.

However, using gel-filtration chromatography we demonstrated that following estrogen treatment there was a small but consistent increase in cyclin E migrating in higher molecular-weight complexes, i.e., >250 kDa, and these complexes contained the majority of cyclin E/Cdk2 kinase activity (Fig. 8B). Consequently, the specific activity of these higher molecular-weight complexes

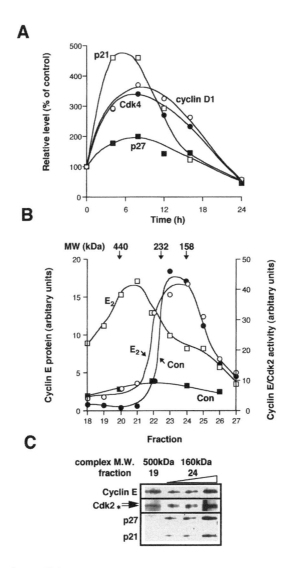

Fig. 8. Effects of estradiol on cyclin D1- and cyclin E-complex formation. (**A**) MCF-7 cells were rescued with estradiol as described in Fig. 1 and at intervals thereafter whole-cell lysates were prepared and immunoprecipitated with anti-cyclin D1 antiserum. Relative levels of cyclin D1 (○), Cdk4 (●), p21 (□), and p27 (■) were determined by densitometry of Western blots and are expressed relative to the vehicle-treated controls. (**B**) Cell lysates were prepared 8 h after estrogen (E_2) or vehicle (Con) treatment and fractionated on a Superose 12 gel-filtration column. Fractions were precipitated with acetone and Western blotted for cyclin E or assayed for cyclin E-Cdk2 kinase activity. The elution of known markers (ferritin, 440 kDa; catalase, 232 kDa; aldolase, 158 kDa) are indicated at the top of the graph. (**C**) Cyclin E immunoprecipitates from fractions 19 and 24 of the E2-treated lysate were analysed by Western blot for cyclin E, Cdk2, p21, and p27. Various quantities of the cyclin E immunoprecipitate from fraction 24 were analyzed to permit comparison of equivalent levels of cyclin E complexes with fraction 19. The asterisk marks the more mobile, active form of Cdk2 that is phosphorylated on Thr-160. From ref. *(17)*.

was 10-fold greater than the bulk of the cyclin E eluting as lower molecular-weight forms. Comparison of the composition of cyclin E immunoprecipitates eluting at these different molecular weights revealed that the larger complexes were markedly depleted of both p21 and p27 (Fig. 8C) in contrast to previous results for cyclin E immunoprecipitates from whole-cell lysates. In different experiments, we and others have demonstrated that estrogen relieves a cyclin E-Cdk2 inhibitory activity that is present in antiestrogen-treated cells, which is attributable to p21 *(15,17)*. Therefore, in contrast to estrogen-induced activation of cyclin D1-Cdk4 by increasing cyclin D1 expression, estradiol-mediated activation of cyclin E-Cdk2 appears to result from decreased association with p21. A potential mechanism for the loss of p21 from these complexes is its sequestration by cyclin D/Cdk4-6 induced by estradiol as suggested by Planas-Silva and Weinberg *(15)*. However, more recent data from this laboratory demonstrate a similar mechanism of activation of cyclin E/Cdk2 following induction of c-Myc but in the absence of increased cyclin D1 gene expression and cyclin D1/Cdk4 complex formation *(16)*. These data point to a more direct effect of estrogen/antiestrogen on p21 perhaps via a c-Myc-mediated mechanism.

4.6. Involvement of c-Myc in Antiestrogen Action

Among the first candidate genes to be investigated as potential targets of estrogen-induced mitogenesis was the immediate early gene c-*myc* which encodes a nuclear phosphoprotein (c-Myc). Regulation of this gene is among the earliest detectable responses to estrogens and has been identified in a number of target tissues including rat uteri in vivo *(79,80)* and both normal breast-epithelial cells and breast-cancer cells in vitro *(17,81)*. Increased expression of c-*myc* was attributed to estrogen-induced transcriptional regulation, but not necessarily via a classical estrogen response element (ERE), and demonstrated kinetics similar to those following growth factor stimulation of serum-starved cells *(81,82)*. Furthermore, inhibition of c-*myc* expression by antisense oligonucleotides was accompanied by inhibition of estrogen-induced cell proliferation identifying a critical role for c-*myc* in estrogen action *(83)*. In fibroblasts, c-Myc is both necessary and sufficient for G_1-S phase progression *(58)* and activation of conditional alleles of c-*myc* is followed by the activation of both cyclin D1-Cdk4 and cyclin E-Cdk2 *(59–61)*.

Rapid decreases in c-*myc* mRNA and protein levels are observed in response to a variety of antiestrogens in both in vivo and in vitro models *(21,63,84,85)*, being apparent within 30 min (Fig. 9A). Therefore in addition to cyclin D1 and p21, c-Myc may be a major target molecule through which antiestrogen mediates cell-cycle control. In order to test whether c-Myc expression was critical to antiestrogen arrest, we constructed MCF-7 cell lines stably transfected with c-Myc cDNA under the control of a metal-responsive metallothionein promoter *(16)*. Cells were treated with ICI 182780 resulting in

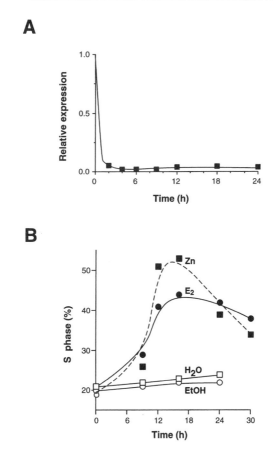

Fig. 9. Effects of estrogen and antiestrogen on c-myc expression in breast-cancer cells. **(A)** T-47D cells proliferating in insulin-supplemented serum-free medium were treated with 500 nM ICI 164384 and harvested at intervals for Northern analysis. Densitometric analysis of data for mRNA expression is presented relative to exponentially growing control cells. From ref. *(21)*. **(B)** An MCF-7 cell line stably transfected with the zinc-inducible p_MT vector containing c-myc cDNA was growth-arrested for 48 h with 10 nM ICI 182780. Cells were treated at time 0 with either 65 μM Zn (■) or vehicle (H_2O,), or 100 nM estradiol (E_2, ●) or vehicle (EtOH, ○). At intervals thereafter, cells were harvested, stained for DNA content and the proportion of cells in S phase determined by flow cytometry. From ref.

G_1-phase arrest. c-Myc expression was induced by Zn treatment and this was sufficient for subsequent S-phase entry (Fig. 9B). This gives strong support to a role for downregulation of c-Myc in antiestrogen action. An analysis of the molecular events preceding S-phase entry demonstrated that c-Myc induction resulted in the formation of high molecular-weight, high specific activity cyclin E/Cdk2 complexes devoid of p21, apparently identical to those induced

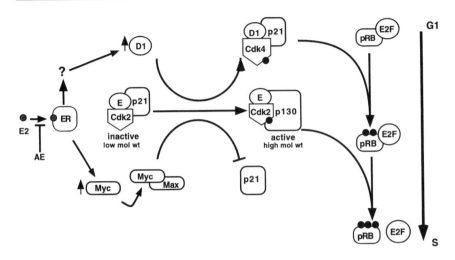

Fig. 10.   A model of estrogen and antiestrogen effects on molecules regulating G_1-phase progression. Estrogen (E_2) binding to ER initiates a cascade of events including transcriptional activation of c-Myc and cyclin D1 gene expression, the latter occuring indirectly through the induction of an intermediary factor (?), which in turn regulates cyclin D1 gene expression. The increased expression of cyclin D1 stimulates the formation of active cyclin D1-Cdk4 complexes containing p21, here acting as an assembly factor rather than an inhibitor of the kinase. Activation of cyclin E-Cdk2 involves conversion to a high molecular-weight form lacking p21 and containing p130. Neither induction of cyclin D1 nor activation of the cyclin D1-Cdk4 complex appear to be c-Myc dependent in this model system, but both cyclin D1-Cdk4 (via sequestration of p21) and c-Myc (via an unknown mechanism) appear to contribute to cyclin E-Cdk2 activation. Antiestrogens inhibit binding of estrogen to the ER and act by opposing the downstream effects of estrogen on gene transcription and activation. E_2, estrogen; AE, antiestrogen; D1, cyclin D1; E, cyclin E; ●, phosphorylation sites.

by estradiol. This occurred in the absence of any detectable changes in cyclin D1/Cdk4 complexes and activity *(16)*.

Together these data identify c-Myc and cyclin D1 as major downstream targets of estrogen/antiestrogen action; these pathways are initially separate but converge at or before the formation of active cyclin E/Cdk2 complexes devoid of p21. Thus the movement of p21 into and out of cyclin E/Cdk2 complexes appears to be a critical event in antiestrogen/estrogen regulated G_1- to S-phase progression. The mechanism responsible for this effect is a major unanswered question in estrogen/antiestrogen action.

5. CONCLUSION

Recent research in this and other laboratories has given us a much clearer understanding of the molecular events that mediate the antiproliferative effects of antiestrogens in ER-positive breast cancer cells. In summary, current evidence suggests that antiestrogens achieve their acute effects on inhibition of breast-cancer cell-cycle progression in G_1 phase via a sequence of events including decreased cyclin D1 and c-*myc* expression, decreased cyclin D1-Cdk4 and cyclin E-Cdk2 activities, at least partially via a redistribution of p21, and finally decreased RB protein phosphorylation. Ectopic expression of either c-*myc* or cyclin D1 is sufficient to overcome antiestrogen arrest in these cells, confirming the critical role of these genes in antiestrogen action. The development of an in vitro model system, where breast-cancer cells are growth-arrested with a pure antiestrogen and cell-cycle progression re-initiated with estrogen, has also contributed to understanding antiestrogen action by allowing much better definition of early molecular events in estrogen action. Current knowledge developed from this model and the results of others is presented in Fig. 10. In summary, mitogenic effects of estrogen appear to be mediated by at least two apparently distinct pathways, involving transcriptional activation of c-*myc* and cyclin D1, the latter requiring *de novo* protein synthesis and leading to formation of active complexes with Cdk4. Both pathways then lead to early activation of cyclin E-Cdk2 by the formation of cyclin E-Cdk2 complexes deficient in the CDK inhibitor p21, and of high molecular weight, presumably due to association with other proteins including p130 *(16)*. Phosphorylation of pRB is a primary action of these active cyclin D1-Cdk4 and cyclin E-Cdk2 complexes, resulting in release of E2F transcription factors necessary for DNA synthesis, and progression from G_1 to S phase of the cell cycle. Antiestrogens act as competitive antagonists of the binding of estrogen to its receptor and appear able to reverse the downstream effects of estrogen at each step along these pathways.

Major questions remain unanswered, however. Further studies on cyclin/CDK complex formation are required to establish the precise mechanisms involved in antiestrogen inhibition of CDK activity, particularly the factors involved in movement of CDKIs in and out of these complexes. In addition, the pathway linking alterations in c-Myc expression to cyclin E-Cdk2 activation needs definition as does the indirect transcriptional regulation of cyclin D1. The latter studies should lead us to the earliest and primary events in antiestrogen/estrogen action.

Growth inhibition by a number of other agents appears to occur by mechanisms different from those responsible for antiestrogen action. Like antiestrogens, the antiprogestin RU 486 and retinoic acid are both potent inhibitors of breast cancer cell proliferation. However, we found that neither appears to downregulate cyclin D1 prior to effects on S phase, despite changes in pRB phosphorylation *(70,86)*. Instead, increased p21 abundance appears to be an important mechanism mediating the antiproliferative effects of antiprogestins *(86)*. CDKIs appear to play a central role for several other growth inhibitors, suppressing CDK function and consequently pRB phosphorylation. TGF-β, for example, which arrests cells in mid- to late- G_1, promotes association of p27 with Cdk2 *(87)* and can also transcriptionally upregulate expression of p15^{INK4}, a Cdk4/Cdk6 inhibitor. p27 is also implicated in the G_1 arrest of murine macrophages by cAMP, where it prevents cyclin D1/Cdk4 activation *(88)* and in progestin-mediated, long-term growth inhibition of breast cancer cells *(89)*. p21 induction is involved in growth inhibition by diverse stimuli, including serum deprivation *(90)* and DNA damage *(74)*.

The evidence presented here for the key roles of c-Myc and cyclin D1 suggest potential roles for overexpression of these molecules in constitutive activation of estrogen-regulated growth pathways and in the important problem of clinical antiestrogen resistance. The common amplification and overexpression at the mRNA and protein levels of these genes in breast tumors *(see* refs. *50,91* and references therein) suggest that these might confer a growth advantage to breast epithelial cells and contribute to the development and progression of breast cancer. In support of this concept, we have demonstrated increments in cyclin D1 protein levels with progression from normal epithelium through hyperplasias to intraductal and invasive carcinomas *(49)*. Thus cyclin D1 overexpression is an early event in the evolution of breast cancer and may play a causative role. Our demonstration that ectopic expression of c-Myc *(16)* or cyclin D1 *(16,70)* can overcome the growth inhibitory effects of antiestrogens in vitro, suggests a mechanism for antiestrogen resistance in clinical breast cancer that needs further investigation. Further research into the mechanisms of cell-cycle control in breast cancer should aid in the refinement of current procedures for the management of this disease. It is hoped that such knowledge will ultimately also contribute to a better understanding of tumorigenesis and progression in breast cancer, providing useful markers of prognosis and therapeutic response and leading to new molecular targets for therapeutic and preventative intervention. The knowledge gained from in vitro models of antiestrogen and estrogen action in breast cancer should also facilitate the exploration of mechanisms underlying hormone action in the normal breast and other estrogen-target tissues.

ACKNOWLEDGMENTS

Research in this laboratory is supported by grants from the National Health and Medical Research Council of Australia and the New South Wales Cancer Council. O.W.J.P. is supported by a post-graduate medical scholarship from the NHMRC. E.M.R. is supported by the US Army Medical Research and Materiel Command under DAMD17-98-1-8087.

REFERENCES

1. Beatson G. On the treatment of inoperable cases of carcinoma of the mamma: suggestions for a new method of treatment, with illustrative cases. *Lancet* 1896; ii:104–107.
2. Lerner LJ, Jordan VC. Development of antiestrogens and their use in breast cancer: Eighth Cain Memorial Award lecture. *Cancer Res* 1990; 50:4177–4189.

3. Early Breast Cancer Trialists' Collaborative Group. Systemic treatment of early breast cancer by hormonal, cytotoxic, or immune therapy. *Lancet* 1992; 339:1–15, 71–85.

4. Early Breast Cancer Trialists' Collaborative Group. Tamoxifen for early breast cancer: an overview of the randomised trials. *Lancet* 1998; 351:1451–1467.

5. Wakeling AE, Bowler J. Steroidal pure antioestrogens. *J Endocrinol* 1987; 112:R7–R10.

6. Wakeling AE. The future of new pure antiestrogens in clinical breast cancer. *Breast Cancer Res Treat* 1993; 25:1–9.

7. Lippman ME, Bolan G. Oestrogen-responsive human breast cancer in long term tissue culture. *Nature* 1975; 256:592–593.

8. Lippman M, Bolan G, Huff K. The effects of estrogens and antiestrogens on hormone-responsive human breast cancer in long term tissue culture. *Cancer Res* 1976; 36:4595–4601.

9. Musgrove EA, Wakeling AE, Sutherland RL. Points of action of estrogen antagonists and a calmodulin antagonist within the MCF-7 human breast cancer cell cycle. *Cancer Res* 1989; 49:2398–2404.

10. Wakeling AE, Newboult E, Peters SW. Effects of antioestrogens on the proliferation of MCF-7 human breast cancer cells. *J Mol Endocrinol* 1989; 2:225–234.

11. Taylor IW, Hodson PJ, Green MD, et al. Effects of tamoxifen on cell cycle progression of synchronous MCF-7 human mammary carcinoma cells. *Cancer Res* 1983; 43:4007–4010.

12. Sutherland RL, Reddel RR, Green MD. Effects of oestrogens on cell proliferation and cell cycle kinetics. A hypothesis on the cell cycle effects of antioestrogens. *Eur J Cancer Clin Oncol* 1983; 19:307–318.

13. Sutherland RL, Hall RE, Taylor IW. Cell proliferation kinetics of MCF-7 human mammary carcinoma cells in culture and effects of tamoxifen on exponentially growing and plateau-phase cells. *Cancer Res* 1983; 43:3998–4006.

14. Reddel RR, Murphy LC, Sutherland RL. Factors affecting the sensitivity of T-47D human breast cancer cells to tamoxifen. *Cancer Res* 1984; 44:2398–2405.

15. Planas-Silva MD, Weinberg RA. Estrogen-dependent cyclin E-cdk2 activation through p21 redistribution. *Mol Cell Biol* 1997; 17:4059–4069.

16. Prall OWJ, Rogan EM, Musgrove EA, et al. c-Myc or cyclin D1 mimics estrogen effects on cyclin E-Cdk2 activation and cell cycle reentry. *Mol Cell Biol* 1998; 18:4499–4508.

17. Prall OWJ, Sarcevic B, Musgrove EA, et al. Estrogen-induced activation of Cdk4 and Cdk2 during G1-S phase progression is accompanied by increased cyclin D1 expression and decreased cyclin-dependent kinase inhibitor association with cyclin E-Cdk2. *J Biol Chem* 1997; 272:10882–10894.

18. Musgrove EA, Sutherland RL. Steroids, growth factors, and cell cycle controls in breast cancer, in *Regulatory Mechanisms in Breast Cancer* (Lippman ME, Dickson RB, eds). Kluwer Academic Publishers, Boston, 1991; pp. 305–331.

19. Watts CKW, Sweeney KJE, Warlters A, et al. Antiestrogen regulation of cell cycle progression and cyclin D1 gene expression in MCF-7 human breast cancer cells. *Breast Cancer Res Treat* 1994; 31:95–105.

20. Musgrove EA, Sutherland RL. Acute effects of growth factors on T-47D breast cancer cell cycle progression. *Eur J Cancer* 1993; 29A:2273–2279.

21. Musgrove EA, Hamilton JA, Lee CSL, et al. Growth factor, steroid and steroid antagonist regulation of cyclin gene expression associated with changes in T-47D human breast cancer cell cycle progression. *Mol Cell Biol* 1993; 13:3577–3587.

22. Daly RJ, Darbre PD. Cellular and molecular events in loss of estrogen sensitivity in ZR-75-1 and T-47-D human breast cancer cells. *Cancer Res* 1990; 50:5868–5875.

23. Furuya Y, Kohno N, Fujiwara Y, et al. Mechanisms of estrogen action on the proliferation of MCF-7 human breast cancer cells in an improved culture medium. *Cancer Res* 1989; 49:6670–6674.

24. Glover JF, Irwin JT, Darbre PD. Interaction of phenol red with estrogenic and antiestrogenic action on growth of human breast cancer cells ZR-75-1 and T-47-D. *Cancer Res* 1988; 48:3693–3697.

25. Katzenellenbogen BS, Kendra KL, Norman MJ, et al. Proliferation, hormonal responsiveness, and estrogen receptor content of MCF-7 human breast cancer cells grown in the short-term and long-term absence of estrogens. *Cancer Res* 1987; 47:4355–60.

26. Vignon F, Bouton MM, Rochefort H. Antiestrogens inhibit the mitogenic effect of growth factors on breast cancer cells in the total absence of estrogens. *Biochem Biophys Res Commun* 1987; 146:1502–1508.

27. Philips A, Chalbos D, Rochefort P. Estradiol increases and anti-estrogens antagonize the growth factor-induced Activator Protein-1 activity in MCF7 breast cancer cells without affecting c-*fos* and c-*jun* synthesis. *J Biol Chem* 1993; 268:14103–14108.

28. Pham TA, Elliston JF, Nawaz Z, et al. Antiestrogen can establish nonproductive receptor complexes and alter chromatin structure at target enhancers. *Proc Natl Acad Sci USA* 1991; 88:3125–3129.

29. Dauvois S, Danielian PS, White R, et al. Antiestrogen ICI 164,384 reduces cellular estrogen receptor content by increasing its turnover. *Proc Natl Acad Sci USA* 1992; 89:4037–4041.

30. Brünner N, Bronzert D, Vindeløv LL, et al. Effect on growth and cell cycle kinetics of estradiol and tamoxifen on MCF-7 human breast cancer cells grown in vitro and in nude mice. *Cancer Res* 1989; 49:1515–1520.

31. Osborne CK, Hobbs K, Clark GM. Effect of estrogens and antiestrogens on growth of human breast cancer cells in athymic nude mice. *Cancer Res* 1985; 45:584–590.

32. Gottardis MM, Jordan VC. Development of tamoxifen-stimulated growth of MCF-7 tumors in athymic mice after long-term antiestrogen administration. *Cancer Res* 1988; 48:5183–5187.

33. Kyprianou N, English HF, Davidson NE, et al. Programmed cell death during regression of the MCF-7 human breast cancer following estrogen ablation. *Cancer Res* 1991; 51:162–166.

34. Cameron DA, Ritchie AA, Langdon S, et al. Tamoxifen induced apoptosis in ZR-75 breast cancer xenografts antedates tumour regression. *Breast Cancer Res Treat* 1997; 45:99–107.

35. Warri AM, Huovinen RL, Laine AM, et al. Apoptosis in toremifene-induced growth inhibition of human breast cancer cells in vivo and in vitro. *J Natl Cancer Inst* 1993; 85:1412–1418.

36. Ellis PA, Saccani-Jotti G, Clarke R, et al. Induction of apoptosis by tamoxifen and ICI 182780 in primary breast cancer. *Int J Cancer* 1997; 72:608–613.

37. Osborne CK, Boldt DH, Estrada P. Human breast cancer cell cycle synchronization by estrogens and antiestrogens in culture. *Cancer Res* 1984; 44:1433–1439.

38. Grana X, Reddy EP. Cell cycle control in mammalian cells: role of cyclins, cyclin dependent kinases (CDKs), growth suppressor genes and cyclin-dependent kinase inhibitors (CKIs). *Oncogene* 1995; 11:211–219.

39. Sherr CJ. Cancer cell cycles. *Science* 1996; 274:1672–1677.

40. Sutherland RL, Prall OWJ, Watts CKW, et al. Estrogen and progestin regulation of cell cycle progression. *J Mammary Gland Biol Neoplasia* 1998; 3:63–72.

41. Sherr CJ. G1 phase progression: cycling on cue. *Cell* 1994; 79:551–555.

42. Nevins JR. Towards an understanding of the functional complexity of the E2F and retinoblastoma families. *Cell Growth Differ* 1998; 9:585–593.

43. Dyson N. The regulation of E2F by pRB-family proteins. *Genes Dev* 1998; 12:2245–2262.

44. Riley DJ, Lee EY-HP, Lee W-H. The retinoblastoma protein: more than a tumor suppressor. *Annu Rev Cell Biol* 1994; 10:1–29.

45. Weinberg RA. The retinoblastoma protein and cell cycle control. *Cell* 1995; 81:323–330.

46. Morgan DO. Principles of CDK regulation. *Nature* 1995; 374:131–134.

47. Fantl V, Stamp G, Andrews A, et al. Mice lacking cyclin D1 are small and show defects in eye and mammary gland development. *Genes Dev* 1995; 9:2364–2372.

48. Sicinski P, Donaher JL, Parker SB, et al. Cyclin D1 provides a link between development and oncogenesis in the retina and breast. *Cell* 1995; 82:621–630.

49. Alle KM, Henshall SM, Field AS, et al. Cyclin D1 protein is over expressed in hyperplasia and intraductal carcinoma of the breast. *Clin Cancer Res* 1998; 4:847–856.

50. Buckley MF, Sweeney KJE, Hamilton JA, et al. Expression and amplification of cyclin genes in human breast cancer. *Oncogene* 1993; 8:2127–2133.

51. Morgan DO. The dynamics of cyclin dependent kinase structure. *Curr Opin Cell Biol* 1996; 8:767–772.

52. Reynisdottir I, Massague J. The subcellular locations of p15(Ink4b) and p27(Kip1) coordinate their inhibitory interactions with cdk4 and cdk2. *Genes Dev* 1997; 11:492–503.

53. Sherr CJ, Roberts JM. Inhibitors of mammalian G1 cyclin-dependent kinases. *Genes Dev* 1995; 9:1149–1163.

54. Russo AA, Jeffrey PD, Patten AK, et al. Crystal structure of the p27Kip1 cyclin-dependent-kinase inhibitor bound to the cyclin A-Cdk2 complex [see comments]. *Nature* 1996; 382:325–331.

55. LaBaer J, Garrett MD, Stevenson LF, et al. New functional activities for the p21 family of cdk inhibitors. *Genes Dev* 1997; 11:847–862.

56. Soos TJ, Kiyokawa H, Yan JS, et al. Formation of p27-cdk complexes during the human mitotic cell cycle. *Cell Growth Differ* 1996; 7:135–146.

57. Zhang H, Hannon GJ, Beach D. p21-containing cyclin kinases exist in both active and inactive states. *Genes Dev* 1994; 8:1750–1758.

58. Henriksson M, Luscher B. Proteins of the Myc network: essential regulators of cell growth and differentiation. *Adv Cancer Res* 1996; 68:109–182.

59. Steiner P, Philipp A, Lukas J, et al. Identification of a Myc-dependent step during the formation of active G_1 cyclin-cdk complexes. *EMBO J* 1995; 14:4814–4826.

60. Rudolph B, Saffrich R, Zwicker J, et al. Activation of cyclin-dependent kinases by Myc mediates induction of cyclin A, but not apoptosis. *EMBO J* 1996; 15:3065–3076.

61. Perez-Roger I, Solomon DL, Sewing A, et al. Myc activation of cyclin E/Cdk2 kinase involves induction of cyclin E gene transcription and inhibition of p27(Kip1) binding to newly formed complexes. *Oncogene* 1997; 14:2373–2381.

62. Watts CKW, Brady A, Sarcevic B, et al. Antiestrogen inhibition of cell cycle progression in breast cancer cells is associated with inhibition of cyclin-dependent kinase activity and decreased retinoblastoma protein phosphorylation. *Mol Endocrinol* 1995; 9:1804–1813.

63. Wilcken NRC, Sarcevic B, Musgrove EA, et al. Differential effects of retinoids and antiestrogens on cell cycle progression and cell cycle regulatory genes in human breast cancer cells. *Cell Growth Diff* 1996; 7:65–74.

63a. Carroll JS, Prall OWJ, Musgrove EA, et al. A pure estrogen antagonist inhibits cyclin E-Cdk2 activity in MCF-7 breast cancer cells and induces accumulation of p130-E2F4 complexes characteristic of quiescence. *J Biol Chem* 2000; 275:38221–38229.

64. Sweeney KJ, Swarbrick A, Sutherland RL, et al. Lack of relationship between CDK activity and G_1 cyclin expression in breast cancer cells. *Oncogene* 1998; 16:2865–2878.

65. Matsushime H, Quelle DE, Shurtleff SA, et al. D-type cyclin-dependent kinase activity in mammalian cells. *Mol Cell Biol* 1994; 14:2066–2076.

66. Matsushime H, Roussel MF, Ashmun RA, et al. Colony-stimulating factor 1 regulates novel cyclins during the G1 phase of the cell cycle. *Cell* 1991; 65:701–713.

67. Altucci L, Addeo R, Cicatiello L, et al. 17b-Estradiol induces cyclin D1 gene transcription, p36D1-p34cdk4 complex activation and p105Rb phosphorylation during mitogenic stimulation of G1-arrested human breast cancer cells. *Oncogene* 1996; 12:2315–2324.

68. Foster JS, Wimalasena J. Estrogen regulates activity of cyclin-dependent kinases and retinoblastoma protein phosphorylation in breast cancer cells. *Mol Endocrinol* 1996; 10:488–498.

69. Albanese C, Johnson J, Watanabe G, et al. Transforming p21ras mutants and c-Ets-2 activate the cyclin D1 promoter through distinguishable regions. *J Biol Chem* 1995; 270:23589–23597.

70. Wilcken NRC, Prall OWJ, Musgrove EA, et al. Inducible overexpression of cyclin D1 in breast cancer cells reverses the growth-inhibitory effects of antiestrogens. *Clin Cancer Res* 1997; 3:849–854.

71. Musgrove EA, Sarcevic B, Sutherland RL. Inducible expression of cyclin D1 in T-47D human breast cancer cells is sufficient for CDK2 activation and pRB hyperphosphorylation. *J Cell Biochem* 1996; 60:363–378.

72. Musgrove EA, Lee CSL, Buckley MF, et al. Cyclin D1 induction in breast cancer cells shortens G_1 and is sufficient for cells arrested in G_1 to complete the cell cycle. *Proc Natl Acad Sci USA* 1994; 91:8022–8026.

73. Lukas J, Bartkova J, Bartek J. Convergence of mitogenic signalling cascades from diverse classes of receptors at the cyclin D-cyclin-dependent kinase-pRb-controlled G1 checkpoint. *Mol Cell Biol* 1996; 16:6917–6925.

74. Harper JW, Adami GR, Wei N, et al. The p21 Cdk-interacting protein Cip1 is a potent inhibitor of G_1 cyclin dependent kinases. *Cell* 1993; 75:805–816.

75. Xiong Y, Hannon GJ, Zhang H, et al. p21 is a universal inhibitor of cyclin kinases. *Nature* 1993; 366:701–704.

76. Won K-A, Xiong Y, Beach D, et al. Growth regulated expression of D-type cyclin genes in human diploid fibroblasts. *Proc Natl Acad Sci USA* 1992; 89:9910–9914.

77. Dulic V, Lees E, Reed SI. Association of human cyclin E with a periodic G_1-S phase protein kinase. *Science* 1992; 257:1958–1961.

78. Koff A, Giordano A, Desai D, et al. Formation and activation of a cyclin E-cdk2 complex during the G1 phase of the human cell cycle. *Science* 1992; 257:1689–1694.

79. Murphy LJ, Murphy LC, Friesen HG. Estrogen induction of N-myc and c-myc proto-onco-gene expression in the rat uterus. *Endocrinology* 1987; 120:1882–1888.

80. Weisz A, Bresciani F. Estrogen induces expression of c-*fos* and c-*myc* protooncogenes in rat uterus. *Mol Endocrinol* 1988; 2:816–824.

81. Dubik D, Dembinski TC, Shiu RPC. Stimulation of c-*myc* oncogene expression associated with estrogen-induced proliferation of human breast cancer cells. *Cancer Res* 1987; 47:6517–6521.

82. Dubik D, Shiu RP. Mechanism of estrogen activation of c-*myc* oncogene expression. *Onco-gene* 1992; 7:1587–1594.

83. Watson PH, Pon RT, Shiu RPC. Inhibition of c-*myc* expression by phosphorothioate anti-sense oligonucleotide identifies a critical role for c-*myc* in the growth of human breast cancer. *Cancer Res* 1991; 51:3996–4000.

84. Wong MS, Murphy LC. Differential regulation of c-*myc* by progestins and antiestrogens in T-47D human breast cancer cells. *J Steroid Biochem Mol Biol* 1991; 39:39–44.

85. Santos GF, Scott GK, Lee WMF, et al. Estrogen-induced post-transcriptional modulation of c-*myc* proto-oncogene expression in human breast cancer cells. *J Biol Chem* 1988; 263:9565–9568.

86. Musgrove EA, Lee CSL, Cornish AL, et al. Antiprogestin inhibition of cell cycle progression in T-47D breast cancer cells is accompanied by induction of the CDK inhibitor p21. *Mol Endocrinol* 1997; 11:54–66.

87. Polyak K, Kato J-Y, Solomon MJ, et al. p27^{Kip1}, a cyclin-Cdk inhibitor, links transforming growth factor-b and contact inhibition to cell cycle arrest. *Genes Dev* 1994; 8:9–22.

88. Kato J-Y, Matsuoka M, Polyak K, et al. Cyclic AMP-induced G_1 phase arrest mediated by an inhibitor (p27^{KIP1}) of cyclin-dependent kinase 4 activation. *Cell* 1994; 79:487–496.

89. Musgrove EA, Swarbrick A, Lee CSL, et al. Mechanisms of cyclin-dependent kinase inacti-vation by progestins. *Mol Cell Biol* 1998; 18:1812–1825.

90. Sheikh MS, Li XS, Chen JC, et al. Mechanisms of regulation of WAF1/CIP1 gene expression in human breast carcinoma: role of p53-dependent and independent signal transduction pathways. *Oncogene* 1994; 9:3407–3415.

91. Hui R, Cornish AL, McClelland RA, et al. Cyclin D1 and estrogen receptor gene expression are positively correlated in primary breast cancer. *Clin Cancer Res* 1996; 2:923–928.

92. Sweeney KJE, Musgrove EA, Watts CKW, et al. Cyclins and breast cancer, in *Breast Cancer: Cellular and Molecular Biology* (Dickson R, Lippman M, eds). Kluwer Academic Publishers, Dordrecht, The Netherlands 1996, pp 141–170.

3 Drug Resistance to Antiestrogens

*Ruth M. O'Regan, Anait S. Levenson,
Gale M. England, Kathy A. Yao,
Henry D. Muenzner, Hiroyuki Takei,
and V. Craig Jordan*

CONTENTS

1. INTRODUCTION

Tamoxifen (Nolvadex®) (Fig. 1), a nonsteroidal antiestrogen, is the endocrine treatment of choice for all stages of breast cancer. The drug has ten million women years of clinical experience and is described by the World Health Organization (WHO) as an essential treatment for breast cancer. The clinical pharmacology of tamoxifen has been studied in great detail because it is continuing to be tested as a preventive for breast cancer in high-risk women

From: *Hormone Therapy in Breast and Prostate Cancer*
Edited by: V. C. Jordan and B. J. A. Furr © Humana Press Inc., Totowa, NJ

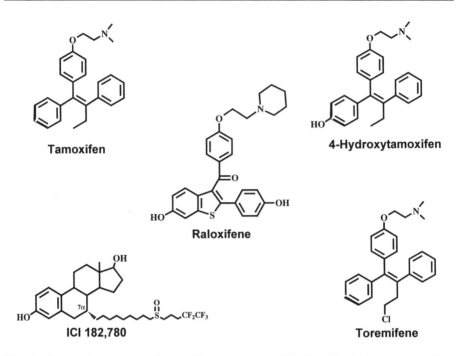

Fig. 1. Chemical structures of tamoxifen, raloxifene, ICI 182,780, 4-hydroxytamoxifen, and toremifene.

(1). This strategy is based on three important facts. Firstly, tamoxifen prevents rat mammary carcinogenesis *(2,3).* Secondly, tamoxifen reduces the incidence of contralateral breast cancer *(4)* and thirdly, when the preliminary studies were started in 1986 *(5),* tamoxifen was believed to have a low incidence of side effects *(6).*

As a prelude to the testing of tamoxifen in healthy women, studies were conducted to evaluate the effect of antiestrogens on bone density. Remarkably, tamoxifen exhibits target site-specific effects in animals; bone density is maintained in ovariectomized rats but estrogen-stimulated uterine weight is blocked *(7)* The action in bone translated to the clinic *(8)* but regrettably our finding of the target site-specific effects of tamoxifen to stimulate endometrial-cancer growth while preventing the estrogen-stimulated growth of breast cancer *(9)* also translated to the clinic. There is a documented two fold increase in the incidence of endometrial cancer in breast-cancer patients who take tamoxifen *(10).* Although no woman being treated for breast cancer with tamoxifen should have the drug stopped because of concerns about endometrial cancer, this troublesome side effect is unacceptable if tamoxifen is to be used by the general population to prevent breast cancer. In the late 1980s, we suggested a paradigm change for the preventions of breast cancer. Targeted drugs should be identified as preventives for osteoporosis but with the beneficial side effects of preventing breast and endometrial cancer *(11)*. The widespread use of the therapy in postmenopausal women would have a significant impact on the incidence of breast cancer.

Raloxifene (Evista®) has recently been approved by the Food and Drug Administration (FDA) in the USA for the prevention of osteoporosis in postmenopausal women. Raloxifene (originally named LY156,750 or keoxifene) (Fig. 1) is a nonsteroidal antiestrogen with a high affinity for the estrogen receptor (ER) *(12)*. Drug development was originally targeted towards breast-cancer therapy but was discontinued in the late 1980s. However, the finding that raloxifene maintained bone density in rats *(7)*, prevented rat mammary carcinogenesis *(13)*, and inhibited tamoxifen-stimulated endometrial carcinoma growth *(14)*, laid the foundation for drug development as a preventive for osteoporosis in the mid 1990s.

The drugs, originally classified as antiestrogens, are having an enormous impact on therapeutics. Raloxifene and tamoxifen are now classified as selective ER modulators because of their diverse pharmacology. An examination of their molecular biology is not only providing a remarkable insight into the mechanism of antiestrogen action but also the mechanism of drug resistance to tamoxifen.

2. DRUG RESISTANCE TO TAMOXIFEN

A decade ago the perceived wisdom was that drug resistance to tamoxifen developed when ER-positive disease converted to ER-negative disease. It was known that tamoxifen was more effective in ER-positive disease *(6)* so the hypothesis was logical.

In the laboratory, the dimethylbenzanthracene (DMBA)-induced rat mammary carcinoma model was used to define the optimal strategy for adjuvant therapy. In the mid 1970s the clinical plan was to use one year of tamoxifen because one year, on average, was effective in controlling advanced disease and there was also a concern that longer treatment would cause the premature development of drug resistance *(15–17)*. It was believed that the early development of ER-negative disease would be a catastrophic outcome of extending adjuvant tamoxifen therapy. In 1977, we proposed that a strategy of longer rather than shorter therapy would be more beneficial to patients *(18)*. Simply stated, we demonstrated that short-term tamoxifen therapy given to rats with subclinical disease produced by DMBA did not control the development of mammary tumors as well as continuous therapy (Fig. 2). If therapy was stopped, tumors developed *(19–21)*. However, the tumors that developed were responsive to a second endocrine modality *(20)*. Tumors

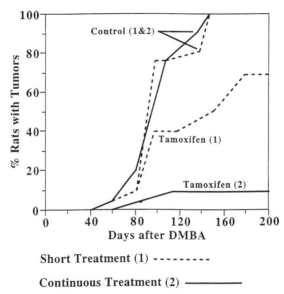

Fig. 2. Rats with DMBA-induced breast tumors. Short-term tamoxifen therapy failed to control breast-cancer growth. Treatment with continuous tamoxifen therapy prevented breast-cancer development compared with animals that did not receive tamoxifen.

induced by DMBA are predominantly ER-positive and we did not detect a significant incidence of ER-negative tumors or drug resistance after months of therapy. We therefore proposed that the strategy of long-term tamoxifen therapy should be tested in clinical trials *(19–21)*. The clinical studies subsequently demonstrated that 2 yr *(22)* and 5 yr *(23)* of adjuvant tamoxifen therapy produced a significant survival advantage for node-positive breast-cancer patients. These conclusions were supported by the overview of clinical trials *(24)* and we now know that 5 yr of adjuvant tamoxifen is superior to 2 yr of tamoxifen *(25)*.

Since we were acutely aware of the fact that tamoxifen was not a cure for breast cancer, and that drug resistance would eventually occur, we decided to address the question by establishing a model of human disease. Our strategy was to establish a model system to evaluate new agents to use when tamoxifen failed. Additionally, we believed it was important to understand the molecular events that occurred so that new agents could be rationally designed.

The ER-positive MCF-7 breast cancer-cell line requires estradiol to grow into tumors when inoculated into the mammary fat pads of athymic mice. Cell lines that are ER-negative grow without estrogen supplementation. Dr. Kent Osborne's group in San Antonio demonstrated that tamoxifen would control estrogen-stimulated MCF-7 tumor growth for prolonged periods, but was ineffective against ER-negative tumor growth *(26)*. We replicated these findings *(27)* but took the studies a step further by developing a transplantable model of tamoxifen-stimulated tumor growth *(28)*. Remarkably, the tumors remain ER-positive and grow in response to estradiol or tamoxifen in athymic rats or mice *(28,29)*. Since there was the possibility that species specific metabolism of tamoxifen might be causing enhanced growth of tumors in mice (where the drug is classified as an estrogen in mouse target tissues [6]), these studies were critical. We subsequently demonstrated that the direct, estrogen-like properties of tamoxifen causes selection of a tamoxifen-stimulated tumor and that local metabolism to estrogens does not play a role in the support of the tamoxifen stimulated phenotype *(30)*.

We had, therefore, developed a unique model of drug resistance that was, in fact, tamoxifen-stimulated for growth. Indeed, if tamoxifen was withdrawn tumor growth slowed but we found that estradiol could then re-activate the ER-positive tumors *(28)*. It was clear therefore that an additional therapy was necessary, after tamoxifen, to block re-activation of tumor growth by estrogen through the ER. Currently two alternatives are available: peripheral aromatase inhibitors, like anastrozole (Arimidex®) or the pure antiestrogens, like ICI 182,780 (Faslodex®) (Fig. 1). Specific inhibitors of aromatase prevent the synthesis of estradiol or estrone thereby denying the tumor a growth stimulus. However, we know that ER-positive breast-cancer cells can retain the ER-positive phenotype in the absence of estrogen and continue to grow *(31,32)*. The tumor cells have become adapted to grow in response to another stimulus *(33)*. Antiestrogens, however, continue to block tumor growth so the developments of new antiestrogenic drugs with novel properties is a reasonable second-line strategy.

The pure antiestrogens were discovered by Wakeling and coworkers in the mid 1980s *(34)*. The compounds are only weakly active orally and must be administered by depot injection. However, there is no reported estrogenic activity; the drugs are complete or pure antiestrogens. Pure antiestrogens were first tested in the tamoxifen-stimulated breast-cancer model prior to clinical evaluation, and the compounds did not support tumor growth *(35,36)*. Currently a clinical study has demonstrated that Faslodex® is effective in controlling a significant proportion of disease that fails tamoxifen *(37,38)* and large international clinical trials are complete (see Chapter 18).

3. TAMOXIFEN AND ENDOMETRIAL CANCER

The development of a laboratory model of endometrial cancer provided the basis for the subsequent clinical examination of, and association between, tamoxifen and endometrial cancer. In 1984, a transplantable human endometrial carcinoma was reported to be partially growth-stimulated by tamoxifen under laboratory conditions *(39)*. Since we were recommending long-term adjuvant therapy *(21)*, we were concerned that pre-existing endometrial cancer could be encouraged to grow by tamoxifen *(9)*. To illustrate the target-site specificity of tamoxifen, athymic mice were transplanted with an ER-positive breast tumor on one side and an endometrial tumor on the other. Animals were treated with tamoxifen and estradiol to determine whether tamoxifen would control the estrogen-stimulated growth of both tumors. Tamoxifen controlled the growth of the breast cancer but not the endometrial cancer so we recommended that patients being treated with long-term tamoxifen therapy should be screened for endometrial cancer *(9)*. The principle was confirmed by the Stockholm group in their adjuvant trial of tamoxifen vs placebo in postmenopausal patients. Patients receiving long-term tamoxifen therapy had a decrease in contralateral breast cancer but an increased incidence of endometrial cancers *(40)*.

During the past decade there has been intense interest in determining the association between tamoxifen and endometrial cancer. We have reviewed the world database *(10,41)* and it is now possible to offer several conclusions. The risk of detecting endometrial cancer in women taking tamoxifen is increased two- to threefold but the stage and grade of the disease is the same as the general population. As a result, there are no strict recommendations for the routine screening of patients taking adjuvant tamoxifen but patients should be followed up immediately if they present with spotting or bleeding.

At present, there is no consensus that tamoxifen is causing endometrial cancer in the human uterus as it is believed to do by producing liver cancer in rats *(42)*. In the rat liver, tamoxifen is metabolized to specific reactive compounds that cause DNA adducts to initiate the process of carcinogenesis *(43)*. These metabolic pathways are not present in human cells *(43)* and DNA adducts have not been detected in human liver biopsies *(44)*. In the uterus, one group of investigators has found no adducts *(46)*, whereas another group has detected an unidentified adduct *(46)*. Unfortunately there has been no progress in the identification of the unknown adduct or in an understanding of its relevance to the genesis of endometrial cancer. However, based on current knowledge of the genesis of cancer, we can estimate that in humans it takes about a decade for the process to occur from initiation to detection. By contrast, endometrial cancer is detected equally before or after the first 2 yr from starting tamoxifen treatment *(10)*. Indeed there are over ten million women-years of experience with tamoxifen worldwide but the number of reported endometrial cancers remains well below a thousand cases of early-stage disease despite a decade of intense investigation.

All of the data pertaining to the carcinogenic potential of tamoxifen has recently been evaluated by the International Agency for Research on Cancer (IARC), but despite the fact that tamoxifen is listed as a carcinogen, there are some specific qualifications. The agency wished to re-assure the clinical and patient community that the benefits of tamoxifen far outweigh the risks and no women should consider stopping taking tamoxifen based on a concern about the slight risk of detecting an endometrial cancer *(47)*.

4. TOREMIFENE: A TAMOXIFEN DERIVATIVE
FOR THE TREATMENT OF ADVANCED BREAST CANCER

Toremifene (Fareston®) (Fig. 1) is approved for the treatment of advanced breast cancer. Clinical results demonstrated a therapeutic equivalence with tamoxifen *(48)* (20 mg daily) using 60 mg daily of toremifene. Side effects are similar but two clinical questions arise that are extremely important: endometrial cancer and cross-resistance with tamoxifen. At present, there have been no reports of an association between toremifene and endometrial cancer. This would be expected because the clinical development of toremifene is approximately where tamoxifen was in 1981. Despite rigorous evaluation of the clinical trials data during the 1980s, an association between tamoxifen and endometrial cancer was only established after 1989.

We have addressed this issue in the same way we did for tamoxifen in 1988 *(9)*. We have now developed two endometrial cancer models to replicate different clinical scenarios. Tumors have been passaged for several years in animals treated either with tamoxifen or estradiol. The first model is designed to mimic patients who have been treated with tamoxifen and have occult endometrial disease that grows in response to the antiestrogens. In contrast, the endometrial tumor passaged in estradiol-treated animals replicates the tamoxifen-naive patient. In Fig. 3, we have compared and contrasted the growth potential of estradiol, tamoxifen, and toremifene in the two different models of endometrial cancers. Toremifene continues to enhance the growth of a tamoxifen-stimulated tumor; there is complete cross-resistance at all doses tested. Therefore, a patient with occult endometrial cancer who switches her breast-cancer therapy from tamoxifen to toremifene would not gain any safety advantage. By contrast, neither tamoxifen nor toremifene produce much of a growth enhancement of tamoxifen-naive endometrial cancers. Most importantly though, both compounds are estrogen-like, not estrogens, in the endometrial-cancer models. In both studies estradiol was superior to the antiestrogens as a growth stimulator. Since we have found that tamoxifen can block the full estrogenic stimulation of tumors, there is every reason to believe that tamoxifen and its analogues will slow the growth of estrogen-stimulated endometrial cancer in patients. Indeed, we see no reason to suppose that these antiestrogens would not be appropriate treatments for endometrial cancer.

It is the standard of practice to offer adjuvant tamoxifen therapy to all node positive or negative ER-positive patients with breast cancer. Therefore the question must be asked "Should toremifene now be used if a breast tumor fails during tamoxifen therapy?" Using our model of tamoxifen-stimulated breast cancer, we now report that tamoxifen and toremifene are completely cross-resistant (Fig. 4). Indeed clinical studies have confirmed this important point *(49,50)* but it should be stressed that if a patient recurs several years after adjuvant tamoxifen, they should be rechallenged with tamoxifen because they have not failed tamoxifen. If

A

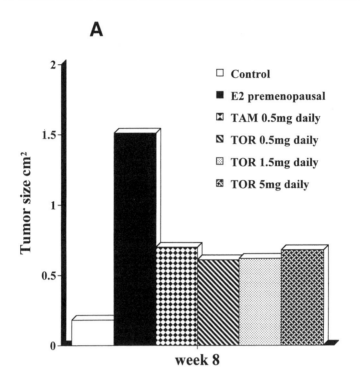

B

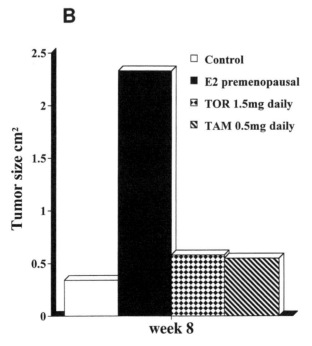

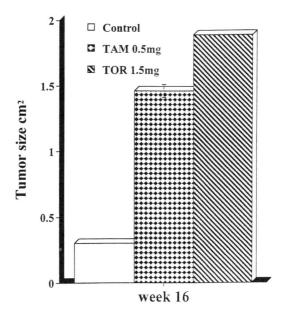

Fig. 4. Athymic mice were implanted with tamoxifen-stimulated breast tumors and treated with vehicle (control), estrogen (premenopausal levels), tamoxifen 0.5 mg or toremifene 1.5 mg daily, for 5 d each week. Clinical trials have demonstrated that tamoxifen 20 mg is equivalent to toremifene 60 mg. There was no significant difference in the effects of either antiestrogen on tumor growth and both agents stimulated tumor growth compared with control, suggesting that they are cross-resistant.

the original tumor was ER-positive, then it is more than likely that micrometastatic disease has grown in response to the patients own estrogen in the years after tamoxifen was stopped *(51)*. In fact, we have noted, in our laboratory studies, that low-dose tamoxifen treatment is more likely to stimulate tamoxifen-stimulated tumors than high-dose therapy. It is therefore possible that higher doses of tamoxifen will control disease better than lower doses. Our observation may explain the

Fig. 3. *(left)* **(A)** Athymic mice were implanted with tamoxifen-stimulated endometrial tumors and treated with vehicle (control), estrogen (premenopausal levels), tamoxifen 0.5 mg or toremifene 0.5 mg, 1.5 mg, or 5 mg daily for 5 d each week. A wide range of toremifene doses were chosen to simulate clinical trials. Estrogen and both antiestrogens stimulated tumor growth compared to control. There was no significant difference between the effects of tamoxifen or any of the three doses of toremifene on tumor growth, suggesting that the two agents are cross-resistant in this model. **(B)** Athymic mice were implanted with tamoxifen-naive endometrial tumors and treated with vehicle (control), estrogen (premenopausal levels), tamoxifen 0.5 mg or toremifene 1.5 mg daily for 5 d each week. Clinical trials have demonstrated that tamoxifen 20 mg is equivalent to toremifene 60 mg. Estrogen significantly stimulated tumor growth but neither antiestrogen significantly stimulated tumor growth, compared to control.

sporadic reports of the isolated successes of high-dose toremifene treatment to cause tumor stasis after tamoxifen failure *(49,52)*. It is the dose and not the drug that is responsible for the tumor stasis.

Overall toremifene has only limited applications and no advantages over tamoxifen for the treatment of advanced breast cancer. By contrast, since toremifene does not produce liver tumors in rats *(53)*, it may be a reasonable agent to consider for the next generation of clinical trials to prevent breast cancer in high-risk women.

5. A MOLECULAR MECHANISM OF ANTIESTROGEN ACTION

The ER was first identified by Jensen and Jacobson in 1962 *(54)* and isolated from the rat uterus by Gorski's group in the mid 1960s *(55)*. However, Jensen subsequently suggested that ER determinations could be used as a marker for the hormone dependency of breast cancer *(56)* and for two decades the ER protein has had a central role in the management of breast cancer as the target for antiestrogen action *(57)*.

For the past 30 years there has been a quest to solve the crystal structure of the estradiol-ER complex and define the molecular events of estrogen action. In 1997, the ligand-binding domain of the ER was crystallized with estradiol and raloxifene *(58)*. Estradiol forms a complex in the hydrophobic ligand-binding pocket through hydrogen bonding at amino acids Glu 353 and Arg 394 with the 3-phenolic hydroxyl and amino acid His 524 with the 17β hydroxyl (Fig. 5A). As a result, there is a conformational change in the protein that re-orients helix 12 to snap shut on the ligand-binding pocket and to seal the steroid inside the protein (Fig. 5A). Helix 12 contains the important AF-2 region and three amino acids (Asp 538, Glu 542, Asp 545) *(59,60)* have been identified that are essential for the subsequent activation of the receptor complex as a transcription unit at an estrogen-sensitive gene. Site-directed mutagenesis in this region destroys AF-2 activity and nonsteroidal antiestrogens also silence AF-2 activity *(61)*.

Raloxifene is anchored at the same two amino acids as estradiol (Fig. 5B), however the aminoethoxy side chain extends away from the molecule. The alkylaminoethoxy side chain is known to be the essential structural feature of all antiestrogens *(62)*. Changes in the distance between the oxygen and the nitrogen *(63)*, restriction in the conformation of the side chain *(64)*, or the basicity of the nitrogen *(65)* all result in a decrease in antiestrogenic activity. Indeed, removal of the side chain results in either an increase in estrogenic properties or a complete loss of activity *(66)*.

An earlier model of estrogen and antiestrogen action, based on experimental evidence with polyclonal antibodies to the ER, described estradiol as being "locked" into the ligand-binding site but that antiestrogens were wedged into the site because of multipoint attachment via the alkylaminoethoxy side chain

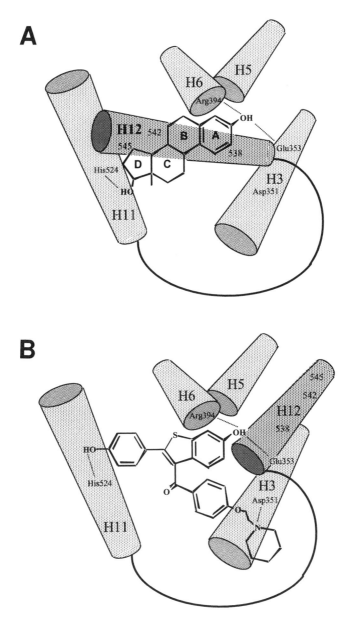

Fig. 5. A molecular mechanism of estrogen and antiestrogen action. **(A)** Helix 12 snaps shut on the ligand binding pocket and seals the steroid inside the protein. This allows co-activators to bind to the critical amino acids (538, 542, 545) to complete the formation of a transcriptional complex. By contrast. **(B)** Raloxifene causes a shift in helix 12 because the piperazine ring binds to amino acid 351. This repositions the helix and masks the AF-2 site.

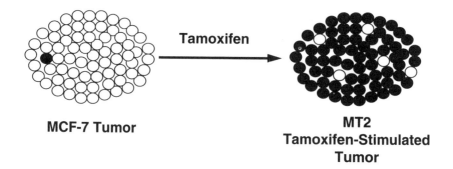

Fig. 6. Selection pressure with tamoxifen to enrich for cells containing mutant ER (black cells).

(67). Similarly a model of antiestrogen action based on the structure-function assays of antiestrogens in cell culture, proposed that the aminoethoxy side chain would bind to an "antiestrogenic region" of the ligand-binding domain to prevent the closure of the ligand-binding pocket *(68).* That interaction was the key to antiestrogen action.

By reference to the crystal structure of the raloxifene ER complex the alkylaminoethoxy side chain binds to amino acid 351 (Aspartate) (Fig. 5B). The consequences of this interaction is a macromolecular perturbation in the complex that moves helix 12 to a new position, thereby masking the critical three amino acids in the AF-2 region: Asp 538, Glu 542, Asp 545 *(60).* Raloxifene has silenced AF-2 activity (Fig. 5B). It is proposed that the co-activators that are needed to form a transcription complex can no longer bind to ER. However, the most compelling evidence to support the molecular model of antiestrogen action for raloxifene comes from the study of drug resistance to tamoxifen.

6. A MUTANT RECEPTOR
IN TAMOXIFEN-STIMULATED TUMORS

Based on the crystal structure of the raloxifene-ER complex, two pathways merit consideration: a mutant receptor or a selective increase in co-activator molecules (or both). During the early 1990s, a popular theory to explain drug resistance to tamoxifen was the selection of breast-cancer cells containing a mutant receptor that translates an antiestrogenic response to an estrogenic response. The concept is illustrated in Fig. 6. Mahfoudi and coworkers *(69)* proposed a mutation hypothesis for the AF-2 region based on their work with the mouse ER. However sequencing of the AF-2 region of tamoxifen-stimulated breast and endometrial tumors demonstrated that this was not the cause of tamoxifen-stimulated growth in reproducible laboratory models *(70).* None of the appropriate mutations were found. By contrast, we addressed the hypothesis by developing different transplantable MCF-7 tumor lines in athymic mice, describing their biological characteristics *(71)* and sequencing the whole receptor in each tumor line *(72)*.

We noted one tumor line that contained a codon 351 asp→tyr mutation as the majority of receptor present *(72)*. However, the problem was to test the efficacy of the receptor appropriately. We chose not to test the biology in animal or yeast cells because of our concern that the results would reflect the wrong cellular context with either inappropriate or insufficient levels of supporting transcription factors. We chose to prepare stable transfectants with clone 10A of the ER-negative breast cancer-cell line MDA-MB-231. We reasoned that receptors would function optimally in the correct context, i.e., a breast-cancer cell, replete with co-activators.

In 1992, we reported the creation of stable transfectants of MDA-MB-231 cells with cDNA's from wild-type and codon 400 gly→val mutant ERs *(73)*. Our goal of that time was to determine whether re-introduction of the ER into receptor negative breast cancer would reassert control by estrogen. We found that estrogen decreased growth rather than increased growth. The pure antiestrogen ICI 164,384 blocked estrogen action. Although we did not determine the precise mechanism for the phenomenon, we used the end point of growth inhibition as an assay for the "estrogenicity" of any ligand receptor complex.

We noted that 4-hydroxytamoxifen (Fig. 1) and a steroidal antiestrogen RU 39,411 with a structural similarity to 4-hydroxytamoxifen *(74)* were more estrogenic in cells transfected with the codon 400 gly→val mutant ER cDNA. Raloxifene, by contrast, is an antiestrogen in transfectants with either wild-type or codon 400 gly→val mutant cDNAs *(74)*. 4-hydroxytamoxifen, therefore, appears to be more promiscuous with estrogen-like activity in the codon 400 gly→val mutant transfectants *(75)*. Although the data with the 400 mutant ER were of interest, the receptor is a cloning artifact rather than a natural mutant *(76)*. By contrast, the codon 351 asp→tyr mutant is the first natural mutant to be identified that could possibly have a role in drug resistance. We prepared stable transfectants with the cDNA for the mutant receptor in MDA-MB-231 cells *(77)* and discovered that an analogue of 4-hydroxytamoxifen was a potent estrogen and inhibited cell growth. We devised a strategy of using single, double, and triple vitellogenin estrogen-response elements *(78)* with a luciferase reporter gene to show that the mutant receptor was more estrogenic than the wild-type receptor. However, it is extremely hard to re-transfect our transfectants so we searched for a gene target *in situ*.

7. THE KEY TO THE ANTIESTROGENIC ACTIVITY OF RALOXIFENE

Estradiol increases the transcription of transforming growth factor α (TGF-α) mRNA in MDA-MB-231 cells transfected with the cDNA for the ER *(79)*. This

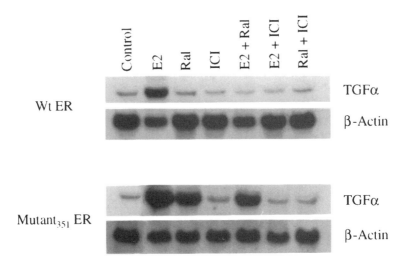

Fig. 7. Effects of estradiol and antiestrogens, or combinations of compounds on TGF-α mRNA expression in ER-transfectants analyzed by Northern blot. The sources for RNAs were following: Control, cells treated with EtOH vehicle; E2, cells treated with 10^{-9} M estradiol (wt ER), and 10^{-8} M estradiol (mutant$_{351}$ER); Ral, cells treated with 10^{-6} M raloxifene; ICI, cells treated with 10^{-6} M ICI 182,780; E2 + Ral, cells treated with 10^{-9} M or 10^{-8} M estradiol (depending on the cell line) and 10^{-6} M raloxifene; E2 + ICI, cells treated with 10^{-9} M or 10^{-8} M estradiol (depending on the cell line) and 10^{-6} M ICI 182,780; Ral + ICI, cells treated with 10^{-} M raloxifene and 10^{-6} M ICI 182,780. β-Actin was used as a loading control.

action of estradiol is blocked by the pure antiestrogen ICI 164,384 *(80)*. Since the regulation of TGF-α is well-recognized as an estrogen-dependent event, we chose this gene to use as a precise assay, in human cells, to document the efficacy of ligand ER complexes. Raloxifene is a complete antiestrogen in the wild-type ER transfectant *(81)* (Fig. 7). However, when raloxifene is liganded to the 351 mutant receptor, raloxifene induces TGF-α mRNA. The pure antiestrogen ICI 182,780 blocks the induction of TGF-α mRNA by both estradiol and raloxifene. It is therefore clear that the specific mutation at amino acid 351 changes the pharmacology of raloxifene from an antiestrogen to an estrogen. The data derived from a natural mutant ER are extremely important as they confirm the key role of amino acid 351, aspartate, which is identified in the crystal structure as interacting with the alkylaminoethoxy side chain. Additionally, our studies identify, for the first time, a specific mechanism for the development of drug resistance to tamoxifen. The mutation clearly provides a growth advantage for breast-cancer cells by exploiting the increased estrogenicity of the receptor complex. Nevertheless, it is important to appreciate that the mutation does not compromise the effectiveness of the pure antiestrogen ICI 182,780 as an appropriate second-line breast-cancer therapy following tamoxifen-treatment failure.

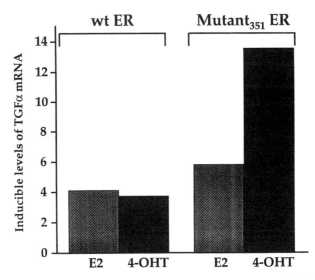

Fig. 8. Induction of TGF-α mRNA expression by estradiol (E2) and 4-hydroxytamoxifen (4-OHT) in cells with wild-type (wt) ER and mutant$_{351}$ ER. Cells were treated with $10^{-7}\,M$ of E2 or 4-OHT for 24 h and analyzed by Northern blot. The graph shows inducible levels of TGF-α mRNA (ratio of normalized TGF-α mRNA in cells treated with compounds to normalized levels in untreated cells) as determined by densitometric analyses.

8. FUTURE ADVANCES IN UNDERSTANDING DRUG RESISTANCE TO TAMOXIFEN

Although we have identified a mechanism of drug resistance to tamoxifen and described the molecular mechanism for the antiestrogen raloxifene, the molecular mechanism of action of tamoxifen or 4-hydroxytamoxifen is subtly different. This in turn has implications for the eventual development of tamoxifen-stimulated tumor growth. The great majority of tamoxifen-stimulated tumors in the laboratory have a wild-type ER so a growth mechanism other than mutation must be amplified in these tumor cells.

We have developed our current hypothesis based on evidence we have recently published using the stable transfectants with cDNAs from either wild-type or 351 mutant ER. Unlike raloxifene, that exhibits estrogen-like activity only with the 351 mutant ER *(81)*, 4-hydroxytamoxifen exhibits estrogen-like properties to initiate TGF-α mRNA synthesis with either wild-type or 351 mutant ER *(82)* (Fig. 8). The 4-hydroxytamoxifen-ER complex is more promiscuous than the raloxifene-ER complex. We suggest that the 4-hydroxytamoxifen-ER complex is subtly different from the raloxifene-ER complex so that it is able to bind with the large concentration of co-activators in the MDA-MB-231 cells. Indeed, the stable transfectant containing the 351 mutant is supersensitive to the action of

4-hydroxytamoxifen *(82)*. The enhanced efficacy of the receptor complex would provide a clear-cut growth advantage in the development of a tumor from the original MCF-7 cells. These data support the proposition *(83)* that antiestrogen-receptor complexes are subtly different in shape and this conclusion should act as a stimulus for investigators to crystallize the 4-hydroxytamoxifen-ER complex. Additionally, it is clearly a priority to determine how the family of co-activator (or co-repressor) proteins regulates gene activation.

9. SUMMARY AND CONCLUSIONS

Laboratory models for breast and endometrial cancer have had an enormous impact on the clinical development of antiestrogens. Results from the DMBA-induced rat mammary-cancer model have provided the scientific principles required to evaluate long-term adjuvant tamoxifen therapy. Similarly, the athymic mouse model allowed the identification of a clinically relevant mechanism of drug resistance to tamoxifen and a model system to test new agents for cross-resistance. Additionally, the endometrial cancer model has allowed the identification of agents that cause a slight increase in the risk of endometrial cancer long before the data were available from clinical studies. However, it should be stressed that this model is really only relevant for agents to be tested as preventives in normal women. The risks of developing endometrial cancer during tamoxifen therapy are slight compared with the survival benefit in controlling breast cancer.

Finally the discovery of the carcinogenic potential of tamoxifen in the rat liver, 20 years after it was first introduced into clinical practice, raises an interesting issue. If the studies of liver carcinogenicity had been completed and published in the early 1970s there might have been no tamoxifen and tens of thousands of women with breast cancer would have died prematurely. In fact, there would have been no incentive to develop new agents as alternatives to tamoxifen or following tamoxifen failure. Most importantly, we would not have any knowledge about the target-site or selective actions of antiestrogens. All the current interest in selective estrogen-receptor modulators (SERMs) is based on the huge clinical data base obtained with tamoxifen. The success of tamoxifen as an agent that preserves bone density, lowers cholesterol, and prevents contralateral breast cancer *(84)* has become a classic example of a multimechanistic drug. These concepts have acted as a catalyst to develop new agents for new applications. The laboratory studies of raloxifene *(13,14,85)* provided the scientific rationale for the use of raloxifene as a preventive for osteoporosis *(86)* but with the goal of preventing breast cancer in postmenopausal women *(87,88)* (Fig. 9). It is clear that the close collaboration between laboratory and clinical research has revolutionized the prospects for women's health care in the 21st century.

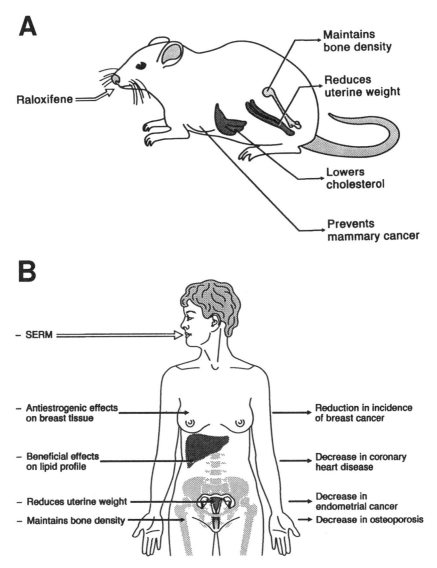

Fig. 9. (A) Known effects of raloxifene in the rat. **(B)** Desired effects of the ideal SERM in women.

ACKNOWLEDGMENT

These studies were supported in part by Breast Cancer Program Development Grant R21CA-65764 and the generosity of the Lynn Sage Breast Cancer Research Foundation of Northwestern Memorial Hospital.

REFERENCES

1. Jordan VC. Current view of the use of tamoxifen for the treatment and prevention of breast cancer. Gaddum Memorial Lecture. *Br J Pharmacol* 1993; 110:507–517.
2. Jordan VC. Antitumour activity of the antioestrogen ICI46,474 (tamoxifen) in the dimethyl-benzanthracene (DMBA)-induced rat mammary carcinoma model. *J Steroid Biochem* 1974; 5:354.
3. Jordan VC. Effect of tamoxifen (ICI46,474) on initiation and growth of DMBA-induced rat mammary carcinoma. *Eur J Cancer* 1976; 12:419–424.
4. Cuzick J, Baum M. Tamoxifen and contralateral breast cancer. *Lancet* 1985; 2:282.
5. Powles TJ, Hardy JR, Ashley SE, Farrington GM. A pilot trial to evaluate the acute toxicity and feasibility to tamoxifen for prevention of breast cancer. *Br J Cancer* 1989; 60:126–133.
6. Furr BJA, Jordan VC. The pharmacology and clinical uses of tamoxifen. *Pharmacol Ther* 1984; 25:127–205.
7. Jordan VC, Phelps E, Lindgren JU. Effects of antiestrogens on bone in castrated and intact female rats. *Breast Cancer Res Treat* 1987; 10:31–35.
8. Love RR, Mazess RB, Barden HS, Epstein S, Newcomb PA, Jordan VC. Effects of tamoxifen on bone mineral density in postmenopausal women with breast cancer. *N Engl J Med* 1992; 326:852–856.
9. Gottardis MM, Robinson SP, Satyaswaroop PG, Jordan VC. Contrasting actions of tamoxifen on endometrial and breast tumor growth in the athymic mouse. *Cancer Res* 1988; 48:812–815.
10. Assikis VJ, Neven P, Jordan VC, Vergote I. A realistic clinical perspective of tamoxifen and endometrial carcinogenesis. *Eur J Cancer* 1996; 32A:1464–1476.
11. Lerner LJ, Jordan VC. Development of antiestrogens and their use in breast cancer. English Cain Memorial Lecture. *Cancer Res* 1990; 50:4177–4189.
12. Black LJ, Jones CD, Falcone JF. Antagonism of estrogen action with a new benzothiophene-derived derived antiestrogen. *Life Sci* 1983; 32:1031–1036.
13. Gottardis MM, Jordan VC. The antitumor action of keoxifene (raloxifene) and tamoxifen in the N-nitrosomethylurea-induced rat mammary carcinoma model. *Cancer Res* 1987; 47:4020–4024.
14. Gottardis MM, Ricchio MD, Satyaswaroop PG, Jordan VC. Effect of steroidal and non-steroidal antiestrogens on the growth of a tamoxifen-stimulated human endometrial carcinoma (EnCa101) in athymic mice. *Cancer Res* 1990; 50:3189–3192.
15. Rose C, Thorpe SM, Andersen KW, Pedersen BV. Beneficial effect of adjuvant tamoxifen therapy in primary breast cancer patients with high oestrogen receptor values. *Lancet* 1985; i:16–19.
16. Ribeiro G, Swindell R. The Christie Hospital Adjuvant Tamoxifen Trial: status at 10 years. *Br J Cancer* 1988; 57:601–603.
17. Hubay CA, Pearson OH, Marshall JS, Stellato TA, Rhodes RS. Adjuvant therapy of stage II breast cancer: 48 month follow-up of a prospective randomized clinical trial. *Breast Cancer Res Treat* 1981; 1:77–82.
18. Jordan VC. Use of the DMBA-induced rat mammary carcinoma system for the evaluation of tamoxifen treatment as a potential adjuvant therapy. *Rev Endo Rel Cancer* 1978; (October Suppl):49–55.
19. Jordan VC, Dix CJ, Allen KE. The effectiveness of long term tamoxifen treatment in a laboratory model for adjuvant hormone therapy of breast cancer, in (Salmon SE, Jones SE, eds.) *Adjuvant Therapy of Cancer II.* Grune & Stratton Inc., Orlando, 1979, pp 19–26.
20. Jordan VC, Allen KE. Evaluation of the antitumour activity of the nonsteroidal antioestrogen monohydroxytamoxifen in the DMBA-induced rat mammary carcinoma model. *Eur J Cancer* 1980; 16:239–251.

21. Jordan VC. Laboratory studies to develop general principles for the adjuvant treatment of breast cancer with antiestrogens: problems and potential for future clinical applications. *Breast Cancer Res Treat* 1983; 3(Suppl):73–86.

22. Baum M, Brinkley DM, Dossett JA, McPherson K, Patterson JS, Rubens RD, et al. Improved survival amongst patients treated with adjuvant tamoxifen after mastectomy for early breast cancer. *Lancet* 1983; ii:450.

23. Scottish Cancer Trials Office. Adjuvant tamoxifen in the management of operable breast cancer: The Scottish Trial. Report from the Breast Cancer Trials Committee, Scottish Cancer Trials Office (MRC), Edinburgh. *Lancet* 1987; ii:171–175.

24. Early Breast Cancer Trialists' Collaborative Group. Systemic treatment of early breast cancer by hormonal, cytotoxic, or immune therapy: 133 randomized trials involving 31,000 recurrences and 24,000 deaths among 75,000 women. *Lancet* 1992; 339:1–15, 71–85.

25. Swedish Breast Cancer Cooperative Group. Randomized trial of two versus five years of adjuvant tamoxifen for postmenopausal early stage breast cancer. *J Natl Cancer Inst* 1996; 88:1543–9.

26. Osborne CK, Hobbs K, Clark GM. Effects of estrogens and anti-estrogens on growth of human breast cancer cells in athymic nude mice. *Cancer Res* 1985; 45:584–590.

27. Gottardis MM, Robinson, SP, Jordan VC. Estradiol-stimulated growth of MCF-7 tumors implanted in athymic mice: a model to study the tumoristatic action of tamoxifen. *J Steroid Biochem* 1988; 20:311–314

28. Gottardis MM, Jordan VC. Development of tamoxifen-stimulated growth of MCF-7 tumors in athymic mice after long-term antiestrogen administration. *Cancer Res* 1988; 48:5183–5187.

29. Gottardis MM, Wagner RJ, Borden EC, Jordan VC. Differential ability of antiestrogens to stimulate breast cancer cell line (MCF-7) growth in vivo and in vitro. *Cancer Res* 1989; 49:4765–4769.

30. Wolf DM, Langan-Fahey SM, Parker CJ, McCague R, Jordan VC. Investigation of the mechanism of tamoxifen-stimulated breast tumor growth using nonisomerizable analogs of tamoxifen and metabolites. *J Natl Cancer Inst* 1993; 85:806–812.

31. Welshons WV, Jordan VC. Adaptation of estrogen-dependent MCF-7 cells to low estrogen (phenol red-free) culture. *Eur J Cancer Clin Oncol* 1987; 23:1935–1939.

32. Pink JJ, Jiang S-Y, Fritsch M, Jordan VC. An estrogen-independent MCF-7 breast cancer cell line which contains a novel 80-kilodalton estrogen receptor-related protein. *Cancer Res* 1995; 55:2583–2590.

33. Jordan VC. The control of hormone-dependent breast cancer growth: are we talking about estrogen alone?. *Eur J Cancer Clin Oncol* 1988; 24:1245–1248.

34. Wakeling AE. Therapeutic potential of pure antiestrogens in the treatment of breast cancer. *J Steroid Biochem Mol Biol* 1990; 37:771–775.

35. Gottardis MM, Jiang SY, Jeng MH, Jordan VC. Inhibition of tamoxifen-stimulated growth of an MCF-7 tumor variant in athymic mice by novel steroidal antiestrogens. *Cancer Res* 1989; 49:4090–4093.

36. Osborne CK, Coronado-Heinsohn EB, Hilsenbeck SG, McCue BL, Wakeling AE, McClelland RA, et al. Comparison of the effects of a pure steroidal antiestrogen with those of tamoxifen in a model of human cancer. *J Natl Cancer Inst* 1995; 87:746–750.

37. Howell A, DeFriend D, Robertson H, Blamey R, Walton P. Response to a specific antiestrogen (ICI 182,780) in tamoxifen-resistant breast cancer. *Lancet* 1995; 345:29–30.

38. Howell A, DeFriend DJ, Robertson JF, Blamey RW, Anderson L, Anderson E, et al. Pharmacokinetics, pharmacological and antitumour effects of the specific anti-oestrogen ICI 182,780 in women with advanced breast cancer. *Br J Cancer* 1996; 74:300–306.

39. Satyaswaroop PG, Zaino RJ, Mortel R. Estrogen-like effects of tamoxifen on human endometrial carcinoma transplanted into nude mice. *Cancer Res* 1984; 44:4006–4010.

40. Fornander T, Rutqvist LE, Cedermark B, Glass U, Mattsson A, Silfverswaard C, et al. Adjuvant tamoxifen in early breast cancer: ocurrence of new primary cancers. *Lancet* 1989; i:117–120.
41. Assikis VJ, Jordan VC. Gynecological effects of tamoxifen and the association, with endometrial cancer. *Int J Gynaecol Obstet* 1995; 49:241–257.
42. Jordan VC, Morrow M. Should clinicians be concerned about the carcinogenic potential of tamoxifen? *Eur J Cancer* 1994; 30A:1714–1721.
43. Phillips DH, Carmichael PL, Hewer A, Cole KJ, Hardcastle IR Poon GK, Deogh A. Activation of tamoxifen and its metabolite alpha-hydroxytamoxifen to DNA-binding products: comparisons between human, rat and mouse hepatocytes. *Carcinogenesis* 1996; 17:89–94.
44. Martin EA, Rich KJ, White IN, Woods KL, Powles TH, Smith LL. 32P-postlabelled DNA adducts in liver obtained from women treated with tamoxifen. *Carcinogenesis* 1995; 16:1651–1654.
45. Carmichael PL, Ugwumadu AH, Neven P, Herwe AH, Poon GK, Phillips DH. Lack of genotoxicity of tamoxifen in human endometrium. *Cancer Res* 1996; 56:1475–1479.
46. Hemminki K, Rajaniemi H, Lindahl B, Moberger B. Tamoxifen-induced DNA adducts in endometrial samples from breast cancer patients. *Cancer Res* 1996; 56:4374.
47. International Agency for Research on Cancer (IARC) Tamoxifen. *IARC Monogr Eval Carcinog Risks Hum* 1996; 66:253–365. (http://www.iarc.fr/preleases/111e.htm)
48. Hayes DF, Van Zyl JA, Hacking A, Goedhals L, Bezwoda WR, Mailliard JA, et al. Randomized comparison of tamoxifen and two separate doses of toremifene in postmenopausal patients with metastatic breast cancer. *J Clin Oncol* 1995; 13:2556–2566.
49. Vogel CL, Shemano I, Schoenfelder J, Gams RA, Green MR. Multicenter phase II efficacy trial of toremifene in tamoxifen refractory patients with advanced breast cancer. *J Clin Oncol* 1993; 11:345–350.
50. Stenbygaard LE, Herrstedt J, Thomsen JF, Svendsen KR, Engelholm SA, Dombernowsky P. Toremifene and tamoxifen in advanced breast cancer- a double-blind cross-over trial. *Breast Cancer Res Treat* 1993; 25:57–63.
51. Merimsky O, Inbar M, Kovner F, Ohaitchik S. Adjuvant tamoxifen: 5 year control of dormant disease. *Eur J Cancer* 1996; 32A:174.
52. Ebbs SR, Roberts J, Baum M. Response to toremifene (Fc-1157a) therapy in tamoxifen failed patients with breast cancer. Preliminary communication. *J Steroid Biochem* 1990; 36:239.
53. Hard GC, Iatropoulos MJ, Jordan K, Radi K, Kaltenberg OP, Imondi AR, Williams GM. Major difference in the hepatocarcinogenicity and DNA adduct forming ability between toremifene and tamoxifen in female Crl:CD(BR) rats. *Cancer Res* 1993; 53:4534–4541.
54. Jensen EV, Jacobson HI. Basic guides to the mechanism of estrogen action. *Recent Prog Horm Res* 1962; 18:378–414.
55. Gorski J, Toft D, Shyamala G, Smith D, Notides A. Hormone receptors: studies on the interaction of estrogen with the uterus. *Recent Prog Horm Res* 1968; 24:45–80.
56. Jensen EV, Block GE, Smith S, Kyser K, PeSombre ER. Estrogen receptors and breast cancer response to adrenalectomy, in Prediction of Response in Cancer Therapy Monogr Natl Cancer Inst. (Hall TC, ed). Washington DC, 1971; 34:55–70.
57. Jordan VC. William L. McGuire Memorial Lecture. "Studies on the estrogen receptor in breast cancer": 20 years as a target for the treatment and prevention of breast cancer. *Breast Cancer Res Treat* 1995; 36:267–285.
58. Brzozowski AM, Pike ACW, Dauter Z, Hubbard RE, Bonn T, Engstom O, et al. Molecular basis of agonism and antagonism in the oestrogen receptor. *Nature (Lond)* 1997; 389:753–758.
59. Danielian PS, White R, Lees JA, Parker MG. Identification of a conserved region required for hormone dependent transcriptional activation by steroid hormone receptors. *EMBO J* 1992; 11:1025–1033.
60. Tzukerman MT, Esty A, Santiso-Mere D, Santiso-Mere D, Danelian D, Parker MG, et al. Human estrogen receptor transactivational capacity is determined by both cellular and pro-

moter context and mediated by two functionally distinct intramolecular regions. *Mol Endocrinol* 1994; 18:21–30.

61. Berry M, Metzger D, Chambon P. Role of the two activating domains of the oestrogen receptor in the cell-type and promoter-context dependent agonistic activity of the anti-oestrogen 4-hydroxytamoxifen. *EMBO J* 1990; 9:2811–2818.

62. Jordan VC. Biochemical pharmacology of antiestrogen action. *Pharmacol Rev* 1984; 36:245–276.

63. Lednicer D, Lyster SC, Aspergren BD, Duncan GW. Mammalian antifertility agents. III. 1-Aryl-2-phenyl-1,2,3,4-tetrahydro-1-naphthols, 1-anyl-2-phenyl-3,4-dihydronaphthalenes and their derivatives. *J Med Chem* 1966; 9:172–176.

64. Clark ER, Jordan VC. Oestrogenic, antiestrogenic and antifertility properties of a series of compounds related to ethamoxytriphetol (MER-25). *Br J Pharmacol* 1976; 57:487–493.

65. Robertson DW, Katzenellenbogen JA, Hayes JR, Katzenellenbogen BS. Antiestrogen basicity-activity relationships: A comparison of the estrogen receptor binding and antituterotrophic potencies of several analogues of (Z)-1,2-diphenyl-1-[4-[2-(dimethylamino)ethoxy]phenyl]-1-butene (Tamoxifen, Nolvadex) having altered basicity. *J Med Chem* 1982; 25:167–171.

66. Jordan VC, Gosden B. Importance of the alkylaminoethoxy side chain for the estrogenic and antiestrogenic actions of tamoxifen and trioxifene in the immature rat uterus. *Mol Cell Endocrinol* 1982; 27:291–306.

67. Tate AC, Greene GL, DeSombre ER, DeSombre ER, Jensen EV, Jordan VC. Differences between estrogen and antiestrogen-estrogen receptor complexes identified with an antibody raised against the estrogen receptor, *Cancer Res* 1984; 44:1012–1018.

68. Lieberman ME, Gorski J, Jordan VC. An estrogen receptor model to describe the regulation of prolactin synthesis by antiestrogens in vitro. *J Biol Chem* 1983; 258:4741–4745.

69. Mahfoudi A, Poulet E, Dauvois S, et al. Specific mutations in the estrogen receptor change the properties of antiestrogens to full agonists. *Proc Natl Acad Sci USA* 1995; 92:4206–4210.

70. Bilimoria MM, Assikis VJ, Muenzner HD, Wolf DM, Satyaswaroop PG, Jordan VC. An analysis of tamoxifen-stimulated human carcinomas for mutations in the AF-2 region of the estrogen receptor. *J Steroid Biochem Mol Biol* 1996; 58:479–488.

71. Wolf DM, Jordan VC. Characterization of tamoxifen stimulated MCF-7 tumor variant grown in athymic mice. *Breast Cancer Res Treat* 1994; 31:117–127.

72. Wolf DM, Jordan VC. The estrogen receptor from a tamoxifen stimulated MCF-7 tumor variant contains a point mutation in the ligand binding domain. *Breast Cancer Res Treat* 1994; 31:129–138.

73. Jiang SY, Jordan VC. Growth regulation of estrogen receptor-negative breast cancer cells transfected with complementary DNAs for estrogen receptor. *J Natl Cancer Inst* 1992; 84:580–591.

74. Jiang SY, Parker CJ, Jordan VC. A model to describe how a point mutation of the estrogen receptor alters the structure function relationship of antiestrogens. *Breast Cancer Res Treat* 1993; 26:139–148.

75. Jiang SY, Langan-Fahey SM, Stella A, McCague R, Jordan VC. Point mutation of the estrogen receptor (ER) in the ligand binding domain changes the pharmacology of antiestrogens in ER-negative breast cancer cells stably expressing cDNAs for ER. *Mol Endocrinol* 1992; 6:2167–2174.

76. Tora L, Mullick A, Metzger D, Ponglikitmongkol M. The cloned human oestrogen receptor contains a mutation which alters its hormone binding properties. *EMBO J* 1989; 8:1981–1986.

77. Catherino WH, Wolf DM, Jordan VC. A naturally occurring estrogen receptor mutation results in increased estrogenicity of a tamoxifen analogue. *Mol Endocrinol* 1995; 9:1053–1063.

78. Catherino WH, Jordan VC. Increasing the number of tandem estrogen response elements increases the estrogenic activity of a tamoxifen analogue. *Cancer Lett* 1995; 92:39–47.

79. Jeng M-H, Jiang S-Y, Jordan VC. Paradoxical regulation of estrogen-dependent growth factor gene expression in estrogen receptor (ER)-negative human breast cancer cells stably expressing ER. *Cancer Lett* 1994; 82:123–128.

80. Jordan VC, Jiang SY, Jeng MH, Catherino WH, Wolf DM. Regulation of cell growth with the transfected estrogen-receptor gene, in *Sex Hormones and Antihormones in Endocrine Dependent Pathology: Basic and Clinical Aspects* (Motta M, Serio M eds.). Elsevier Science BV, Amsterdam, 1994, pp 243–248.

81. Levenson AS, Catherino WH, Jordan VC. Estrogenic activity is increased for an antiestrogen by a natural mutation of the estrogen receptor. *J Steroid Biochem Mol Biol* 1997; 60:261–268.

82. Levenson AS, Tonetti DA, Jordan VC. The estrogen-like effect of 4-hydroxytamoxifen on transforming growth factor alpha mRNA in MDA-MB-231 breast cancer cells stably expressing the oestrogen receptor. *Br J Cancer* 1998; 77:1812–1819.

83. McDonnell DP, Clemm DL, Hermann T, Hermann T, Goldman ME, Pike JW. Analysis of estrogen receptor function in vitro reveals three distinct classes of antiestrogens. *Mol Endocrinol* 1995; 9:659–669.

84. Jordan VC: Fourteenth Gaddum Memorial Lecture. A current view of tamoxifen for the treatment and prevention of breast cancer. *Br J Pharmacol* 1993; 110:507–517.

85. Jordan VC, Phelps E, Lindgren JU. Effects of anti-estrogens on bone in castrated and intact female rats. *Breast Cancer Res Treat* 1987; 10:31–35.

86. Delmas PD, Bjarnason NH, Mitlak BH, Ravoux AC, Shah AS, Huster WJ, et al. Effects of raloxifene on bone mineral density, serum cholesterol concentrations, and uterine endometrium in postmenopausal women. *N Engl J Med* 1997; 337:1641–1647.

87. Jordan VC, MacGregor JI, Tonetti DA. Tamoxifen: from breast cancer therapy to the design of a postmenopausal prevention maintenance therapy. *Osteoporos Int* 1997; 7(S1):S52–57.

88. Jordan VC. Tamoxifen: the herald of a new era of preventive therapeutics. *J Natl Cancer Inst* 1997; 89:747–749.

4 Mechanisms of Liver Carcinogenesis by Antiestrogens

David H. Phillips

1. INTRODUCTION

Tamoxifen (Fig. 1) is a human and animal carcinogen *(1);* it causes endometrial cancer in women and is potent inducer of liver tumors in rats. The structurally related antiestrogen toremifene does not induce liver tumors in rats *(2)* but it has not been in clinical use for sufficiently long for its carcinogenic effects in humans to be assessed. In order to assess fully the long-term risks of tamoxifen therapy or prophylaxis, and of the safety of toremifene and other analogues (such as droloxifene and idoxifene) that are coming into clinical use, it is important to understand its mechanism of tumor induction and to what extent extrapolations between species can be made. A starting point for such assessments is the investigation, commenced relatively recently, of the carcinogenicity of tamoxifen in rat liver.

From: *Hormone Therapy in Breast and Prostate Cancer*
Edited by: V. C. Jordan and B. J. A. Furr © Humana Press Inc., Totowa, NJ

69

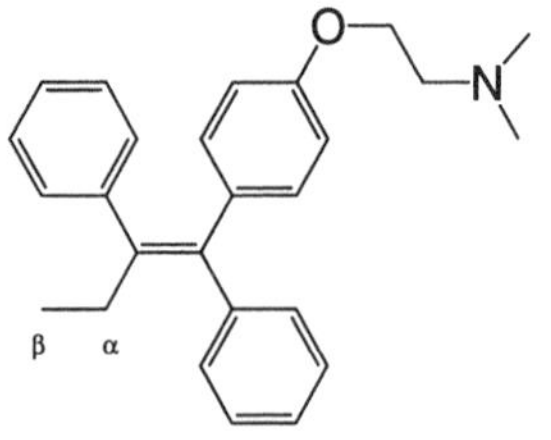

TAMOXIFEN

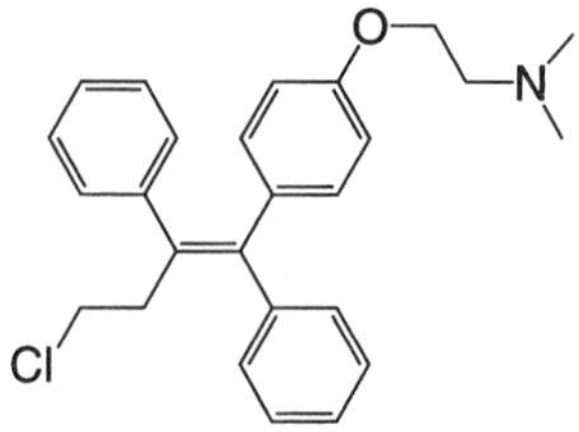

TOREMIFENE

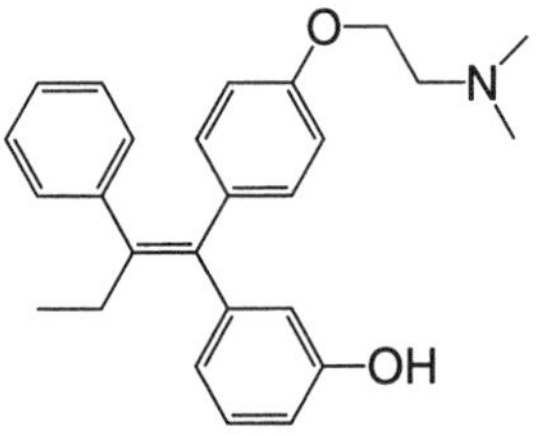

DROLOXIFENE

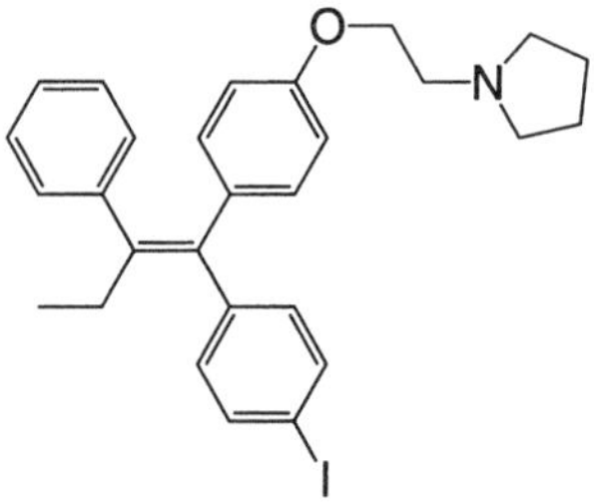

IDOXIFENE

Fig. 1. Structures of antiestrogenic triphenylethylenes.

2. CARCINOGENICITY OF TAMOXIFEN

There are now a number of studies that show clearly that tamoxifen is carcinogenic to rat liver *(2–7)*. The main characteristics are equal susceptibility of both sexes, early onset of tumors, and evidence of a dose response. A high frequency of hepatocellular carcinomas was observed in all studies. These characteristics differentiate the carcinogenic properties of tamoxifen from those of other estrogenic compounds that produce mostly benign adenomas in rat liver, generally at relatively low frequency *(8)*.

There is no evidence, however, that tamoxifen is a hepatocarcinogen in the mouse. This species difference is by no means unusual: aflatoxin B1, an extremely potent liver carcinogen in rats (and humans), does not cause liver tumors in mice *(9)*. Nevertheless, other neoplastic changes have been observed in mice. When administered by gastric instillation for 3 mo, then for a further 12 mo in the diet, tamoxifen caused intestitial cell tumors of the testis in males and granulosa-cell adenomas of the ovary in females *(10)*. When administered neonatally to mice, atypical uterine hyperplasia and malignant lesions, including endometrial adenocarcinoma, developed *(11)*. When administered prenatally to mice, tamoxifen caused proliferative lesions in the oviduct and uterine epithelium of female off-spring, including some tumors, although not endometrial carcinomas *(12)*.

Because tamoxifen has been widely, and successfully, used as adjuvant therapy for breast cancer, information on the carcinogenic properties for humans has emerged. At the present time it is evident that there is an increased occurrence of endometrial cancer in women who have taken tamoxifen. The evidence is sufficient for tamoxifen to be classed as a human carcinogen *(1)*. Tumor induction in other organs remains a possibility: an excess risk of gastrointestinal cancer has been reported *(13)*, but this has not been seen in other studies. Longer periods of follow-up in human studies will address these issues.

The carcinogenicity of tamoxifen in other species has not been tested, so further interspecies comparisons are not possible. Because of its hormonal activity, it is plausible that tamoxifen induces tumor formation in mice by a nongenotoxic mechanism. However, the carcinogenic activity in rats is unusual for a nongenotoxic carcinogen. As described below, there is much experimental evidence to suggest that tamoxifen is a genotoxic carcinogen in rats.

3. EVIDENCE THAT TAMOXIFEN IS A GENOTOXIC CARCINOGEN

Tamoxifen forms covalent DNA adducts in rat liver *(14–16)*. It also forms DNA adducts in the livers of mice *(15)* and of hamsters *(14)*, and it has been shown to bind covalently to protein in the presence of human liver microsomal fractions *(17)*. It also induces micronucleus formation in metabolically competent human cells *(15,18)*, and induces unscheduled DNA synthesis in hepatocytes from tamoxifen-pretreated rats *(15)*. Low doses of tamoxifen result in aneuploidy in rat liver *(19)* and studies in transgenic rats reveal that it causes gene mutations in the liver *(20)*.

Taken together with the rat liver carcinogenicity data, these properties suggest very strongly that the mechanism of carcinogenicity of tamoxifen in rat liver is a genotoxic one, involving direct damage to DNA by reactive metabolites. Less likely, at least in this organ, is the possibility of a purely hormonal, nongenotoxic mechanism, although tamoxifen may have additional mitogenic activity *(21)* that could contribute to tumor promotion by providing a proliferative stimulus to tamoxifen-initiated cells. This possibility is supported by the observation that tamoxifen produces liver tumors more rapidly in rat strains in which cell proliferation is also induced *(7)*.

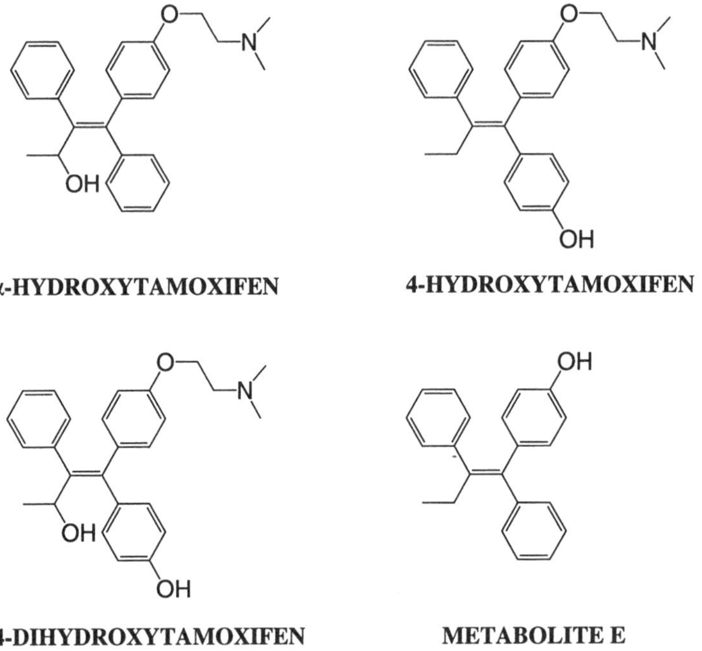

α-HYDROXYTAMOXIFEN   4-HYDROXYTAMOXIFEN

α,4-DIHYDROXYTAMOXIFEN   METABOLITE E

Fig. 2. Metabolites or putative metabolites of tamoxifen with the potential to form DNA adducts.

4. METABOLISM AND ACTIVATION OF TAMOXIFEN IN RAT LIVER

4.1. Phase I Activation

To date, a number of tamoxifen metabolites, or putative metabolites, have been shown to possess DNA binding activity. In some cases chemical activation or incubation with metabolizing enzymes is required to elicit DNA binding. The derivatives in question are α-hydroxytamoxifen (22), 4-hydroxytamoxifen (23), α,4-dihydroxytamoxifen (24), and (Z)-1,2-diphenyl-1,-(4-hydroxyphenyl)but-1-ene (metabolite E) (25) (Fig. 2). Evidence presented that tamoxifen 1,2-epoxide has DNA binding activity (26) has since been discounted (27).

A mechanism of activation of tamoxifen that involves oxidation at the α-position of the ethyl group has been proposed (28). A prediction of this hypothesis is that substituting the hydrogen atoms at the α-position with deuterium will result in a less genotoxic compound. Metabolism studies show that hydroxylation of the α-position is approx three times slower in the deuterated compound than in the isotopically normal tamoxifen (29). Comparison of the DNA binding activity of [D5-ethyl]tamoxifen and tamoxifen showed that the latter formed 2.5-fold higher levels of DNA adducts in rat liver in vivo than the

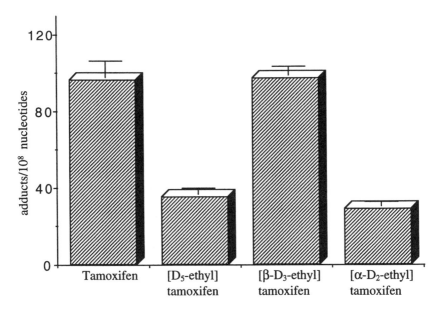

Fig. 3. Formation of DNA adducts in primary cultures of rat hepatocytes incubated with 10μM nondeuterated and deuterated tamoxifen.

former *(30)*. Deuteration resulted in a similar reduction in micronucleus-forming activity in MCL-5 cells *(30)*. Further refinement of this approach has demonstrated that the effect is specific to the α-position: thus [α-D$_2$-ethyl]tamoxifen shows the same reduced DNA binding activity as [D$_5$-ethyl]tamoxifen both in rat liver in vivo and in rat hepatocytes in vitro, while [β-D$_3$-ethyl]tamoxifen has the same DNA binding activity as nondeuterated tamoxifen (Fig. 3) *(31)*.

Binding of tamoxifen to protein in human and rat liver microsomal preparations is reported to be mediated by the cytochrome P450 (CYP) 3A subfamily *(32)*. α-Hydroxytamoxifen is a metabolite of tamoxifen and preliminary evidence suggests that its formation is catalysed by CYP 3A4 (unpublished results). In primary cultures of rat hepatocytes, it forms the same DNA adduct pattern as tamoxifen, but adduct levels are 50-fold higher *(22)*. This is strong evidence that α-hydroxytamoxifen is an intermediate in the metabolic activation of tamoxifen. The metabolite has weak chemical reactivity at neutral pH, forming the same adduct pattern as seen in cells. At acid pH, its chemical reactivity increases dramatically *(27)*. The synthetic derivative α-acetoxytamoxifen is highly reactive towards DNA *(27)*, suggesting that further metabolic activation of α-hydroxytamoxifen occurs in vivo. The main product in DNA formed by reaction with α-acetoxytamoxifen is at the N^2-position of guanine, namely *(E)*-α-(N^2-deoxyguanosinyl)tamoxifen *(27)*, with minor products formed being the *cis*-adduct at the N^2-position of guanine and also the *trans*-adduct formed at the N^6-position of adenine residues in DNA *(33)*. As would be expected, the sulphate ester of α-hydroxytamoxifen is more reactive still than α-acetoxytamoxifen and forms the same pattern of adducts *(34)*.

The Potter hypothesis *(28)* also predicts that oxidation at the 4-position will increase the reactivity of a carbocation formed at the α-position. As 4-hydroxytamoxifen is a major metabolite, this possibility is of great interest. Some studies have shown DNA adduct formation by 4-hydroxytamoxifen in cell-free systems and the tentative identification of a minor adduct formed by it in rat liver in vivo *(23)*, but in our own studies DNA adduct formation by this metabolite has not been detected either in rat liver in vivo or in rat hepatocytes in vitro *(35)*. 4-Hydroxytamoxifen may be further oxidized to a quinone methide. Generation of this intermediate chemically and reaction *in situ* with DNA results in DNA adduct formation at the N^2-position of guanine *(36)*. Another route to the same product is by reaction of α,4-dihydroxytamoxifen with DNA at acid pH *(24,35)*. However, despite the high chemical reactivity of this putative tamoxifen metabolite, DNA adducts were not observed when the compound was incubated with primary cultures of rat hepatocytes or administered to rats *(35)*. Other studies confirm this finding *(37)*. This implies that an efficient detoxification pathway overrides any potential pathway leading to reactive intermediates capable of binding to DNA in cells. This may explain why the major metabolic pathway leading to DNA adduct formation in liver cells does not involve 4-hydroxylation.

Recently, other studies have demonstrated that *N*-demethylation accompanies α-hydroxylation in the metabolic activation of tamoxifen, resulting not only in the formation of DNA adducts in which tamoxifen remains di-substituted with methyl groups at the amino function but also in adducts in which it is mono-methylated and, to a minor extent, unmethylated *(31,38,39)*.

4.2. Phase II Activation

The low chemical reactivity of α-hydroxytamoxifen at neutral pH implies that its potent DNA binding activity in cells is mediated by further metabolism. This could involve phase II metabolism at the α-position to provide a good leaving group for the formation of a carbocation. As stated earlier, both α-acetoxytamoxifen and the analogous sulphate ester react extensively with DNA to give adducts that are indistinguishable from those formed by tamoxifen and α-hydroxytamoxifen in vivo and in vitro *(27,34)*. Our recent studies show that the further activation of α-hydroxytamoxifen to DNA binding products in rat hepatocytes is highly dependent on sulphate *(40)*. DNA binding of both tamoxifen (10 μ*M*) and α-hydroxytamoxifen (1 μ*M*) was 10-fold higher with medium containing 10 μ*M* sulphate than in sulphate-free medium, and the level of DNA adduct formation

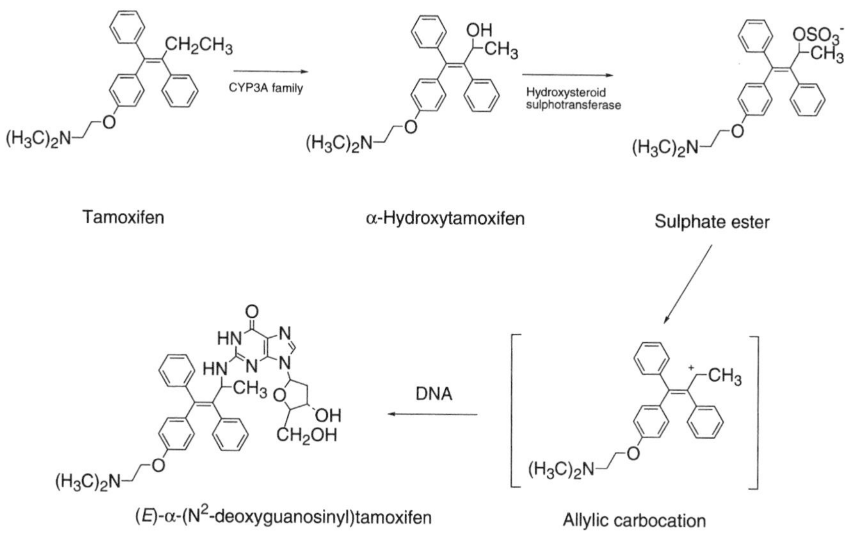

Fig. 4. Pathway of metabolic activation of tamoxifen in rat liver. The major adduct formed at guanine bases in DNA is shown. Analogous pathways in which tamoxifen is *N*-demethylated also occur (*see* text).

was directly proportional to concentration of sulphate in the medium. Furthermore, inclusion of dehydroisoandrosterone-3-sulphate (0.1 m*M*), an inhibitor of hydroxysteroid sulphotransferase (hST), reduced DNA binding of both compounds by up to 80%. It is concluded that the activation of tamoxifen in rat liver cells proceeds predominantly through hydroxylation followed by sulphate ester formation at the α-position of the ethyl group. The proposed scheme for the metabolic activation of tamoxifen in rat liver is shown in Fig. 4.

Although hydroxysteroid sulphotransferase is expressed at much higher levels in the liver of female rats than in males *(41)*, tamoxifen is equipotent as a carcinogen to both sexes *(3)*. An explanation for this apparent paradox has recently been found. In male rat hepatocytes and in male rat liver in vivo following a single oral dose, tamoxifen forms much lower levels of DNA adducts than in female cells *(42)*. However, after multiple doses of tamoxifen to rats, liver DNA adduct levels in males become similar to those in females, and this rise is accompanied by a sharp increase in sulphotransferase activity in male liver. Significantly, only one isoform is induced in males, hydroxysteroid sulphotransferase rHSTa, which is the one form that conjugates α-hydroxytamoxifen to a reactive ester *(42)*. Thus, tamoxifen induces its own activation in the male rat. When the conditions of the carcinogenicity experiment are reproduced, there is a close correlation observed between DNA adduct formation and carcinogenicity, and between adduct formation and sulphotransferase activity.

5. COMPARISONS BETWEEN RODENTS AND HUMANS

α-Hydroxytamoxifen is a human metabolite, detected in blood plasma *(43)* and is also formed when primary cultures of human hepatocytes are incubated with tamoxifen *(44)*. However, the concentration of the metabolite formed in cultures of rat hepatocytes is at least 50-fold higher than in cultures of human cells *(44)*.

In a comparison of the metabolic activation of tamoxifen and α-hydroxy-tamoxifen in primary cultures of rat, mouse, and human hepatocytes, it was found that tamoxifen formed detectable DNA adducts in rat and mouse cells, but not in human cells. Adducts were formed by α-hydroxytamoxifen in all three, but the levels in the human cells were 300-fold lower than in rat hepatocytes *(44)*.

Thus, there are very large quantitative differences between human and rodent cells in adduct formation. Studies with subcellular fractions show less interspecies variation in tamoxifen activation *(45,46)*, but it must be borne in mind that such systems as microsomal fractions do not accurately represent the balance between activation and detoxification pathways found in vivo. A small study of liver DNA obtained from women taking tamoxifen and from controls found a relatively high level of adducts in both groups *(47)*, but did not show significantly different levels of adducts between the two groups.

Our recent studies suggest reasons for the apparent interspecies differences. Studies of the metabolism and DNA binding of tamoxifen and α-hydroxy-tamoxifen in bacteria and mammalian cells genetically engineered to express specific enzymes indicate that tamoxifen is metabolized, as mentioned earlier, to α-hydroxytamoxifen by CYP3A4, which is further activated by hydroxy-steroid sulphotransferase. However α-hydroxytamoxifen is a much better substrate for the rat isoform of the sulphotransferase than for the human form. Thus, adducts are formed and mutant colonies are generated in *S. typhimurium* TA1538 and in V79 cells expressing rat hST treated with α-hydroxytamoxifen, but not in cells expressing human hST (Table 1) *(48)*.

The question of genotoxicity of tamoxifen in the uterus is at present controversial. A low level of DNA adduct formation was reported to occur in rat uterus after administration of tamoxifen at high dose *(49)*, but to date our own studies have failed to confirm these findings (unpublished results). Exposure of human endometrium to tamoxifen in explant culture did not result in detectable tamoxifen-DNA adducts *(50)*. In one study of DNA isolated from the endometrium of women taking tamoxifen, tamoxifen-related adducts were not detected *(50)*, while

Table 1
Mutagenicity of α-Hydroxytamoxifen

Cell type	Mutations	DNA adducts
Bacterial		
S. typhimurium TA1538	No	No
TA1538 expressing rat hydroxysteroid ST	**YES**	**YES**
TA1538 expressing human hydroxysteroid ST	No	No
Mammalian		
V79 cells	No	No
V79 cells expressing rat hydroxysteroid ST	**YES**	**YES**
V79 cells expressing human hydroxysteroid ST	No	No

in another study a low level of adduct formation was reported *(51)*. However, this latter finding has been questioned *(52)* and, although another group has reported the detection of tamoxifen-DNA adducts in some human endometrial samples *(53)*, our own further studies have still not revealed the presence of tamoxifen-DNA adducts in endometrium from women taking tamoxifen *(54)* (and further unpublished results). Whether or not it transpires that some women form DNA adducts in this tissue, the biological significance of the low levels claimed to be formed is unclear. If the mechanism of carcinogenicity of tamoxifen in the human endometrium was deemed to be genotoxic, then it would imply that analogues that are not genotoxic carcinogens in rat liver (*see* Subheading 6.) would be less of a carcinogenic risk to women; however, if the mechanism of tamoxifen-associated endometrial carcinogenesis was nongenotoxic, no such prediction about the safety of the analogues can be made.

6. ANALOGUES OF TAMOXIFEN

Toremifene is not a rat liver carcinogen *(2)*. Its DNA adduct formation in this organ is reported either to be undetectable *(2,16)* or at least a 100-fold lower level than that formed by tamoxifen *(15)*. Studies with sub cellular fractions or purified enzymes indicate a DNA binding potential of toremifene closer to that of tamoxifen *(46,55)*, but again it is not clear to what extent these systems represent the balance between activation and detoxification operating in intact cells.

Droloxifene is also reported to be noncarcinogenic for rat liver *(56)*. Similarly, DNA adducts were not detected in droloxifene-treated rats *(15)*.

Idoxifene has not been tested for carcinogenicity. However, when administered to rats for 6 mo, DNA adducts were observed in only 3 of 5 treated animals, at levels at least 100 times lower than in rats treated with an equimolar dose of tamoxifen *(57)*. This suggests that idoxifene is unlikely to be a carcinogen in rat liver. Studies of the chemical reactivity and DNA adduct-forming ability in human and rat hepatocytes of idoxifene metabolites and derivatives indicate that they are significantly less genotoxic than the corresponding tamoxifen compounds *(58)*.

7. CONCLUSIONS

The mechanism of tamoxifen carcinogenicity in rat liver has been established as a genotoxic process involving, principally, activation at the α-position of the ethyl side-chain. Biochemical evidence suggests that tamoxifen and its metabolites are much poorer substrates for the human isoforms of the enzymes that carry out this biotransformation in the rat. This is reassuring, given the potent carcinogenicity of tamoxifen in rats. However the mechanism of tamoxifen-associated endometrial cancer in women and whether there are additional long-term risks to other organs from treatment with tamoxifen have yet to be established. Consequently the long-term carcinogenic potential of other antiestrogens remains to be determined.

ACKNOWLEDGMENTS

I am indebted to the following collaborators and members of my research team for their invaluable contributions to our studies: Paul Carmichael, Kathy Cole, Warren Davis, Hansruedi Glatt, Ian Hardcastle, Alan Hewer, Martin Horton, Mike Jarman, Walter Meinl, Martin Osborne, Grace Poon, Gerry Potter, Krzysztof Rajkowski, Alastair Strain, and Stan Venitt. The support of the Cancer Research Campaign is gratefully acknowledged.

REFERENCES

1. IARC. Some Pharmaceutical Drugs, IARC Monographs on the Evaluation of the Carcinogenic Risks to Humans, vol. 66. International Agency for Research on Cancer, Lyon, 1996.
2. Hard GC, Iatropoulos MJ, Jordan K, Radi L Kaltenberg OP, Imondi AR, Williams GM. Major difference in the hepatocarcinogenicity and DNA adduct forming ability between toremifene and tamoxifen in female Crl:CD(BR) rats. *Cancer Res* 1993; 53:4534–4541.
3. Greaves P, Goonetilleke R, Nunn G, Topham J, Orton T. Two-year carcinogenicity study of tamoxifen in Alderley Park Wistar-derived rats. *Cancer Res* 1993; 53:3919–3924.
4. Williams GM, Iatropoulos MJ, Djordjevic MV, Kaltenberg OP. The triphenylethylene drug tamoxifen is a strong liver carcinogen in the rat. *Carcinogenesis* 1993; 14:315–317.
5. Hirsimaki P, Hirsimaki Y, Nieminen L, Payne BJ. Tamoxifen induces hepatocellular carcinoma in rat liver: a 1-year study with two antiestrogens. *Arch Toxicol* 1993; 67:49–54.

6. Carthew P, Martin EA, White INH, De Matteis F, Edwards RE, Dorman BM, et al. Tamoxifen induces short-term cumulative DNA damage and liver tumors in rats: promotion by phenobarbital. *Cancer Res* 1995; 55:544–547.

7. Carthew P, Rich KJ, Martin EA, De Matteis F, Lim C-K, Manson MM, et al. DNA damage as assessed by ^{32}P-postlabelling in three rat strains exposed to dietary tamoxifen: the relationship between cell proliferation and liver tumour formation. *Carcinogenesis* 1995; 16:1299–1304.

8. IARC. Sex Hormones (II), IARC Monographs on the Evaluation of the Carcinogenic Risk of Chemicals to Humans, vol. 21. International Agency for Research on Cancer, Lyon, 1979.

9. IARC. Some Naturally Occurring Sustances: Food Items and Constituents, Heterocyclic Aromatic Amines and Mycotoxins, IARC Monographs on the Evaluation of the Carcinogenic Risks to Humans, vol. 56. International Agency for Research on Cancer, Lyon, 1993.

10. Tucker MJ, Adam HK, Patterson JS. Tamoxifen. In *Safety Testing of New Drugs* (Lawrence DR, McClean AEM, Wetherall M, eds). Academic Press, London, 1984, pp 125–161.

11. Newbold RR, Jefferson WN, Padilla-Burgos E, Bullock BC. Uterine carcinoma in mice treated neonatally with tamoxifen. *Carcinogenesis* 1997; 18:2293–2298.

12. Diwan BA, Anderson LM, Ward JM. Proliferative lesions of oviduct and uterus in CD-1 mice exposed prenatally to tamoxifen. *Carcinogenesis* 1997; 18:2009–2014.

13. Rutqvist LE, Johansson H, Signomklao T, Johansson U, Fornander T, Wilking N. Adjuvant tamoxifen therapy for early stage breast cancer and second primary malignancies. *J Natl Cancer Inst* 1995; 87:645–651.

14. Han X, Liehr JG. Induction of covalent DNA adducts in rodents by tamoxifen. *Cancer Res* 1992; 52:1360–1363.

15. White INH, de Matteis F, Davies A, Smith LL, Crofton-Sleigh C, Venitt S, et al. Genotoxic potential of tamoxifen and analogues in female Fischer F344/n rats, DBA/2 and C57B1/6 mice and in human MCL-5 cells. *Carcinogenesis* 1992; 13:2197–2203.

16. Montandon F, Williams GM. Comparison of DNA reactivity of the polyphenylethylene hormonal agents diethylstilbestrol, tamoxifen and toremifene in rat and hamster liver. *Arch Toxicol* 1994; 68:272–275.

17. Mani C, Kupfer D. Cytochrome P-450-mediated activation and irreversible binding of the antiestrogen tamoxifen to proteins in rat and human liver: possible involvement of flavin-containing monooxygenases in tamoxifen activation. *Cancer Res* 1991; 51:6052–6058.

18. Crofton-Sleigh C, Doherty A, Ellard S, Parry, EM, Venitt S. Micronucleus assays using cytochalasin-blocked MCL-5 cells, a proprietary human cell line expressing five human cytochromes P-450 and microsomal epoxide hydrolase. *Mutagenesis* 1993; 8:363–372.

19. Sargent LM, Dragan YP, Bahnub N, Wiley JE, Sattler CA, Schroeder P, et al. Tamoxifen induces hepatic aneuploidy and mitotic spindle disruption after a single in vivo administration to female Sprague-Dawley rats. *Cancer Res* 1994; 54:3357–3360.

20. Davies R, Oreffo VIC, Martin EA, Festing MFW, White INH, Smith LL, Styles JA. Tamoxifen causes gene mutations in the livers of lambda/*lacI* transgenic rats. *Cancer Res* 1997; 57:1288–1293.

21. Dragan YP, Vaughan J, Jordan VC, Pitot HC. Comparison of the effects of tamoxifen and toremifene on liver and kidney tumor promotion in female rats. *Carcinogenesis* 1995; 16:2733–2741.

22. Phillips DH, Carmichael PL, Hewer A, Cole KJ, Poon GK. α-Hydroxytamoxifen, a metabolite of tamoxifen with exceptionally high DNA-binding activity in rat hepatocytes. *Cancer Res* 1994; 54:5518–5522.

23. Pathak DN, Pongracz K, Bodell WJ. Microsomal and peroxidase activation of 4-hydroxytamoxifen to form DNA adducts: comparison with DNA adducts formed in Sprague-Dawley rats treated with tamoxifen. *Carcinogenesis* 1995; 16:11–15.

24. Hardcastle IR, Horton MN, Osborne MR, Hewer A, Jarman M, Phillips DH. Synthesis and DNA reactivity of putative metabolites of non-steroidal antiestrogens. *Chem Res Toxicol* 1998; 11:369–374.

25. Pongracz K, Pathak DN, Nakamura T, Burlingame AL, Bodell WJ. Activation of the tamoxifen derivative metabolite E to form DNA adducts: comparison with the adducts formed by microsomal activation of tamoxifen. *Cancer Res* 1995; 55:3012–3015.

26. Phillips, DH, Hewer A, White INH, Farmer PB. Co-chromatography of a tamoxifen epoxide-deoxyguanylic acid adduct with a major DNA adduct formed in the livers of tamoxifen-treated rats. *Carcinogenesis* 1994; 15:793–795.

27. Osborne MR, Hewer A, Hardcastle IR, Carmichael PL, Phillips DH. Identification of the major tamoxifen-deoxyguanosine adduct formed in the liver DNA of rats treated with tamoxifen. *Cancer Res* 1996; 56:66–71.

28. Potter GA, McCague R, Jarman M. A mechanistic hypothesis for DNA adduct formation by tamoxifen following hepatic oxidative metabolism. *Carcinogenesis* 1994; 15:439–442.

29. Jarman M, Poon GK, Rowlands MG, Grimshaw R, Horton MN, Potter GA, McCague R. The deuterium isotope effect for the α-hydroxylation of tamoxifen by rat liver microsomes accounts for the reduced genotoxicity of [D_5-ethyl]tamoxifen. *Carcinogenesis* 1995; 16:683–688.

30. Phillips DH, Potter GA, Horton MN, Hewer A, Crofton-Sleigh C, Jarman M, Venitt S. Reduced genotoxicity of [D_5-ethyl]-tamoxifen implicates α-hydroxylation of the ethyl group as a major pathway of tamoxifen activation to a liver carcinogen. *Carcinogenesis* 1994; 15:1487–1492.

31. Phillips DH, Hewer A, Horton MN, Cole KJ, Carmichael PL, Davis W, Osborne MR. N-Demethylation accompanies α-hydroxylation in the metabolic activation of tamoxifen in rat liver cells. *Carcinogenesis* 1999; 20:2003–2009.

32. Mani C, Pearce R, Parkinson A, Kupfer D. Involvement of cytochrome P4503A in catalysis of tamoxifen activation and covalent binding to rat and human liver microsomes. *Carcinogenesis* 1994; 15:2715–2720.

33. Osborne MR, Hardcastle IR, Phillips DH. Minor products of reaction with DNA of α-acetoxytamoxifen. *Carcinogenesis* 1997; 18:539–543.

34. Dasaradhi L, Shibutani S. Identification of tamoxifen-DNA adducts formed by α-sulfate tamoxifen and α-acetoxytamoxifen. *Chem Res Toxicol* 1997; 10:189–196.

35. Osborne MR, Davis W, Hewer AJ, Hardcastle IR, Phillips DH. 4-Hydroxytamoxifen gives DNA adducts by chemical activation, but not in rat liver cells. *Chem Res Toxicol* 1999; 12:151–158.

36. Marques MM, Beland FA. Identification of tamoxifen-DNA adducts formed by 4-hydroxytamoxifen quinone methide. *Carcinogenesis* 1997; 18:1949–1954.

37. Beland FA, McDaniel LP, Marques MM. Comparison of the DNA adducts formed by tamoxifen and 4-hydroxytamoxifen in vivo. *Carcinogenesis* 1999; 20:471–477.

38. Brown K, Heydon RT, Jukes R, White INH, Martin EA. Further characterisation of the DNA adducts formed in rat liver after the administration of tamoxifen, N-desmethyltamoxifen or N,N-didesmethyltamoxifen. *Carcinogenesis* 1999; 20:2011–2016.

39. Rajaniemi H, Rasanen I, Koivisto P, Peltonen K, Hemminki K. Identification of the major tamoxifen-DNA adducts in rat liver by mass spectroscopy. *Carcinogenesis* 1999; 20:305–309.

40. Davis W, Venitt S, Phillips DH. The metabolic activation of tamoxifen and α-hydroxytamoxifen to DNA binding species in rat hepatocytes proceeds via sulphation. *Carcinogenesis* 1998; 19:861–866.

41. Rajkowski KM, Robel P, Baulieu EE. Hydroxysteroid sulfotransferase activity in the rat brain and liver as a function of age and sex. *Steroids* 1997; 62:427–436.

42. Davis W, Hewer A, Rajkowski KM, Meinl W, Glatt HR, Phillips DH. Sex differences in the activation of tamoxifen to DNA binding species in rat liver in vivo and in rat hepatocytes in vitro: role of sulphotransferase induction. *Cancer Res* 2000; 60:2887–2891.

43. Poon GK, Walter B, Lønning PE, Horton MN, McCague R. Identification of tamoxifen metabolites in human Hep G2 cell line, human liver homogenate, and patients on long-term therapy for breast cancer. *Drug Metab Disp* 1995; 23:377–382.

44. Phillips DH, Carmichael PL, Hewer A, Cole KJ, Hardcastle IR, Poon GK, et al. Activation of tamoxifen and its metabolite α-hydroxytamoxifen to DNA-binding products: comparisons between human, rat and mouse hepatocytes. *Carcinogenesis* 1996; 17:88–94.

45. Pathak DN, Bodell WJ. DNA adduct formation by tamoxifen with rat and human liver microsomal activation systems. *Carcinogenesis* 1994; 15:529–532.

46. Hemminki K, Widlak P, Hou S-M. DNA adducts caused by tamoxifen and toremifene in human microsomal system and lymphocytes in vitro. *Carcinogenesis* 1995; 16:1661–1664.

47. Martin EA, Rich KJ, White INH, Woods KL, Powles TJ, and Smith LL. ^{32}P-Postlabelled DNA adducts in liver obtained from women treated with tamoxifen. *Carcinogenesis* 1995; 16:1651–1654.

48. Glatt H, Davis W, Meinl W, Hermersdorfer H, Venitt S, Phillips DH. Rat, but not human, sulfotransferase activates a tamoxifen metabolite to produce DNA adducts and gene mutations in bacteria and mammalian cells in culture. *Carcinogenesis* 1998; 19:1709–1713.

49. Pathak DN, Pongracz K, Bodell WJ. Activation of 4-hydroxytamoxifen and the tamoxifen derivative metabolite E by uterine peroxidase to form DNA adducts: comparison with DNA adducts formed in the uterus of Sprague-Dawley rats treated with tamoxifen. *Carcinogenesis* 1996; 17:1785–1790.

50. Carmichael PL, Ugwumadu AHN, Neven P, Hewer A, Poon GK, Phillips DH. Lack of genotoxicity of tamoxifen in human endometrium. *Cancer Res* 1996; 56:1475–1479.

51. Hemminki K, Rajaniemi H, Lindahl B, Moberger B. Tamoxifen-induced DNA adducts in endometrial samples from breast cancer patients. *Cancer Res* 1996; 56:4374–4377.

52. Orton TC, Topham JC. Correspondence re: K. Hemminki et al. Tamoxifen-induced DNA adducts in endometrial samples from breast cancer patients. *Cancer Res* 1996; 56:4374–4377. *Cancer Res* 1997; 57:4148.

53. Shibutani S, Suzuki N, Terashima I, Sugarman SM, Grollman AP, Pearl ML. Tamoxifen-DNA adducts detected in the endometrium of women treated with tamoxifen. *Chem Res Toxicol* 1999; 12:646–653.

54. Carmichael PL, Sardar S, Crooks N, Neven P, Van Hoof I, Ugwumadu A, et al. Lack of evidence from HPLC ^{32}P-post-labelling for tamoxifen-DNA adducts in the human endometrium. *Carcinogenesis* 1999; 20:339–342.

55. Davies AM, Martin EA, Jones RM, Lim CK, Smith LL, White INH. Peroxidase activation of tamoxifen and toremifene resulting in DNA damage and covalently bound protein adducts. *Carcinogenesis* 1995; 16:539–545.

56. Hasmann M, Rattel B, loser R. Preclinical data for droloxifene. *Cancer Lett* 1994; 84:101–116.

57. Pace P, Jarman M, Phillips DH, Hewer A, Bliss JM, Coombes RC. Idoxifene is equipotent to tamoxifen in inhibiting mammary carcinogenesis but forms lower levels of hepatic DNA adducts. *Br J Cancer* 1997; 76:700–704.

58. Osborne MR, Hewer A, Davis W, Strain AJ, Keogh A, Hardcastle IR, Phillips DH. Idoxifene derivatives are less reactive to DNA than tamoxifen derivatives, both chemically and in human and rat liver cells. *Carcinogenesis* 1999; 20:293–297.

5 The Effects of Triphenylethylene Antiestrogens on Parameters of Multistage Hepatocarcinogenesis in the Rat

Yvonne P. Dragan and Henry C. Pitot

1. INTRODUCTION

Knowledge of environmental factors that are causative of human cancer has been gained primarily from epidemiologic studies. Since neoplastic disease occurs spontaneously in lower mammals and can be induced in at least one species by virtually all of the agents shown to be carcinogenic by epidemiologic studies *(1)*, animals may be appropriate counterparts for the assessment of human disease. Since the earliest studies demonstrating the chemical induction of cancer in mice and rats, the use of such rodents for determining the carcinogenicity of chemical agents has represented the "gold standard" in classifying an agent as a carcinogen. However, since the numbers of new chemicals entering our environment every year are in the thousands *(2)*, the "gold standard" cannot be applied to every chemical for reasons of expense and time. As a result, a number of more rapid and less expensive tests indicative of the carcinogenicity of a test agent have been devel-

From: *Hormone Therapy in Breast and Prostate Cancer*
Edited by: V. C. Jordan and B. J. A. Furr © Humana Press Inc., Totowa, NJ

Table 1
Short-Term Tests for Carcinogen Identification

Gene mutation assay
    Bacterial: Ames assay (histidine reversion assay in *Salmonella*)
    Mammalian: mouse lymphoma thymidine kinase assay
        Chinese hamster ovary hypoxanthine-guanine phosphoribosyltransferase
Chromosome aberration
    In vitro assay in cell lines
    Mouse micronuclei
    Rat bone marrow cytogenetics
Primary DNA damage
    DNA adducts-^{32}P postlabeling
    Strand breakage
    Induction of DNA repair
        Bacteria: SOS response
        Rat liver: unscheduled DNA synthesis (UDS) induction
    Sister chromatid exchange (SCE)
Morphological transformation
    Syrian hamster embryo (SHE)
    Balb/c 3T3

oped. A listing of some of the more commonly used short-term tests that can be indicative of carcinogenicity is provided in Table 1. As noted, these tests are carried out both in bacteria and in mammalian cells in vitro, and some short-term tests for mutagenesis and clastogenicity are performed in whole animals (mouse micronuclei and rat bone-marrow cytogenetics). All of these short-term tests, with the exception of those involving morphological transformation of cells in culture, are concerned directly with induced structural changes in the genome. The basis for this is that cancer is considered to be a genetic disease, the cancer genotype inherited from mother to daughter cell. A positive result with a specific compound in these short-term tests can not be used to classify the test compound as carcinogenic. However, because of the expense involved in performing a chronic 2-yr bioassay for carcinogenicity, many chemicals found to be positive in one or more of the short-term tests, especially the Ames assay, may never be further developed. In contrast, other chemicals that test negative in several short-term tests but that are later positive in the chronic bioassay have posed significant problems with respect to assessment of their potential for human cancer induction.

2. METHODS OF CARCINOGENICITY TESTING

Carcinogenicity testing is a necessary aspect of the therapeutic use of chemicals in humans. While knowledge of causative factors for human cancer is based on epidemiological data, other animals are susceptible to both spontaneous and chemically induced neoplasia. Since known human carcinogens can induce neo-plasia in at least one species of rodent, these mammals are useful surrogates of human disease *(1)*. Because animals are physiologically and biochemically similar to humans, they are used to assess the potential risk to humans from chemical exposure. The initial studies for assessment of potential carcinogenicity resulted in the use of two species of rodents (rats and mice). These studies consisted of life-time exposure (young adult to later age) to the maximally tolerated dose of the compound. This is a stringent test of potential carcinogenicity, requiring that the test organism be similar (with respect to metabolic capacity, disease status, genetic background) to the intended human population. Moreover, the nature of therapy— acute, intermittent, or chronic—during specific periods of life and within certain disease states with induced changes in physiological processes and responses may or may not be well mimicked by these assessments in animals. Nonetheless, epi-demiological studies are the gold standard for assessment of carcinogenicity in humans, while animal studies provide the gold standard for risk-assessment processes *(1)*. Interpretation of animal carcinogenicity data and their use for risk determination for use in humans requires an understanding of both the similarities and the differences between humans and biological test species *(3,4)*.

Specifically, the pharmacokinetic and pharmacodynamic properties of the agent under consideration in the rodent after chronic, "high-dose" administra-tion or therapeutic administration to a specific population of humans with a variety of genetic backgrounds, disease states, and lifestyle considerations may impact on differences in biological activity of the compound of interest *(5,6)*. Cross-species extrapolation requires an understanding of the pharmacology and metabolism of the agent in question and the differences in metabolism that arise as serum and tissue concentrations vary with both dose and duration of exposure. Both the biology of the organism at risk and the chemistry of the test agent are necessary components in appropriate risk assessment *(7)*.

Epidemiological analysis of familial susceptibility to cancer provides the pri-mary basis for the somatic mutation theory of human cancer development. Stud-ies performed by Knudson and his colleagues led to a description of tumor-suppressor genes *(8)*. Syndromes in the human that occur in individuals with a mutation in one allele of a tumor-suppressor gene have indicated that a minimum of two rate-limiting events is necessary for the induction of certain cancers *(9,10)*. Epidemiological analysis of the age-related incidence of certain human cancers supports experimental observations that cancer is a multistage process in both animals and humans *(11)*. The somatic mutation theory is the pri-mary basis for current cancer risk assessment strategies, although the incorpora-tion of mechanistic and pharmacokinetic data is implied. Additionally, processes that are separate from mutagenic activity may contribute to the carcinogenicity of a compound. One factor other than mutation that is important in human cancer development is enhanced cell proliferation *(12–15)*. A role for epigenetic processes in carcinogenesis is becoming more apparent *(16,17)*. In addition, cancer is a multistep *(18,19)*, a multi-stage *(20)*, and a multi-path *(21)* process, and pathogenesis has implications for carcinogen testing and human risk assessment.

Based primarily on the linear genotoxic response of certain cells to radiation and on the two-hit, somatic mutation theory of carcinogenesis, most rapid screens for carcinogenic potential have equated mutagenicity with carcinogenic potential *(2)*. A number of rapid genotoxicity screens have been established (Table 1). These short-term tests are performed in both bacterial *(22,23)* and mammalian cells *(24)* in vitro. In addition, a number of tests *(25)* for aneuploidy, chromosomal aberrations, and clastogenesis induction are performed in vivo (mouse micronuclei and rat bone-marrow cytogenetics). These tests are based on the induction of structural changes in DNA, but they have limitations (Table 2). It is known that epigenetic mechanisms contribute to carcinogenesis and control gene-expression patterns including those irreversible processes of development and differentiation. One short-term test that may detect both genetic and epigenetic changes in the genome assesses morphological transformation. However, human cancer is frequently epithelial in origin *(26)*, and these tests are generally performed in fibroblasts. The Syrian hamster embryo (SHE) transformation test overcomes this particular problem in that all three germ-cell layers are potentially targeted *(27)*. It is not clear to what extent morphologic changes are true predictors of carcinogenic potential. While a positive result in a short-term test is not sufficient to classify an agent as carcinogenic, such tests are indicative of potential mode of action *(2)*. Because of the expense of performing 2-yr bioassays for carcinogenicity, many compounds that are positive in one or more of these short-term tests, specifically the Ames assay, will not be developed further. In contrast, chemicals which test negative in several short-term tests but that prove positive in a chronic bioassay pose significant problems with respect to determination of their potential risk for human cancer induction.

The limitations of the chronic bioassay are of considerable significance and may be greater than for the individual short-term tests *(28)*. Perhaps the greatest limitation of the bioassay as it is currently performed is the statistical power of the test. Specifically, the use of 50 animals fed ad libitum per test condition (dose, sex, etc.) requires a relatively large number of animals with induced neoplasms for a statistically detectable effect even when the background incidence is low. For example, with a background incidence of neoplasia of 1% in the control animals, at least a 10% incidence in the treated groups would be necessary to detect a statistical difference. The background incidence of neoplasia is generally greater than 1% in any one tissue, indicating that a fairly potent carcinogenic action would be required for detection in this system. Ames and his colleagues *(29,30)* have pointed out the fallacies of administering extreme doses of a test agent, which may cause tissue destruction and compensatory hyperplasia *(5,6)*. With such excessive doses, the induction of neoplasia may

Table 2
Limitations of Some Short-Term Tests for Carcinogen Identification

Test	Limitation
Mutagenesis	
Ames test	Unique bacterial metabolism of chemical
	S_9 metabolism of chemical to ultimate form not found in human
	Bacterial flora needed to metabolize chemical
Mammalian cell mutagenesis	S_9 may not work effectively in culture, or ultimate carcinogenic form is not produced or does not diffuse to nucleus
Clastogenesis	
In vitro in cell lines	Aneuploidy of cell line may not reflect clastogenic effects in stable diploid cells
	S_9 etc. $\rightarrow$ ultimate form not effective
Micronuclei in vitro	Difficult to distinguish toxicity from clastogenesis
Micronuclei formation and clastogenesis in vivo	Ultimate form may not be produced in or reach the target site, of interest
	In vivo difference(s) in metabolism of chemical in rodent and human
DNA damage	
Adducts and ^{32}P postlabeling	Adduct may be species-specific—relative to metabolism as above
	Adducts (^{32}P) may be indirectly related to test chemical or to other conditions of the test employed
Strand breakage	Spontaneous occurrence – low levels near back ground
UDS	Mechanisms may be indirect; S_9 metabolism not effective
	Background may be high
SCE	Mechanism unknown; not good stand-alone test
Morphologic transformation	
Syrian hamster embryo (SHE)	Difficult to interpret: metabolism limited
3T3	Meaning of transformation in an aneuploid fibroblast cell line

reflect the response to the toxicity of the compound and not its potential for the induction of neoplasia. Furthermore, because of unique hormonal feedback mechanisms and specific metabolic pathways, the induction of neoplasms in certain tissues by selected compounds is due to effects unique to animals and not seen in humans (4,31,32).

Despite the limitations of both short-term tests and the chronic bioassay, these tests continue in routine use as indicators of the potential of therapeutics, foodstuffs, and industrial chemicals *(7,33)*. By combining the results of these classic short-term and chronic tests with cell proliferation *(34,35)*, pharmacokinetic *(36–38)* and pharmacodynamic *(38)* data, a rational and scientifically based assessment of the potential for carcinogenic risk to the human population is established. One aspect of understanding the potential for risk with administration of different doses and durations of exposure is to examine the effect of the test agent on the different stages in cancer development. Another factor is in the integration of biological data into the risk-assessment process *(39,40)*.

Epidemiological analysis of human cancer incidence has provided several key pieces of information regarding the cancer-development process. Specifically, the age-related incidence of certain human cancers *(10,11)*, in concert with analysis of individuals with familial cancer syndromes *(11,12)*, provides evidence for the somatic mutation theory of cancer development. These studies provide insight into the requirement for a minimum of two rate-limiting steps in the cancer development process in many tissues *(10)*. Later studies provided evidence that this could involve two inactivating events within certain genes, those associated with a tumor-suppressor function *(41,42)*. In addition, epidemiological studies supported observations in other animals that a long latency period separated the initial exposure of a chemical from the ultimate clinical detection of neoplasia *(9,10)*. Furthermore, epidemiological studies of cancer induction suggest that cancer is a dynamic process that is multistage *(20)*, multistep *(18,19)*, and multipath *(21)*. Laboratory studies provide evidence that the neoplastic process may be operationally divided into the stages of initiation, promotion, and progression *(20)*. Biochemical and molecular changes associated with the pathogenesis of neoplasia development during these stages have been examined in experimental systems of mouse skin *(43–46)* and rat liver *(47–50)*. The natural history for cancer development is reflected in age-incidence patterns of several human cancers *(10)*. In addition, altered patterns of cell proliferation also clearly contribute to an increased risk of cancer development, even though such increases in proliferation are not strictly one of the rate-limiting events in cancer development *(12)*. Carcinogenic agents can affect the neoplastic process at any or each of the steps in the natural history of cancer development.

3. THE MULTISTAGE NATURE OF CARCINOGENESIS

Neoplasia is characterized by a long latency period between first contact with the carcinogenic agent and the ultimate development of neoplasia. A better understanding of the biology and ultimately the mechanism of this latency period and its role in carcinogenesis resulted from studies in animals, especially in the mouse skin *(51)* and the rat liver *(52)*, and from human epidemiology *(11)*. These studies have led to the current concept that the pathogenesis of neoplasia develops through at least three operationally defined stages, beginning with the stage of initiation, followed by an intermediate stage termed promotion from which evolves, the ultimate stage of progression with the appearance of frank malignancy. We *(53)* and others *(54,55)* have defined several biochemical and molecular characteristics of these three stages, as a result of studies of the pathogenesis of neoplastic development in mouse skin and rat liver.

3.1. Initiation

Until recently, the stage of initiation had been characterized and quantitated well after the process of carcinogenesis had begun. As with mutational events, initiation requires cell division for the "fixation" of the process *(56,57)*. The quantitative parameters of initiation—dose response and relative potency—have been demonstrated in a variety of experimental systems *(55,58,59)*. These parameters may be modulated by alteration of xenobiotic metabolism *(60)* or DNA repair *(61)* and by trophic hormones *(62)*. In addition, the metabolism of initiating agents to nonreactive forms and the high efficiency of DNA repair can also alter the process of initiation.

A major characteristic of the stage of initiation is its irreversibility in the sense that the phenotype is established at the time of initiation. There is accumulating evidence that not all initiated cells survive over the period of an experiment or the lifespan of the organism. The demise of initiated cells appears to be due to the process of programmed cell death or apoptosis *(63)*.

Spontaneous preneoplastic lesions have been described in a number of experimental systems *(64,65)* as well as in the human *(65–67)*. Thus, it would appear that the spontaneous or fortuitous initiation of cells in a variety of tissues is a very common occurrence. It follows then that the development of neoplasia can result from the action of agents at the stages of promotion and/or progression.

3.2. Promotion

As is true of the initiation stage of carcinogenesis, a variety of chemicals have been shown to induce the promotion stage of cancer development. However, unlike chemicals that induce the stage of initiation, promoting agents and their metabolites do not interact with DNA directly. For certain promoting agents, metabolism is not required for their effectiveness. A target tissue specificity of promoting agents has included tetradecanoyl phorbol acetate (TPA) in mouse skin-tumor promotion *(51)*, and saccharin for the bladder *(68)*, while phenobarbital is an effective promoting agent for rodent hepatocarcinogenesis *(52)*. Agents such as 2,3,7,8-tetrachlorodibenzo-*p*-dioxin (TCDD) are very effective promoting agents for rat liver carcinogenesis *(69)* and mouse lung and skin *(70,71)*. Endogenous agents including both androgens and estrogens are effective promoting agents in their target end organs, as well as in liver *(72–74)*. In addition, cholic acid enhances preneoplastic and neoplastic lesions in the rat colon *(75)*. Agents that induce the synthesis of peroxisomes in liver are effective promoting agents and induce hepatic neoplasms upon chronic high-dose administration *(76)*. Multiple other agents including polypeptide hormones, dietary factors including total calories, halogenated hydrocarbons, and numerous other chemicals have been found to enhance the development of preneoplastic and neoplastic lesions in one or more systems of carcinogenesis including the human *(53,77)*.

The distinctive characteristic of promotion as contrasted with initiation or progression is the reversible nature of this stage *(77)*. Boutwell *(51)* first demonstrated that by decreasing the frequency of application of the promoting agent after initiation in mouse skin there was a lower yield of papillomas than was obtained by more frequent application of the promoting agent. Other investigators *(78,79)* later demonstrated that papillomas developing during promotion in mouse epidermal carcinogenesis regress in large numbers both on removal of the promoting agent and during its continued application. The regression of preneoplastic lesions upon withdrawal of the promoting agents may be due to apoptosis *(63)*. This proposed mechanism is supported by the demonstration that certain promoting agents inhibit apoptosis in preneoplastic lesions *(80,81)*. Another potential pathway of this operational reversibility is "redifferentiation" or remodeling *(82)*. Thus, cells in the stage of promotion are dependent on continued administration of the promoting agent *(83)*, as implied by the early studies of Furth *(84)* on hormonally dependent neoplasia.

Another characteristic of promotion is its susceptibility to modulation by physiologic factors. The stage of promotion may be modulated by the aging process *(85)*, as well as by dietary and hormonal factors *(86)*. For example, the promotion of hepatocarcinogenesis *(87)* and chemically induced rat mammary cancer are modulated by dietary *(88)* and hormonal *(89)* factors. Several hormones can be carcinogenic and are effective promoting agents *(90–92)*. Thus, hormones may serve as an exogenous or endogenous source for modulation of cell proliferation during carcinogenesis *(77)*. Such physiological agents may be one factor underlying endogenous promotion of initiated cells.

The dose-response relationships of promoting agents exhibit sigmoid-like curves with an observable threshold and maximal effect *(93–95)*. The relative potency of promoting agents may be determined as a function of their ability to induce the clonal growth of initiated cells. Thus, the net rate of growth of preneoplastic lesions can be employed to determine relative potencies of promoting agents *(58,96)*.

3.3 Progression

The transition from the early progeny of initiated cells to a malignant-cell population constitutes the major part of the natural history of neoplastic development. Foulds recognized the importance of the development of neoplasia beyond the appearance of any initial identifiable lesions *(97)*. The characteristics of malignant progression that he observed—growth rate, invasiveness, metastatic frequency, hormonal responsiveness, and morphologic characteristics—vary independently as neoplasia develops. The stage of progression is distinguished from the stage of promotion by its irreversibility and evolving karyotypic instability *(98)*; however, environmental alterations may influence the stage of progression. For example, exposure to promoting agents can alter gene expression and induce cell proliferation. As growth of the neoplasm continues and karyotypic instability evolves, responses to environmental factors may be lost or altered *(98,99)*. Agents that act only to effect the transition of a cell from the stage of promotion to that of progression may be termed progressor agents. Such agents would presumably have the characteristic of inducing chromosomal aberrations, but may not necessarily be capable of initiation. In some cases, progressor agents may serve to enhance the clastogenesis associated with evolving karyotypic instability. Mechanisms during progression that may contribute to an evolving karyotypic instability include the inhibition of DNA repair *(100)*, including altered topoisomerase activity *(101)*, gene amplification *(102)*, and altered telomere integrity *(103)*. As with initiation and promotion, spontaneous progression may also occur. In fact, spontaneous progression would be highly fostered by increased cell replication *(104)*.

3.4. Evidence of the Multistage Nature of Carcinogenesis from Animal Studies

As noted earlier, the definition and characteristics of the three stages of carcinogenesis – initiation, promotion, and progression – have been derived from animal studies. The first experimental system in which initiation and promotion were investigated was mouse epidermis *(51)*. In the early 1970s, several investigators *(55,105)*, but notably Dr. Carl Peraino and his associates *(106)*, demonstrated initiation and promotion in rat liver. Since that time a number of multistage models of carcinogenesis in the rodent have been described *(52)*. Furthermore, the distinction between the stages of promotion and progression, which was not appreciated in the early studies of multistage carcinogenesis *(84)*, has been demonstrated from investigations in the mouse epidermal and rat liver systems *(107–109)*. Most other multistage experimental carcinogenesis systems have not rigorously distinguished between the stages of promotion and progression, although such a distinction could be made. On the other hand, there are numerous examples of preneoplastic lesions indicative of the multistage nature of carcinogenesis. In addition, both genotypic and phenotypic distinctions between the stages of promotion and progression can be made. While the characteristics of reversibility, euploidy, and the selective enhancement of growth and inhibition of apoptosis by promoting agents in these lesions have not been applied in most cases, it is reasonable to argue on the basis of their biological behavior that such lesions are the precursors of malignancy, even though the frequency is low *(110)*. Furthermore, in all cases, such lesions pre-cede the appearance of the malignant state.

Since it has been argued that the genetic changes occurring in the stages of initiation and progression are analogous if not equatable to the first and second "genetic hits" postulated as rate-limiting events for the malignant state *(111)*, the multistage nature of neoplasia is probably ubiquitous in animals and humans. In this way, the multistage nature of induced carcinogenesis and the evolution of Mendelian-inherited cancer can readily be accommodated.

3.5. Evidence of the Multistage Nature of Carcinogenesis in Humans

Even prior to the demonstration of the more general applicability of the mul-tistage model of carcinogenesis exemplified by mouse epidermis, the concept was applied to an understanding of human neoplasia through the use of a num-ber of multistage models of carcinogenesis, especially those patterned after the Armitage and Doll model *(112)*. In this and related models, the effect of carcino-genic agents was described as altering the rates at which cells pass from one stage to the next. Through such concepts, some agents effective as carcinogens for the human were proposed to effect transitions primarily at an early stage, whereas others would affect the process at a later stage. From this model, it was possible to separate carcinogens into those acting at an "early stage" and those at a "late stage" of the process. It is clear that numerous factors are very important in the determination of such actions by carcinogenic agents, the most useful relating exposure to duration and age of the exposed individual. In particular, the time since the initial exposure, the duration of exposure, the time following ces-sation of exposure, and the age at first exposure to the agent all become impor-tant considerations. Unfortunately, in many cases, it may not be possible to determine each of these parameters with confidence for the human. If the agent were an "early stage" carcinogen, both the increase in incidence beginning with and during exposure and the decrease in incidence following cessation of expo-sure will be delayed. However, in the case of a late-stage carcinogen, responses both to starting and ceasing exposure will be much more rapid. Such relation-ships have been discussed by Day and Brown *(113)*. Through such reasoning, ionizing radiation may be considered as an early-stage carcinogen in the induc-tion of a number of solid tumors in the human. In several known examples of neoplasia induced by ionizing radiation, an increased incidence of clinically detected cancer tends to occur only about 10 yr after exposure and continues to increase for several decades thereafter *(114)*. In contrast, the marked excess of reticulum-cell sarcomas after organ transplantation is evident within 6 mo after the transplant, so that the process may be considered a late-stage carcinogen by the reasoning describe earlier *(115)*. Exposure to sunlight and its relation to nonmelanoma skin cancer in the average individual would classify it as an early-stage carcinogen, but exposure of patients with the genetic disease xeroderma pigmentosum to the same agent would classify sunlight as a late-stage carcinogen, in view of the extremely rapid appearance of skin neoplasms in such individuals *(116)*. This latter finding emphasizes the critical nature of the genetic background of the individual when such a carcinogen classification is utilized. From these examples and others, it is clear that the terms "early" and "late" as used in attempting to correlate multistage models with epidemiologic findings may not necessarily relate directly to the stages of initiation, promotion, and progression, as discussed previously.

By comparing the findings in human epidemiology with experimental results in multistage models in animals, it is possible to define other evidence in support of a multistage development of neoplasia in the human. In most histogenetic types of human neoplasia, it is possible to demonstrate a pathologically characteristic preneoplastic and/or premalignant lesion that occurs prior in time to the malignant process *(117)*. In some of these examples, the premalignant form or carcinoma-*in-situ* can be seen to arise in the preneoplastic lesion. Furthermore, the incidence of cancer in the human clearly increases with age, but different neoplasms exhibit different peak incidences during the lifespan of the human *(118)*. The major incidence of many cancers that exhibit a Mendelian type of inheritance occurs in early childhood, whereas the peak incidence of breast and cervical cancer is usually in the fifth and sixth decades, and that of prostatic cancer after the age of 65. These observations may be reconciled with the multistage nature of neoplastic development in that those neoplasms that occur primarily late in life require a prolonged process of promotion for their development. As has been previously pointed out *(53)*, the major causes of human cancer as identified by Doll and Peto *(119)* are related primarily to the action of promoting agents and account for the vast majority of the most common human neoplasms occurring in older age groups. In those neoplasms exhibiting an autosomal dominant pattern of inheritance, the multistage nature of their development may be related to the concept that all cells of the organism may be considered as initiated, exhibiting a single genetic alteration or "hit" as originally proposed by Knudson *(111)*. The second hit, which results primarily from chromosomal or other global genetic changes resulting in homozygosity of the altered genetic locus associated with tumor development, is comparable to the stage of progression *(120)*. Although our definitive knowledge of specific carcinogenic agents for the human is not nearly so extensive as that in the animal, there are sufficient data for a number of human neoplasms that some of the factors involved in the multistage nature of several types of human neoplasms can be proposed (Table 3). For the most part, in this table the identity of the initiating agent is not clear and thus is presumed as occurring "spontaneously." The evidence for the stage of promotion is emphasized in this tabulation, while in most cases the stage of progression may

Table 3
Multistage Factors in Human Carcinogenesis

Neoplasm/tissue	Preneoplastic lesion	Promoting/progressor agent(s)	Reversibility of risk and/or precursor lesion	References
Carcinoma/esophagus	Dysplasia	Croton oil components	ND*	(121,122)
		Alcohol/smoking	Yes	(123,124)
Carcinoma/stomach	Intestinal metaplasia, dysplasia	Smoking	Yes	(125–128)
Carcinoma/colon	Aberrant crypts	Bile acids, fat, protein	ND	(129,130)
Carcinoma/breast	Atypical lobular hyperplasia	Calories (fat?), alcohol	ND	(131–134)
Carcinoma/respiratory tract	Dysplasia	Cigarette smoke	Yes	(135–138)
Carcinoma/liver	Dysplasia, adenomatous hyperplasia	Synthetic estrogens, alcohol	Yes	(139–142)
Carcinoma/bladder	Dysplasia	Cigarette smoke	Yes	(143,144)
Carcinoma/endometrium	Atypical hyperplasia	Estrogens, antiestrogens	Yes	(145)
Carcinoma/cervix	Dysplasia	Cigarette smoke, synthetic estrogens	Yes	(146–149)
Carcinoma/prostate	Atypical hyperplasia, intraepithelial neoplasia	Androgen, dietary fat	ND	(150–152)

* ND, Not determined.

be spontaneous. Thus, one may tentatively conclude that the natural history of neoplastic development in the human, as in other animals, occurs through the stages of initiation, promotion, and progression. This concept has profound implications in the prevention, therapy, and management of neoplastic disease in the human, as examined for a class of chemicals therapeutically useful in the human, the triphenylethylene antiestrogens.

4. THE TRIPHENYLETHYLENE ANTIESTROGENS: A PARADIGM OF DRUG DEVELOPMENT IN ANIMALS AND HUMANS

The demonstration of the effectiveness of surgical oophorectomy for the treatment of breast cancer *(153)*, coupled with an increasing understanding of the ovarian hormones responsible for vaginal cornification *(154)*, laid the foundation for the use of antiestrogens to treat and prevent breast cancer in the human. The discovery of the estrogen receptor as the endogenous protein to which the active component of the ovary responded and which, if present in the breast cancer, predicted response to endocrine manipulations *(155,156)* was a major breakthrough in understanding ovarian-hormone action. Even prior to the discovery and appreciation of the estrogen receptor, there was great interest in the structural attributes of estrogen and antiestrogen action.

The triphenylethylene derivatives have a very complex pharmacology, with both estrogenic and antiestrogenic activity, as exemplified by studies of the species, strain, hormonal status, tissue, and gene specificity of its action *(157)*. Since ovarian hormones and presumably estrogens are necessary for the maturation of the immature female reproductive tract, the effects of estrogenic and antiestrogenic agents have been classified with this as an end point *(154)*. Early studies established that the phenanthrene ring is not necessary for estrogenic activity in the mouse vaginal cornification test *(158,159)*. However, a bisphenolic structure is sufficient for estrogenic action. The presence of a diethyl substitution of the ethylenic bond of stilbesterol resulted in the potent estrogen, diethylstilbesterol *(160)*. The triphenylethylene structure is a weak estrogen in such systems *(161)*; however, replacement of the free ethylenic hydrogen in the triphenylethylene structure by a halogen increased the potency and duration of action of the estrogenic action. For example, the chlorinated compound TACE (Tri-p-anisylchloroethylene) is an effective estrogen in the Allen-Doisey test *(162)*. In 1958, Lerner and his colleagues synthesized the first nonsteroidal antiestrogen ethamoxytriphetol, MER 25 *(163)*. Importantly, MER25 was antiestrogenic in every species tested *(163,164)*; however, it was withdrawn from the clinic because of central nervous system (CNS) side effects. When MER 25 was removed from development, other triphenylethylenes were developed. Clomiphene, while more potent than MER 25, had a mixed agonist/antagonist activity at the estrogen receptor *(165)*. Nonetheless, several triphenylethylenes including clomiphene, nafoxidine, and tamoxifen were tested in both laboratory animals and in the clinic for activity against breast cancer (cf. *166*). The triphenylethylenes have an intrinsic antiestrogenicity *(167)*, but their metabolism to a 4-hydroxy derivative is advantageous as demonstrated by the increased antiestrogenic activity of compounds halogenated at the 4 hydroxy position *(168,169)*. Interestingly, the triphenylethylenes, while potent antagonists of the estrogen receptor, also have a partial agonist activity *(170,171)*. In addition, striking species differences in response to triphenylethylenes exist *(172)*. Antiestrogens that are potent but have a low intrinsic estrogenicity have been developed, such as the benzothiophene antiestrogens *(173)*. Antiestrogens with less intrinsic estrogenic action are being developed, and these include the polyhydroxylated antiestrogen, raloxifene. The in vivo effectiveness of the triphenylethylenes is a function of the intrinsic estrogen/antiestrogen action of the agent, its metabolic activation or inactivation, and the concentration attained at the target tissue. The ability of tamoxifen to inhibit the estrogen-dependent growth of specific tumors, including the breast, and to lower the risk of osteoporosis and of cardiovascular disease has resulted in widespread interest in establishing safe and effective therapeutics with target-specific action *(166,174)*.

Determination of structure activity relationships after in vivo administration are fraught with concerns over the pharmacokinetics and pharmacodynamics of the different compounds, and this is particularly true for the triphenylethylenes. These agents have an extremely complex pharmacology. Structure activity assessments of the triphenylethylenes differ with respect to the end point and the tissue (including species, strain, and hormonal status) examined. Compounds that have a genotoxic potential in vitro differ in this respect between tissues that have different complements of metabolic capabilities including both phase 1 and phase 2 enzyme systems, DNA repair activities, and proliferative rates. The structural basis of genotoxic action of a compound may differ from its ability to stimulate proliferation, effect tumor promotion, and induce tumors.

4.1. Metabolism

Tamoxifen undergoes extensive oxidative metabolism resulting in a pattern of metabolites that reflect the tissue and species under examination (c.f. *175–179*). The metabolism of tamoxifen includes demethylation, deamination, and hydroxylation pathways mediated by cytochrome P450s *(176,180–185)*, flavin monooxygenase *(186)*, and peroxidase *(187)* enzymes. The three primary serum metabolites of tamoxifen are the N-desmethyl *(188)*, 4-hydroxy tamoxifen *(189)*, and N-oxide tamoxifen *(190,191)*. Further metabolism of tamoxifen can occur including deamination to Metabolite Y *(192,193)* and didemethylation to Metabolite Z *(194)*. Various combination steps in tamoxifen metabolism have been detected including products such as 4-hydroxy N-desmethyl tamoxifen and α-hydroxy, N-oxide tamoxifen *(195,196)*. Both glucuronidated and sulfated derivatives have also been detected after in vivo administration *(197)*. In addition, low levels of didesmethyl and 3,4-dihydroxy tamoxifen and compounds E and Y have been detected as have α-hydroxy tamoxifen, α-hydroxy N-desmethyl tamoxifen, 4-hydroxy desmethyl tamoxifen, and 4-hydroxy, N-oxide tamoxifen *(198)*. In the rat, males have a higher rate of N-demethylation than females, while female rats have a higher rate of 4-hydroxylation. In males, CYP1A2 and CYP3A2 may contribute to N-demethylation of tamoxifen, while CYP3A1 predominates in the female. The predominance of 4-hydroxylation may be due to CYP2C12 or CYP2A1 in the female rat *(176)*. Metabolic differences between species and different tissues are of interest since tamoxifen is carcinogenic to the rat liver, the immature mouse uterus, and potentially the human uterus. Comparative analysis of metabolism has been made between microsomes, cultured cells, and after in vivo administration *(175,179,185,195,198)*.

At least three lines of evidence indicate that tamoxifen is metabolized to its primary serum metabolite, N-desmethyl tamoxifen, through the action of CYP3A. First, molecular modeling analyses indicate that CYP3A is involved in this metabolic route of tamoxifen *(199)*. Mani and his co-workers *(176,185)* have indicated the involvement of CYP3A and possibly CYP1A, CYP2C11, and CYP2C6 in the metabolism of tamoxifen to its N-desmethyl metabolite in the rat. Jacolot and co-workers have further demonstrated the importance of CYP3A in the generation of N-desmethyl tamoxifen in isolated rat hepatic microsomes *(184)*, and Mani et al. *(185)* have indicated that CYP3A is the predominant form active in human microsomes. Metabolic activation of tamoxifen has been determined from analysis of the covalent binding of tamoxifen derivatives to proteins *(185,200–202)* and to DNA *(203–209)*. The activation of tamoxifen is partially P450 dependent and may occur through the CYP3A pathway *(85,201–202)*. White and his coworkers have suggested that CYP3A4 and CYP2B6 mediate activation of tamoxifen in the human, while CYP3A1 and CYP2B1 may mediate its activation in the rat *(202)*. Data from Mani and Kupfer would support the predominant role of the CYP3A family in this process *(185)*. The flavin mono-oxygenase has likewise been implicated in the activation of tamoxifen for protein binding *(200)*, and it is potentially responsible for metabolism of tamoxifen to the N-oxide *(186)*. The 4-hydroxylation of tamoxifen is through an as yet uncharacterized pathway believed due to a constitutive P450 *(186)*. A constitutive P450, possibly of the CYP2C class, has been suggested to be involved in this metabolism *(186)*, while other studies implicate the inducible CYP1A1 or CYP2B1/2 forms. These latter findings on the P450 pathway responsible are not supported by antibody-inhibition studies *(186)*, while the involvement of 3A1 in activation of tamoxifen in rat liver has been confirmed. One modeling study implicates CYP2C9 or CYP2D6 *(199)*, while a separate study that examined a limited number of human samples suggests that CYP2D6 is not involved *(210)*. Studies by White et al. *(202)* indicate that CYP3A4 and CYP2B6 may be involved in protein binding detected in human microsomes incubated with tamoxifen. In vitro studies indicate that tamoxifen is metabolized to the N-desmethyl, the 4-hydroxy, and under certain circumstances the N-oxide. In microsomal preparations, various epoxides have been detected *(177)* including the 3,4 epoxide, which has been suggested to bind to microsomal protein under these conditions *(201)*.

A mechanistic hypothesis implicates the α-hydroxy derivative of the allylic carbon of the ethyl side chain as the reactive intermediate which results in formation of the DNA adduct *(211)*. This hypothesis is supported by the enhanced chemical reactivity of the α-hydroxy metabolite compared with the parent tamoxifen molecule and the decreased reactivity of the deuterated [D_5ethyl] tamoxifen derivative *(212,213)*, and while the P450(s) responsible for this metabolism have not been determined, the CYP3A family has been implicated *(185)*. The metabolic route responsible for generation of the α-hydroxy tamoxifen is unknown, but the CYP3A gene family is probably involved based on the role of CYP3A in the generation of the procarcinogenic form. Species differences in the rate of tamoxifen metabolism have been established, with the mouse a more rapid metabolizer than the rat, which is more rapid than the human *(177,202)*. In the mouse, the detoxification pathways of N-oxidation and 4-hydroxylation predominate, in contrast to the N-demethylation route observed in the rat and human. Certain tamoxifen metabolites are observed in the mouse, but not the rat or human, including the 4-hydroxy N-oxide and 3,4 dihydroxy tamoxifen. In the rat, the 3′4′ epoxide was detected in addition to the 3,4 epoxide formed by both mouse and human microsomes. The rat hepatic microsomes synthesized more epoxide than did those from either the mouse or human *(177)*. The biological reactivity of epoxides and the lack of information on the metabolic pathway involved in their generation suggest that this pathway should be further explored. A quinone hypothesis has been put forward in which 4-hydroxy tamoxifen is subsequently oxidized to the electrophilic methide quinone *(187,214)* from which detected DNA adducts have been deduced to arise *(215)*.

Importantly, toremifene is metabolized by this family of enzymes (CYP3A), and in vitro but not in vivo data indicate that toremifene may have a genotoxic potential under certain conditions. At least one modeling paper indicates that toremifene has structural correlates indicative of carcinogenic potential *(216)*. Similar to tamoxifen, toremifene is extensively metabolized in both the rat and the human *(217,218)* to numerous metabolites including N-desmethyltoremifene. The N-desmethyltoremifene is further metabolized to didesmethyl toremifene, carboxylic acids, and deaminohydroxy derivatives *(219)*. Under certain conditions 4-hydroxy toremifene is also detected (cf. *220–225*). Two newer triphenylethylene derivatives, droloxifene *(226–228)* and idoxifene *(229,230)*, have enhanced clearance rates compared with tamoxifen.

Species comparisons of tamoxifen metabolism have been performed in microsomal preparations and in vivo. The pathways of metabolism that contribute to the genotoxic and carcinogenic potential of tamoxifen are not entirely delineated *(179)*. While certain pathways are believed to be involved in the generation of tamoxifen-derived adducts *(179,231)*, other pathways may contribute to additional biological activities that impact on cancer development. The biotransformation pathways available at high and low doses may differ within an individual and different tissues, as clearly occurs between species. In addition, the accumulation of tamoxifen and its metabolites in tissue relative to serum may contribute to less well-described patterns of metabolism *(232)*. Furthermore, distinct metabolic pathways may exist in different tissues and between species.

Although evidence of adduct generation has been observed for acute toremifene administration, a lower number and quantity of DNA adducts are produced than by tamoxifen *(202,204,205);* structural alerts imply a genotoxic potential for toremifene *(216)*, as had been suggested from in vitro studies *(205,233,234)*. Idoxifene is purported to be without adduct-forming ability; however, pyrrolidino-tamoxifen results in the formation of adducts *(205)*, indicating a genotoxic potential for idoxifene. Clinically relevant antiestrogens may be genotoxic with chronic exposure *(235)*, and the mechanism for this carcinogenic potential needs to be assessed prior to their use in chronic treatment strategies for nonmalignant indications.

Distinct mechanisms of activation may occur in different organs with, for example, tamoxifen *(185,236)* and toremifene *(187,237)* undergoing peroxidative metabolism in the uterus but not in the liver *(238)*. In addition, a low level of kidney adducts has been observed in the rat with tamoxifen treatment *(203,207,209,238)*. One study did not detect uterine adducts in humans *(236)*, while others have detected uterine adducts in both rats *(187)* and humans *(239)* treated with tamoxifen. Numerous adducts have been detected upon administration of tamoxifen, indicating that more than one pathway contributes to the adduct load detected after tamoxifen administration, as has been demonstrated in the mouse *(207)*. The observation of mutations in the p53 gene in hepatic neoplasms of tamoxifen-treated rats *(240)* and the suggestion of p53 mutations in samples from tamoxifen-treated patients *(241)* indicate that these adducts may also have a mutagenic potential. In addition, mutations in the Ki-ras gene have been detected at a higher frequency in endometrial tumors of tamoxifen-treated breast-cancer patients than in other endometrial neoplasms *(241)*. Recently, a mutagenic action of tamoxifen has been demonstrated in Fischer lacI transgenic rats administered tamoxifen *(242,243)*. It will be important to identify those adducts that arise from activation of the triphenylethylene structure, as well as those which result from alteration of the endogenous modifications present in DNA *(209)*.

Metabolism of tamoxifen and its phase 1 metabolites by phase 2 conjugation enzymes may also be an important component of its bioactivation *(211)*. The DNA adduct-forming activity of α-hydroxy tamoxifen *(207,212,213)* necessitates protonation or conjugation *(211)*. Importantly, inhibition of sulfotransferase inhibits detection of selected DNA adducts while enhancing the detection of other adducts, implicating phase 2 reactions in its in vivo bioactivation *(207,244)*. In vitro, both α-acetoxytamoxifen *(234,245)* and α-sulfate *(245)* tamoxifen react with DNA to form adducts. In addition, glucuronidation *(246–248)*, sulfation *(207,244)*, and conjugation with glutathione *(247,248)* influences excretion rates and tissue and species specificity of tamoxifen action, including its potential for toxicity.

4.1.1. DNA ADDUCTS

The identity of the activated electrophilic metabolite(s) of tamoxifen has not been completely determined, but α-hydroxy tamoxifen has been implicated as the reactive intermediate. Several lines of evidence support this contention; specifically, D_5-ethyl tamoxifen is less DNA reactive than the parent tamoxifen compound *(249,250)*. In addition, α-hydroxy tamoxifen is more reactive than the parent tamoxifen *(233,234)*. However, the α-hydroxy group must first be protonated or conjugated to create a good leaving group *(211)*, thus creating a very reactive intermediate. The loss of this leaving group would create a very reactive carbon center resulting in DNA adduct formation *(211)*. An important study performed by Randerath et al. *(207,244)* indicates that two pathways exist for the formation of DNA adducts from tamoxifen, at least in mice. In these studies, pentachlorophenol, an inhibitor of sulfotransferase enzymes (as well as other enzyme activities), limits the formation of one subset of tamoxifen-induced DNA adducts, while enhancing the formation of a second set of adducts.

The α-hydroxy tamoxifen derivative is formed in vitro from derivatives of tamoxifen such as the N-oxide, which retain nitrogen group basicity *(190,251)*. Importantly, microsomes from mice, rats, and humans synthesize α-hydroxy tamoxifen. Furthermore, the α-hydroxyglucuronide has been detected in the liver of rats treated with tamoxifen *(246)*. Other studies have implicated the CYP3A pathway and possibly the flavin-mono-oxygenase in the generation of the electrophile(s) from tamoxifen *(200)*. The 3,4 epoxide of tamoxifen has also been suggested as a precursor of tamoxifen-induced DNA adducts *(201,208,237,252)*, as have the 4-hydroxy tamoxifen *(214,237)* and Metabolite E derivatives *(253)*. Interestingly, droloxifene (3-hydroxy tamoxifen) does not appear to induce DNA adducts with in vivo administration *(205)*. Phillips et al. *(213)* initially suggested that the 1,2 epoxide of tamoxifen may account for up to 40% of the detected DNA adducts, but it has been suggested that this metabolite is not formed in vivo; were it to be formed under physiological conditions, it is metabolically stable. The 3,4 epoxide of tamoxifen has likewise been suggested as a potential source of DNA adducts *(201,205,237,252)*, and this metabolite is formed by rat, mouse, and to a lesser extent human *(177,198)*. Several other hypotheses exist with respect to the identity of the precursor metabolite including modification of the basic ether side chain *(200,216)* and the substitution of the alkyl side chain of ethylene with an α-hydroxyl group *(211)*. In addition, the quinone methide has been suggested as an alternative pathway for tamoxifen activation primarily by Pathak and Boddell *(206)* with supporting evidence from the work of Moorthy et al. *(214)*. The challenge will be to determine which adducts are formed in vivo, which are mutagenic, and which trigger processes leading to tissue-specific carcinogenesis.

The electrophilic metabolite of tamoxifen that is responsible for genotoxicity is unclear. Several groups have proposed a variety of candidates including α-hydroxy tamoxifen *(234,250)*, 1,2 epoxy tamoxifen *(250)*, 4-hydroxy tamoxifen *(214)*, 3,4 epoxy tamoxifen *(177,254)*, and the 3′,4′ epoxy *(177,254)* tamoxifen metabolites. Lim et al. *(177)* have detected tamoxifen 3,4 epoxide as a metabolite of tamoxifen, while the 1,2 epoxide was not detected. In addition, the 1,2 epoxide is chemically stable and the dihydroxy diol derivative is not observed. Furthermore, both the N-oxide, α-hydroxy metabolite, and the N-desmethyl, α-hydroxy metabolite have been detected in the urine of patients that were administered tamoxifen, suggesting that the α-hydroxylation pathway is a detoxification pathway. The 4-hydroxy, α-hydroxy tamoxifen derivative is additionally formed. While α-hydroxy tamoxifen derivatives are not highly DNA-reactive in vitro *(250)*, the generation of this hydroxyl group when combined with esterification, for example, sulfation or acetylation, can result in the formation of very reactive intermediates, which appear responsible for a portion of the spectrum of tamoxifen-derived DNA adducts *(207,234,244,245)*. Thus, the α-hydroxy metabolite, which is made by mice, humans, and rats *(198)*, can be activated, at least in vitro, to a DNA-reactive form *(243)*. Recent studies have demonstrated that the α-(N^2-deoxyguanosinyl) tamoxifen derivatives in which the trans form predominates are in vivo adducts formed from tamoxifen *(234,240,244)*. In addition, the dG-N^2-tamoxifen adduct epimers have been demonstrated to be miscoding and hence may be responsible for the generation of mutations by tamoxifen in vitro. Since polymerase α can insert a G opposite the dG N^2 adduct, a G-C transversion can arise, as can small deletions. Similarly, polymerase β can result in both G-C and G-T transversions from dG-N^2 tamoxifen adducts *(255)*. Furthermore, the 3,4 epoxide derivative and the 3,4-dihydro-diol have been detected in preparations from microsomes *(177)* and may also result in DNA adduct formation. The hypothesis of Potter and his colleagues indicates a mechanism whereby toremifene and droloxifene would have a limited genotoxic potential based on their relative inability to generate the pro-DNA adduct forming α-hydroxy metabolite *(211)*.

4.2. Evidence for Initiating Activity of Tamoxifen

4.2.1. STANDARD IN VITRO GENOTOXICITY TESTS OF TAMOXIFEN

The in vitro genotoxicity of tamoxifen has been recently reviewed (c.f. *179* and *231,256*). Standard mutational analyses have been performed with tamoxifen, and these have been uniformly negative at up to 1 mg per plate *(257)*. Five strains of *Salmonella typhimurium* (TA 1535, 1537, 1538, 98, and 100) have been used both with and without a rat liver postmitochondrial supernate (S9). Doses up to and including the toxic dose of 50 μg per plate were not mutagenic (c.f. *179*). Furthermore, Tannenbaum *(179)* has indicated that forward mutations at the hypoxanthine phosphoribosyl transferase locus are not induced by the administration of tamoxifen either with or without an activated rat S9 in Chinese hamster ovary (CHO) cells. A dominant lethal study in rats indicated that tamoxifen was also negative at doses of up to 9.6 mg per rat administered for 5 d *(257)*.

Results on the mutagenicity of toremifene in bacterial and mammalian mutagenicity screen have not been published. However, toremifene administration will induce micronuclei in MCL-5 cells that contain exogenous CYP2E1 or CYP3A4 without addition of an activating system *(252,255)*. In addition, a low, but detectable, level of DNA adducts has been observed in rat liver following acute toremifene administration of 33 mg/kg *(258)* to 50 mg/kg *(204,255)* po. Additionally, human lymphocytes incubated in vitro with 100 μg/mL (but not lower concentrations) toremifene were also positive for DNA adduct formation *(259)*. In comparison to tamoxifen, toremifene induced only a low level of DNA adducts in microsomal activation studies *(252,255)* and after in vivo administration *(209,246,252)*. However, horseradish peroxidase-activated toremifene results in the generation of covalent DNA and protein adducts at a level equivalent to that of tamoxifen *(237)*.

4.2.2. UNSCHEDULED DNA SYNTHESIS (UDS) ASSAY

A lower level of unscheduled DNA synthesis occurs in tamoxifen-pretreated rats (45 mg/kg per os for 3 d) than in those that are untreated *(179,257)*, indicating that tamoxifen may induce its own activation. However, unscheduled DNA synthesis in rat hepatocytes has been demonstrated. Incubation with 2 μg tamoxifen/mL was used in hepatocytes from rats induced for 3 d with 45 mg tamoxifen per kg. Alterations were not observed with lower doses of tamoxifen or with microsomes prepared from rats not pretreated with tamoxifen. Thus, neither bacterial nor mammalian mutagenesis assays have demonstrated a positive response with tamoxifen, and only a very weak response was detected in the unscheduled DNA synthesis (UDS) assay. In addition, the results obtained with tamoxifen indicate that some type of genetic damage may be induced by high-dose tamoxifen administration, but that it is not detected in bacterial mutagenesis screens or in a mammalian forward mutagenesis assay as currently performed. These observations are similar to previous findings with diethylstilbesterol, namely, that gene mutations are not observed in the absence of cytotoxicity and that carcinogenesis appears independently of measurable gene mutation *(260)*. However, the inclusion of a metabolic activating system in the assay can result in the detection of mutations following DES exposure *(261,262)*.

4.2.3. EVIDENCE OF THE IN VIVO GENOTOXICITY AND INITIATING ACTIVITY OF TAMOXIFEN

Despite the ability of tamoxifen to induce DNA adducts as detected by ^{32}P-postlabeling *(203–209,212–215,258,259)*, single-dose administration of tamoxifen (40 mg/kg) was insufficient to induce sufficient genotoxic damage to result in focal hepatic lesions as detected with a maximally effective promoting dose of phenobarbital in Fischer rats *(263)*. This lack of initiating action of a single acute dose (100 times the human therapeutic dose) indicates either that the carcinogenic effect of tamoxifen is not entirely related to the induction of DNA adducts, those DNA adducts observed do not give rise to the carcinogenic action of tamoxifen, or the DNA adducts induced by tamoxifen are of an insufficient magnitude to result in carcinogenicity unless administration is prolonged. Other types of genetic damage, with the acute administration of single doses of tamoxifen, also result in the induction of aneuploidy and spindle disturbances. Such genetic damage may instead lead to apoptotic cell death or irreparable damage to the cell, which precludes its ability to divide.

Interestingly, the studies by Yager et al. *(264)* indicated that in rats subjected to a 70% partial hepatectomy and then administered a single dose of 20 mg diethylnitrosamine per kg the chronic administration of tamoxifen resulted in an increase in the number but not the percentage of liver gamma glutamyl transpeptidase (GGT)-positive foci when administered to female Sprague Dawley rats for 4 mo *(264)*. These studies indicated a genotoxic potential for both doses of tamoxifen tested (15 or 50 µg/day). In similar studies, tamoxifen inhibited, in a non-dose-dependent manner, the promotion of GGT-positive focal hepatocytes by ethinyl estradiol in both DEN and non-DEN initiated rats.

Later studies by Ghia and Mereto *(265)* further implicated tamoxifen and a related triphenylethylene, clomiphene, as potentially genotoxic agents in a modified version of the initiation-selection protocol of Solt and Farber *(266)*. In these studies, a clear increase in the number and volume fraction of liver GGT-positive foci was observed when 400 ppm tamoxifen or 1000 ppm clomiphene was administered as either the initiating or selecting agent *(182)*. The ratio of the rat dose to the human dose in these studies was approx 50 for tamoxifen and 20 for clomiphene. In the initiating study, the rats received the equivalent of nearly 5 mg tamoxifen/rat/d for 6 wk for a cumulative dose of approx 200 mg/rat.

Williams et al. *(267)* have demonstrated that tamoxifen but not toremifene initiated the development of altered hepatic foci in female Sprague-Dawley rats. In these studies, rats that were administered 40 mg tamoxifen/kg for 2 wk demonstrated an increase in the number of GST^+ cells, while an increase in this multiplicity was observed for all doses of tamoxifen from 5–40 mg/kg after 12 or 36 wk, but not for 42.5 mg toremifene/kg. Studies in which 20 mg tamoxifen/kg was administered for 12 wk, followed by phenobarbital for an additional 24 wk, resulted in liver neoplasms in Sprague-Dawley but not Fischer rats. Continuous administration of 40 mg tamoxifen/kg for 36 wk was carcinogenic in Sprague Dawley rats, while Fischer rats were, by comparison, resistant during the observation period.

Studies by Carthew et al. *(235)* more definitively demonstrated that 420 ppm tamoxifen induces cumulative genetic damage that can be detected after chronic administration (3 mo), followed by a 6-mo period of recovery or by administration of the promoting agent, phenobarbital. The rats received the equivalent of ~5 mg tamoxifen/rat/d for 12 wk for a cumulative dose of >400 mg/rat. These findings are in keeping with the structural alerts present in the tamoxifen structure *(216)*. In addition, tamoxifen induces gene mutations in the liver of female Fischer lambda/lac I transgenic rats administered either 10 or 20 mg/kg/d for 6 wk *(240,241)*. This corroborates findings by Vancutsem et al. *(240)* of specific p53 mutations in hepatic neoplasms that arise in tamoxifen-treated rats and is provisionally supported by the observation of an increased incidence of Ki-ras mutations in endometrial tumors arising in patients on tamoxifen compared with those not administered this drug *(241)*. Recent studies have demonstrated that the α-(N^2-deoxyguanosinyl) tamoxifens in which the trans form predominates are in vivo adducts formed from tamoxifen *(234,245)*. In addition, the dG-N^2-tamoxifen adduct epimers have been demonstrated to be miscoding and hence responsible for the generation of mutations in vitro *(255)*.

4.3. Metabolism of Triphenylethylene Antiestrogens

4.3.1. CLOMIPHENE

Several studies have examined the effect of chronic administration of antiestrogens on hepatic endpoints including tumor incidence. Newberne et al. *(268)* indicated that 420 ppm clomiphene for 1 yr to rats did not have an effect on the liver despite its potent action to inhibit gonadotrophin activity. The gonadotrophic effects of clomiphene were independent of any progestational, androgenic, or antiandrogenic activity or any action on thyroid-stimulating hormone (TSH) or adrenocorticotropic hormone (ACTH.) Since more than 40 mg clomiphene/kg/d in the diet reduced diet intake, the dose range tested was 5, 15, and 40 mg/kg/d. In the female, ovarian atrophy and endometrial squamous metaplasia were observed, while in male rats, prostate and seminal vesicle dose-dependent atrophy was noted. A decrease in circulating cholesterol and an increase in desmosterol were also reported. At the doses given, consistent organ-to-body weight differences were not observed. The marked effect of clomiphene to inhibit pituitary gonadotropin release in the rat is in contrast to the release of gonadotropins, which has been reported to occur in humans.

4.3.2. CHLOROTRIANISENE

Chlorotrianisene (TACE) has been tested in rats at doses of 0, 0.05, 0.2, and 2 mg/kg for 1 yr in the diet *(269)*. In these studies, a decrease in body-weight gain was observed, as was a slight increase in adrenal and liver weight without any evidence of liver pathology, although gonadal atrophy was observed. Earlier studies had indicated that TACE can induce the formation of protein adducts in a microsomal system *(270)*. Despite this property, TACE did not induce liver neoplasms in the chronic bioassay performed *(269)*.

4.3.3. DROLOXIFENE

Hasmann et al. *(271)* have reviewed some of the toxicology data on droloxifene (3-hydroxy tamoxifen). Specifically, a comparison of the liver changes after 6 mo of administration of 2, 20, or 200 mg droloxifene/kg and 0.6, 6, and 60 mg tamoxifen/kg was performed. In these studies, 60 mg tamoxifen/kg/d induced hepatic neoplasms including adenocarcinomas in the rat, while droloxifene was without effect on proliferative lesions in the liver. In addition, a 2-yr study comparing 36 mg tamoxifen/kg/d with 4–90 mg droloxifene/kg/d was performed. A 100% incidence of hepatic neoplasms was observed in the tamoxifen treated group, while droloxifene inhibited the spontaneous induction of basophilic foci. Systemic toxicity was not observed following administration of 100 mg droloxifene/kg to rats for 4 wk. An atrophy in the gonadal tissue of both male and female rats was observed with this treatment owing to the antiestrogenic activity of droloxifene administration to rats *(272)*. In a separate study, Sprague Dawley rats of both sexes were administered 0, 2, 20, or 200 mg droloxifene/kg for 6 wk without evidence of liver pathology *(273)*.

4.3.4. TOREMIFENE

Several studies have examined the potential carcinogenicity of toremifene. Hirsamaki et al. have compared tamoxifen at 45 mg/kg and toremifene at 48 mg/kg and demonstrated an increase in the incidence of hepatic tumors in the rat with tamoxifen but not toremifene administration *(274)*. This observation has been extended by a number of investigators. In one study in which female Sprague-Dawley rats were administered 12 or 24 mg toremifene/kg and sacrificed at 12 or 15 mo, hepatic tumors were not observed; in addition, neither pituitary tumors not mammary tumors were detected *(204)*. Both Hirsamaki et al. *(275)* and Ahotupa et al. *(276)* have extended previous observations to a larger number of animals with 12 or 48 mg/kg for 12 mo; they were sacrificed or observed for an additional 13 wk. Similarly, Dragan et al. *(277)* have fed diets containing 250, 500, or 750 ppm toremifene for 6 or 18 mo and observed an increase in GGT- but not GST-expressing enzyme-altered foci. In a 2-yr bioassay with Sprague-Dawley rats of both sexes, toremifene when administered at 0.12, 1.2, 5.0, and 12.0 mg/kg was without effect on liver tumor induction and resulted in a reduction in pituitary and mammary tumor incidence *(278)*. Additional studies have been performed with administration of toremifene in the diet at 250, 500, or 750 ppm after the known carcinogen, 10 mg DEN/kg. At the 6-mo sacrifice, the incidence of foci of cellular alteration was increased in the liver, and at 18 mo hepatic carcinomas were observed in the rats receiving 500 or 750 ppm toremifene following DEN-initiation *(277)*.

4.3.5. TAMOXIFEN

In subacute toxicity testing in Sprague-Dawley rats, a dose of 0.007 mg tamoxifen/kg/d represented a no-effect level for various endpoints including body-weight gain at the 5-, 13-, and 26-wk time-points *(279)*. Severe trophic changes of the genitourinary tract in addition to a depression of body-weight gain were observed at doses of 0.7 mg tamoxifen/kg/d and above. Adrenal size was increased in male rats with doses of 0.7 to 70 mg/kg/d, while adrenal weights were depressed in female rats with 0.07–7 mg/kg/d for 5 wk. An increase in lipid in the zona fasiculata was noted with marked hypertrophy of this layer in some animals. Pituitary size was decreased in both sexes when 0.7 to 70 mg tamoxifen/kg was administered for 5 wk. In male but not female rats, the basophilic cells of the pituitary were degranulated and the presence of vacuoles was noted. The number of PAS-positive granules was decreased after 26–35 wk of administration of tamoxifen, while a decrease in PAS-positive cells was not observed. These effects on the pituitary resulting from 5 wk of administration were reversible upon withdrawal of the drug. In male rats receiving 70 mg/kg/d for 5 wk, the size of the pituitary beta cells was reduced. By 26 wk of tamoxifen administration, pituitary size was decreased in both male and female rats. In addition, adrenal size was increased in both sexes at the highest dose. Hepatic nodular hyperplasia was observed in 2 of 6 males and 4 of 6 females administered 35 mg tamoxifen per kg for 26 wk.

Studies in Alderley Park rats used 0, 2, 20, and 100 mg tamoxifen/kg for 3 mo. Histological changes signifying atrophy were observed in gonadal tissue, implying an antiestrogenic effect owing to a blockage of estrogenic action on the hypothalamic-pituitary axis. A depression of body-weight gain was observed in all treatment groups *(257)*. This study was repeated in female rats with 0.5 and 2.0 mg tamoxifen/kg or 4 mg clomiphene/kg for 3 mo followed by immediate sacrifice or sacrifice after an additional 3-mo recovery. In addition, a

6-mo study was performed with 0, 0.5, 0.8, 2.4, 4.8, and 9.6 mg/kg demonstrating a decreased body-weight growth and antiestrogenic effects on the gonads.

4.4. Tumor Promotion by Tamoxifen and Related Antiestrogens

Several studies have demonstrated that estrogenic agents are able to induce hepatocarcinogenesis in the rat. At least two studies in the rat liver indicate that tamoxifen administration can inhibit at least part of this estrogen-induced hepatic tumor promotion (280,281). Further studies have indicated that tamoxifen administration can inhibit the estradiol-induced cell proliferation of hepatocytes (264,282). However, administration of tamoxifen in combination with an estrogenic agent can also result in an additive effect in the liver (182). Under certain circumstances, one can demonstrate a basal effect of tamoxifen to increase hepatic tumor promotion, while inhibiting that of the co-administered estrogenic agent. Fischer rats are more sensitive to the promoting action of tamoxifen than are Sprague-Dawley rats (265). In studies examining the initiating potential of some triphenylethylene antiestrogens, rats were administered 400 ppm tamoxifen (average intake of 206 mg per Sprague-Dawley rat and 50 mg per Fischer rat) for 6 wk with a partial hepatectomy after the first week, after which the rats were administered 0.02% acetylaminofluorene for 2 wk with administration of a necrogenic dose of carbon tetrachloride after 1 wk. Nearly 250 mg clomiphene per rat was administered to Sprague-Dawley rats and 75 mg per rat to Fischer rats in another study.

Carthew et al. (283) have demonstrated that rat strains differ in their sensitivity to tamoxifen-induced hepatocarcinogenesis. In these studies female rats of the Fischer, Wistar, and Lewis strains were administered 420 ppm for 1–6 mo. These studies indicate that Fischer rats are less sensitive than the other two rat strains to the hepatocarcinogenic effects of tamoxifen. In this study, a lower level of DNA adducts was observed at the 1- and 3-mo time points in Fischer compared with the Wistar and Lewis strains. In addition, the level of hepatic-cell proliferation was depressed in the Fischer rat, but enhanced in the Lewis and to an even greater extent in the Wistar rat. Serum tamoxifen levels were not different between strains, but the pattern and level of metabolites that accumulate in the liver did differ, with the Fischer strain maintaining a higher level of tamoxifen than the more sensitive rat strains. The number and area of GST-P lesions was 10-fold lower in Fischer than in the other two strains after 6 mo of tamoxifen administration. Multifocal hyperplastic nodules were observed in the Wistar rats, while an adenoma was observed in the Lewis rat at 6 mo. Hepatic neoplasms were observed in the Fischer rat after 20, but not after 6 mo of tamoxifen administration (283). The relative resistance of female Fischer rats to tamoxifen carcinogenicity may be due to the sulfotransferase dimorphism.

Kim et al. *(284)* have examined the ability of tamoxifen to promote DEN-initiated hepatocytes in the newborn rat model in which female Sprague-Dawley rats were administered saline or 100 mg DEN/kg at 1 d after birth and administered tamoxifen (1 mg/rat/d, s.c.) from 3–12 wk of age. The total tamoxifen citrate intake was ~50 mg/rat and resulted in a significant increase in the number of GST-P positive foci. In the second study, adult female Fischer rats were administered saline or 200 mg DEN/kg and provided tamoxifen 100, 250, or 500 ppm in the diet beginning 3 wk later for a total of 5 wk. A dose-dependent increase in GST-P foci was observed with total cumulative tamoxifen intake of ~60–300 mg/rat.

Six months of administration of 35 mg tamoxifen/kg/d to rats resulted in nodular hyperplasia of the liver *(285)*. Similar results had been previously reported by Watanabe et al. *(279)* with twice the dose of tamoxifen. In addition, administration of tamoxifen at 0.25, 1.0, and 2.5 mg/kg/d for 10 mo resulted in a suppression (from 75% in the controls to 10, 25, and 35% in the three doses, respectively) of the hepatic tumor incidence in male rats administered 100 mg DEN/kg po, and 200 ppm 2 acetylaminofluorene with a partial hepatectomy *(280)*, indicating the estrogen-receptor dependence of the majority of tumors induced by this regimen. A similar result was obtained by Kohigashi et al. *(281)* in male Sprague-Dawley rats administered 200 mg DEN/kg, ip, and 0.5 mg DES/rat/d, 1 mg tamoxifen in the diet per rat/d, or both DES and tamoxifen. Tamoxifen administration increased the size of the lesions in DEN-pretreated rats compared with those receiving DEN but not tamoxifen; whereas tamoxifen administration decreased the size of the lesions in the DEN/DES-treated group.

Ghia and Mereto *(265)* performed initiation-selection studies in both female Sprague Dawley and Fischer rats. These studies indicated that Fischer rats are more sensitive to the promoting action of tamoxifen under the conditions tested than were the Sprague-Dawley strain. In those studies, the rats were fed 200 ppm acetylaminofluorene (AAF) for 2 wk with administration of 1 mL carbon tetrachloride/kg at the midpoint in the AAF administration. After a 1-wk recovery period from the AAF administration, tamoxifen was administered in the diet at 400 ppm for 6 wk, resulting in an efficient promotion of GGT-positive altered hepatic foci. The effective promoting action of tamoxifen in the rat liver had similarly been demonstrated by Yager et al. *(181)*. Female Sprague-Dawley rats were administered 25 mg DEN/kg, ip, 24 h after a partial hepatectomy and 1 wk later provided a silastic capsule to release 15 or 50 µg tamoxifen/kg. After 4 mo of tamoxifen administration, an effective promotion of the GGT-positive foci population was noted.

Dragan et al. *(263)* demonstrated that tamoxifen administration to female Fischer rats at 250 or 500 ppm in a semi-purified diet promoted the development of glucose 6 phosphatase-deficient as well as GGT-positive altered hepatic foci. In female Fischer rats subjected to a 70% partial hepatectomy followed by administration of 10 mg DEN/kg, tamoxifen administration for 15 mo at a concentration of 250 ppm in a semipurified diet resulted in an increased incidence of hepatocellular carcinomas compared with the DEN-initiated control, which was not administered tamoxifen *(286)*. In a study performed in female Fischer rats, rats subjected to a partial hepatectomy were administered the solvent or 10 mg DEN/kg and 2 wk later were administered tamoxifen or one of its nonisomerizable fixed-ring derivatives at 25, 100, or 250 ppm in a cereal-based diet *(287)*. In this study, all three agents were found to be effective promoting agents at the highest dose, although the order of potency was that tamoxifen was greater than the fixed-ring compound, which was greater than the ethylated fixed-ring derivative independent of a pharmacokinetic effect of the parent compound.

In a study performed in female Sprague-Dawley rats *(288)*, rats subjected to a partial hepatectomy were administered the solvent or 10 mg DEN/kg, and 2 wk later were administered tamoxifen at 250 or 500 ppm in a cereal-based diet. Alternatively, the rats were administered 250, 500, or 750 ppm toremifene. The rats were sacrificed at 6 or 18 mo, and some degree of promotion was observed for certain markers with all doses of the triphenylethylenes at both time points. At the 6-mo point, both doses of tamoxifen but none of those of toremifene increased the incidence of neoplastic nodules in the liver in DEN-initiated rats. By 18 mo of tamoxifen administration, 8/15 rats presented with hepatocellular carcinomas in the 500 ppm treatment group, while 18 mo of tamoxifen administration to DEN-initiated rats resulted in 11/18 and 8/8 of the rats with hepatocellular carcinomas in the 250 and 500 ppm groups, respectively. Toremifene in the absence of DEN initiation did not increase the incidence of malignant liver neoplasms. In the presence of DEN initiation, an increased incidence of hepatocellular carcinomas was observed for both 500 ppm (7/16) and 750 ppm (11/18) compared with 2/17 in the DEN-initiated control maintained on the basal diet *(277)*.

4.4.1. CHRONIC BIOASSAY

Greaves et al. *(285)* demonstrated that 2-yr administration of tamoxifen at 5, 20, or 35 mg/kg/d resulted in a dose-related increase in hepatic tumors in Wistar rats. In a separate study performed by Williams et al. *(288)* in female Sprague-Dawley rats, administration of 45.2 mg tamoxifen/kg/d resulted in an increase in hepatic nodule and hepatocellular carcinoma incidence by 6 months (N = 7) with and without a 1-mo recovery. In the recovery group, evidence of progression from adenoma to carcinoma was observed (N = 3). In addition, treatment for 1 yr with 22 mg tamoxifen/kg/d resulted in a 100% incidence of hepatocellular carcinomas, while a 70% incidence was observed with 11 mg tamoxifen/kg. Hepatic tumors were not observed when 2.8 mg tamoxifen/kg/d was administered to female rats for 1 yr *(288)*. Studies by Hirsimaki further confirmed the hepatic carcinogenicity of tamoxifen to rats in a study in which female Sprague-Dawley rats were administered 11.3 or 45 mg tamoxifen/kg/d for 1 yr, in which 3/5 had hepatocellular carcinomas after 1 yr and 5/6 had malignant liver neoplasms after a further 13-wk observation period *(274,275)*. Tamoxifen was not carcinogenic to three different strains of mice including C57B16, DBA, and ICR when administered at 420 ppm in the diet for 2 yr *(289)*. A previous study in Alderley Park strain 1 mice had demonstrated that 5 or 50 mg tamoxifen/kg increased the incidence of interstitial cell tumors of the testes and granulosa cell tumors of the ovary in mice after 1 yr of treatment, but no evidence for hepatic neoplasms was noted *(256)*.

4.5. Progression of Carcinogenesis

4.5.1. SYRIAN HAMSTER EMBRYO (SHE) CELL-TRANSFORMATION ASSAY

Syrian hamster embryo cells have been used to demonstrate that the carcinogenic action of diethylstilbesterol (DES) was due in large part to its action on the induction of aneuploidy *(261,290)*. The induction of aneuploidy by DES and several of its metabolites has been correlated with their ability to transform these cells. At least one group of investigators has demonstrated that tamoxifen and 4-hydroxy tamoxifen (10 μM for 48 hr) can induce transformation of SHE cells in the absence of an exogenous metabolizing system *(256,291)*. Interestingly, the presence of a 3-hydroxy group on the stilbene structure as in droloxifene does not result in the induction of transformation of SHE cells. Droloxifene at a dose of 39 μg/mL did not transform SHE cells in the absence of a metabolic activating system *(291)*. Similarly, covalent binding to DNA was not observed with 47 mg droloxifene/kg p.o. (0.12 mmol/kg) for 4 d as detected by ^{32}P-post labeling *(205)*. Thus, tamoxifen and its 4-hydroxy metabolite can transform SHE cells.

4.6. Micronuclei Formation

Furthermore, tamoxifen can induce micronuclei in a metabolism-competent lymphoblastoid cell line, MCL-5 containing CYP1A1 and transfected with CYP1A2, CYP2A6, CYP2E1, CYP3A4, and epoxide hydrolase *(205,244)*. In addition, 4-hydroxy tamoxifen, 4-hydroxy toremifene, and clomiphene, but not droloxifene, induced micronuclei in these MCL-5 cells. In the parental cell line, which does not contain exogenous drug-metabolizing enzymes, only the 4-hydroxy derivatives of tamoxifen and toremifene induced micronuclei. The induction of micronuclei indicates that an induction of numerical chromosomal changes or spindle disruption has occurred.

In MCL-5 human lymphoblastoid cells that contain a variety of P450s, 4-hydroxy tamoxifen, 4-hydroxy toremifene, and clomiphene increased the incidence of micronuclei, while the 3-hydroxy tamoxifen (droloxifene) did not (0.25–10 μ/mL). Under certain conditions of forced metabolism, clomiphene, 4-hydroxy tamoxifen, and 4-hydroxy toremifene are able to induce micronuclei. These triphenylethylenes may have an intrinsic ability to induce clastogenesis or spindle abnormalities, traits not observed for droloxifene under the conditions used. In cells lacking extensive metabolic activities and in the absence of exogenous metabolizing enzymes, the metabolites 4-hydroxy tamoxifen and 4-hydroxy toremifene were able to induce micronuclei, while the parent compounds were without activity, implicating the 4-hydroxylation pathway in the induction of hepatic aneuploidy or clastogenesis by these agents. Aneuploidy was increased in MCL-5 cells treated with DES, clomiphene, tamoxifen, and toremifene, but not in those cells provided 3-hydroxy tamoxifen (droloxifene). The induction of micronuclei by 4-hydroxy tamoxifen indicates that this metabolite may be responsible for the aneuploidy observed with tamoxifen administration. A statistical increase in chromosomal breakage was observed in hepatocytes of Wistar rats treated once with tamoxifen, while breakage after an equimolar dose of toremifene, droloxifene, and DES did not result in a statistical elevation. When Wistar rats were dosed daily with tamoxifen or toremifene for 4 wk, both agents increased aneuploidy. However, only tamoxifen increased breakage after chronic in vivo administration to female Wistar rats *(292)*. It has been hypothesized that the observed aneuploidy is due to chromosomal nondisjunction. It appears that DES, clomiphene, and 4-hydroxy tamoxifen were aneuplodigens but not clastogens, while both tamoxifen and toremifene can induce structural chromosomal changes under specific experimental conditions. These observations suggest that the 4-hydroxylation pathway may not be the pathway primarily responsible for clastogenesis. Several studies have indicated that DES can induce aneuploidy through a process that in part is due to a disruption of tubulin organization. Loss of tubulin organization may be causal for chromosomal nondisjunction and hence aneuploidy *(205,260,293,294)* through the formation of protein adducts between tamoxifen and tubulin or displacement of an estrogen metabolite from tubulin.

4.6.1. CHROMOSOMAL ABERRATIONS

Tamoxifen has been shown to increase the incidence of structurally abnormal chromosomes after acute administration *(292,295,296)*. In one study, toremifene was shown to increase the incidence of hepatic chromosomal aberrations after in vivo administration *(296),* a result not demonstrated in a second study in a different rat strain *(292)*. Studies on human lymphocytes have not demonstrated an increase in sister chromatid exchange or chromosomal aberrations, although at the highest dose (10 µg/mL, but only in the presence of an S9 activating system, premature chromosome condensation was observed *(179)*.

4.6.2. ANEUPLOIDY INDUCTION

Tamoxifen is structurally related to DES, a known human carcinogen. A causal role for the induction of aneuploidy in the induction of cancer has not been demonstrated. However, the carcinogenic potential of DES best correlates with its ability to induce aneuploidy *(259)*. Progressive nonrandom aneuploidy is a hallmark of malignant neoplasms *(49,297)*. The induction of aneuploidy can occur through numerous mechanisms that are independent of DNA adduction *(293,298)*. These include, but are not limited to, altered microtubule assembly, altered synthesis of the kinetocore proteins, and modulation of calmodulin levels *(293,298)*.

4.6.3. CELL-CYCLE EFFECTS

Tamoxifen can induce a G1 block in breast-cancer cells *(293)*. In addition, tamoxifen can inhibit regenerative cell proliferation after a partial hepatectomy *(282)*, indicative of a hepatic G1 block *(299)*. Furthermore, tamoxifen can induce micronuclei in a metabolism-competent lymphoblastoid cell line *(205,252)*. Similar types of effects have been observed with DES *(291)*, indicating that this class of agents may have several actions that disrupt the tightly coordinated processes of spindle formation and chromosomal integrity *(293,296)*. Both monopolar spindles and shortened spindles have been observed with acute tamoxifen administration *(295)*, suggesting that the mechanism of tamoxifen-induced aneuploidy might be calmodulin inhibition. Tamoxifen and structurally similar compounds are known to inhibit calmodulin *(300–303)* with doses achieved through accumulation in the liver and other tissues. Agents with antiestrogenic action can halt G1 phase, cell-cycle progression in breast-cancer cells *(304)*. One mechanism by which triphenylethylene antiestrogens may inhibit estrogen-induced cell proliferation is through inhibition of protein kinase C (PKC) *(305)* or inhibition of calmodulin *(300,305)*. Calmodulin can bind to the estrogen receptor *(306)*, and this binding mediates the phosphorylation that is required for activation of the estrogen receptor *(307)*. In support of this hypothesis, calmodulin antagonists inhibit estrogen-induced cell proliferation in some tissues *(302)*. The cell cycle changes observed after antiestrogen administration include a decreased expression of cyclin D *(308)*, a decrease in pRB (retinoblastoma) phosphorylation *(309)*, a decreased activity of cyclin-dependent kinases (cdks) that target retinoblastoma (RB) *(309)*, and the increased expression of CDK inhibitors *(310,311)*. Tamoxifen can induce aneuploidy, spindle abnormalities, and altered chromosomal integrity through an alteration of calmodulin activity or an alteration of cell cycle components. Administration of 1 μg of tamoxifen/g at the time of a 70% partial hepatectomy or 6 (but not 12) h later inhibits the compensatory regeneration otherwise observed. Interestingly, these effects of tamoxifen on cell proliferation could be reversed by estradiol, implicating receptor mediation for this effect on the G1 phase of the cell cycle. In addition, tamoxifen inhibits calmodulin, which is an important regulator of cell-cycle effects.

The observation of an apparent threshold for promoting action *(311,312)* suggests that a therapeutic index that maximizes the benefits of breast-tumor suppression while limiting the potential for chronic side effects may be possible with sufficiently low doses of tamoxifen *(313)*. Alternatively, synthesis of structurally or pharmacologically related compounds that are more rapidly cleared (droloxifene *[226–228,314]*, toremifene *[219–225,315,316]*), that are less rapidly metabolized (idoxifene *[229,230,317,318]*), and that have selective target-organ estrogenicity/antiestrogenicity (toremifene *[219,220]*, droloxifene *[226]*, idoxifene *[319]*, and keoxifene *[320,321]*) might overcome this problem. Tamoxifen exhibits a range of estrogen-like activities in laboratory animals *(322,323)* and in postmenopausal women *(324)*. Although some estrogen-like effects may prove beneficial upon long-term therapy, such as decreased serum cholesterol *(324,325)* and reduced osteoporosis *(324–327)*, this pharmacology may promote the development of estrogen-responsive tumors. In the laboratory, tamoxifen administration can promote the growth of human endometrium *(328–330)*.

Several recent findings indicate that a closer look at estrogen-receptor pharmacology needs to be taken. These include the cloning of a second estrogen receptor ERβ *(331–333)*, which has both similarities to and differences from ERα receptor. An exciting finding by Carthew et al. *(334)* demonstrates that ERα expression is not detectable in hepatic neoplasms. Importantly, estrogen-regulated genes containing AP1 sites can respond differently to the same ligand depending upon which estrogen receptor it binds *(335)*. These recent findings indicate the importance of understanding the expression of estrogen receptor(s) in hepatic tissue during the stages of cancer development, including their signaling pathways and regulation of gene expression.

Growth-factor secretion and the altered expression of growth factor receptors have been implicated in the process of cellular growth control *(336)*. Peptide growth factors, specifically IGF-1 and EGF family members, are likely to be involved in estrogen-receptor transduction *(337–342)*. Certain estrogen-regulated genes are induced by nonestrogen response elements including IGF-1 *(343)* and TGF-α *(344)*, which may be important in growth control in tissues with a low estrogen-receptor content. The expression of these genes may also provide a secondary mechanism to induce an "estrogen-like" response in which a liganded estrogen receptor binds to AP1 sites and induces an estrogenic effect *(335,345–347)*. While antiestrogens can competitively inhibit some actions of estrogen, antiestrogens are frequently partial agonists that can activate cell proliferation under certain conditions *(323)*. Tamoxifen can induce TGF-β, which is growth inhibitory and which regulates apoptosis, in several tissues *(348–351)*. The mechanism of tumor promotion involves cell- and tissue-specific changes in proliferation and apoptosis. The perturbation of growth-factor synthesis and action by the triphenylethylene antiestrogens may partially underlie their ability to induce tumor promotion in several tissues.

5. SUMMARY

The finding of a carcinogenic action for tamoxifen in the rat liver suggests a potential for the risk of the induction of secondary cancers following chronic administration to the human. However, the probability that such a risk is relevant to the human at clinically relevant doses or for exposure during the portion of the life cycle during which it is administered needs to be more closely addressed. The similarity and differences of the model used to examine the carcinogenicity of tamoxifen with the human should be very closely examined. Both species and strain differences in the carcinogenic action of tamoxifen have been noted due in part to metabolic and hormonal differences. Gavage administration of tamoxifen in an oil base results in much higher doses on a mg/kg basis than are achievable in standard therapeutic regimens used for breast-cancer therapy or in the clinical trials for chemopreventive measures. Although high-dose tamoxifen administration for reversal of multidrug resistance is practiced, a limited population is exposed to such high-dose effects. With respect to adduct generation, rats generate higher levels of adducts than mice or humans. Since adduct generation correlates with tumor incidence in rats and the lack of effect in mice, the pathways for adduct generation need to be detailed at clinically relevant doses with human tissue. Rodents have a higher metabolic clearance than humans and hence potentially a higher tissue accumulation with comparable serum concentrations *(195)*. Studies by Kohigashi et al. *(281)* indicate that tamoxifen-induced DNA adducts were not detectable in rats treated with 0.5 mg tamoxifen/kg. Similar findings suggest that administration of 2–5 mg tamoxifen/kg to the rat does not result in a significant level of hepatic DNA adducts *(205),* and rat liver carcinogenesis was not induced by administration of 2.8 mg tamoxifen/kg *(288)*. Approximately 5 mg tamoxifen/kg appears to be the threshold for detection of liver tumors in the rat *(288)*. Since women are administered 20 mg tamoxifen/d, they are exposed to 0.3–0.4 mg tamoxifen/kg, demonstrating the need to understand the metabolic pathways (both phase 1 and phase 2) involved in DNA adduct formation and the hormonal factors that contribute to liver carcinogenicity in the rat at 10-fold higher doses. Since both the peak and the total tissue concentration may predicate the metabolic pathway utilized, distinct metabolism routes may be prevalent upon diet administration, gavage administration, and human exposure, implicating these differences in the potential risk of adverse effects in the human at clinically relevant doses. The induction and modulation of DNA adducts with tamoxifen administration indicate that chronic administration, especially at high doses, could lead to mutation and potentially to initiation of the carcinogenic process. In addition, tamoxifen and related compounds can alter cell-cycle kinetics and hence may lead to aneuploidy, altered spindle assembly and function, or to a loss of chromosomal integrity. DNA adducts generated from tamoxifen have been detected infrequently in tissues from individuals treated with tamoxifen, indicating that the increased detection of endometrial cancer in such patients may be due more to its estrogenic action than to its ability to induce adducts or to alter chromosomal stability. The carcinogenicity of tamoxifen and related compounds may reflect the species and tissue specificity of metabolism (both phase 1 and phase 2), cell-proliferative capacity, and DNA repair.

REFERENCES

1. Vainio H, Hemminki K, Wilbourn J. Data on the carcinogenicity of chemicals in the *IARC Monographs* programme. *Carcinogenesis* 1985; 6:1653–1665.
2. Huff J, Haseman J, Rall D. Scientific concepts, value, and significance of chemical carcinogenesis studies. *Annu Rev Pharmacol Toxicol* 1991; 31:621–652.
3. Meijers JMM, Swaen GMH, Bloemen LJN. The predictive value of animal data in human cancer risk assessment. *Reg Toxicol Pharmacol* 1997; 25:94–102.
4. Neumann F. Early indicators for carcinogenesis in sex-hormone-sensitive organs. *Mutat Res* 1991; 248:341–356.
5. Foran JA. Principles for the selection of doses in chronic rodent bioassays. *Environ Health Perspect* 1997; 105:18–20.
6. Apostolou A. Relevance of maximum tolerated dose to human carcinogenic risk. *Reg Toxicol Pharmacol* 1990; 11:68–80.
7. Wiltse J, Dellarco VL. U.S. Environmental Protection Agency guidelines for carcinogen risk assessment: past and future. *Mutat Res* 1996; 365:3–15.
8. Knudson AG Jr. Hereditary cancers disclose a class of cancer genes. *Cancer* 1989; 63:1888–1891.
9. Moolgavkar SH, Knudson AG Jr. Mutation and cancer: a model for human carcinogenesis. *J Natl Cancer Inst* 1981; 66:1037–1052.
10. Moolgavkar SH, Venzon DJ. Two event models for carcinogenesis: incidence curves for childhood and adult tumors. *Math Biosci* 1979; 47:55–77.
11. Moolgavkar SH. Carcinogenesis modeling: from molecular biology to epidemiology. *Annu Rev Public Health* 1986; 7:151–169.
12. Moolgavkar SH, Luebeck EG. Multistage carcinogenesis: population-based model for colon cancer. *J Natl Cancer Inst* 1992; 84:610–618.
13. Cohen SM, Ellwein LB. Genetic errors, cell proliferation, and carcinogenesis. *Cancer Res* 1991; 51:6493–6505.
14. Cohen SM, Purtilo DT, Ellwein LB. Ideas in pathology. Pivotal role of increased cell proliferation in human carcinogenesis. *Mod Pathol* 1991; 4:371–382.
15. Cohen SM, Ellwein LB. Cell proliferation in carcinogenesis. *Science* 1990; 249:1007–1011.
16. Baylin SB. Tying it all together: epigenetics, genetics, cell cycle, and cancer. *Science* 1997; 277:1948–1949.
17. Laird PW, Jaenisch R. The role of DNA methylation in cancer genetics and epigenetics. *Annu Rev Genet* 1996; 30:441–464.
18. Fearon ER, Vogelstein B. A genetic model for colorectal tumorigenesis. *Cell* 1990; 61:759–767.
19. Harris CC. Tumor suppressor genes: at the crossroads of molecular carcinogenesis, molecular epidemiology, and human risk assessment. *Prev Med* 1996; 25:10–12.
20. Pitot HC. Stages in neoplastic development, in *Cancer Epidemiology and Prevention* 2nd ed. (Schottenfeld D, Fraumeni JF, eds). Oxford University Press, NY, 1996, pp 65–79.
21. Nowell PC. Cytogenetic approaches to human cancer genes. *FASEB J* 1994; 8:408–413.
22. Maron DM, Ames BN. Revised methods for the Salmonella mutagenicity test. *Mutation Res* 1983; 113:173–215.

23. Gee P, Maron DM, Ames BN. Detection and classification of mutagens: a set of base-specific *Salmonella* tester strains. *Proc Natl Acad Sci USA* 1994; 91:11606–11610.

24. Swierenga SHH, Heddle JA, Sigal EA, Gilman JPW, Brillinger RL, Douglas GR, Nestmann ER. Recommended protocols based on a survey of current practice in genotoxicity testing laboratories, IV. Chromosome aberration and sister-chromatid exchange in Chinese hamster ovary, V79 Chinese hamster lung and human lymphocyte cultures. *Mutation Res* 1991; 246:301–322.

25. Hoffmann GR. Genetic toxicology, in *Casarett and Doull's Toxicology, The Basic Science of Poisons,* 5th ed. (Klaassen C, ed). McGraw Hill, New York, 1995, pp 269–300.

26. Yamasaki H, Ashby J, Bignami M, Jongen W, Linnainmaa K, Newbold RF, et al. Nongenotoxic carcinogens: development of detection methods based on mechanisms: a European project. *Mutat Res* 1996; 353:47–63.

27. Isfort RJ, LeBoeuf RA. The Syrian hamster embryo (SHE) cell transformation system: a biologically relevant in vitro model – with carcinogen predicting capabilities – of in vivo multistage neoplastic transformation. *Crit Rev Oncogen* 1995; 6:251–260.

28. Sontag JM. Aspects in carcinogen bioassay, in *Origins of Human Cancer* (Hiatt H, Watson J, Winsten J, eds). Cold Spring Harbor Laboratory, 1997, pp 1327–1338.

29. Ames BN, Gold LS. Animal cancer tests and cancer prevention. *J Natl Cancer Inst Monogr* 1992; 12:125–132.

30. Ames BN, Shigenaga MK, Gold LS. DNA lesions, inducible DNA repair, and cell division: three key factors in mutagenesis and carcinogenesis. *Environ Health Perspect* 1993; 101(Suppl 5):35–44.

31. McClain RM. Mechanistic considerations in the regulation and classification of chemical carcinogens, in *Nutritional Toxicology* (Kotsonis FN, Mackey M, Hjelle J, eds). Raven Press, Ltd., NY, 1994, pp 273–304.

32. Green T. Species differences in carcinogenicity: the role of metabolism in human risk evaluation. *Teratogen Carcinogen Mutagen* 1990; 10:103–113.

33. Contrera JF, Jacobs AC, DeGeorge JJ. Carcinogenicity testing and the evaluation of regulatory requirements for pharmaceuticals. *Reg Toxicol Pharmacol* 1997; 25:130–145.

34. Butterworth BE, Eldridge SR. A decision tree approach for carcinogen risk assessment. *Prog Clin Biol Res* 1995; 391:49–70.

35. Goldsworthy TL, Butterworth BE, Maronpot RR. Concepts, labeling procedures, and design of cell proliferation studies relating to carcinogenesis. *Environ Health Perspect* 1993; 5:59–65.

36. Collins JM, Grieshaber CK, Chabner BA. Pharmacologically guided Phase I clinical trials based upon preclinical drug development. *J Natl Cancer Inst* 1990; 82:1321–1326.

37. Monro AM. Interspecies comparisons in toxicology: the utility and futility of plasma concentrations of the test substance. *Reg Toxicol Pharmacol* 1990; 12:137–160.

38. Peck CC, Barr WH, Benet LZ, Collins J, Desjardins RE, Furst DE, et al. Opportunities for integration of pharmacokinetics, pharmacodynamics and toxicokinetics in rational drug development. *Pharmaceut Res* 1992; 9:826–833.

39. Couch DB. Carcinogenesis: basic principles. *Drug Chem Toxicol* 1996; 19:133–148.

40. Clayson DB, Iverson F. Cancer risk assessment at the crossroads: the need to turn to a biological approach. *Reg Toxicol Pharmacol* 1996; 24:45–59.

41. Comings DE. A general theory of carcinogenesis. *Proc Natl Acad Sci USA* 1973; 70:3324–3328.

42. Jacks T. Tumor suppressor gene mutation in mice. *Annu Rev Genet* 1996; 30:603–636.

43. Boutwell RK. Some biological aspects of skin carcinogenesis. *Progr Exp Tumor Res* 1964; 4:207–250.

44. Slaga TJ, Fischer SM, Weeks CE, Klein-Szanto AJP, Reiners J. Studies on the mechanisms involved in multistage carcinogenesis in mouse skin. *J Cell Biochem* 1982; 18:99–119.

45. Hennings H, Glick AB, Greenhalgh DA, Morgan DL, Strickland JE, Tennenbaum T, Yuspa SH. Critical aspects of initiation, promotion, and progression in multistage epidermal carcinogenesis. *Proc Soc Exp Biol Med* 1993; 202:1–8.

46. Nagase H, Bryson S, Fee F, Balmain A. Multigenic control of skin tumour development in mice. *Ciba Foundation Symp* 1996; 197:156–168.

47. Goldsworthy TL, Hanigan MH, Pitot HC. Models of hepatocarcinogenesis in the rat: contrasts and comparisons. *CRC Crit Rev Toxicol* 1986; 17:61–89.

48. Farber E, Sarma DSR. Biology of disease, Hepatocarcinogenesis: a dynamic cellular perspective. *Lab Invest* 1987; 56:4–22.

49. Shackney SE, Shankey TV. Common patterns of genetic evolution in human solid tumors. *Cytometry* 1997; 29:1–27.

50. Dragan YP, Sargent L, Xu YD, Xu YH, Pitot HC. The initiation-promotion-progression model of rat hepatocarcinogenesis. *Proc Soc Exp Biol Med* 1993; 202:16–24.

51. Boutwell RK. Some biological aspects of skin carcinogenesis. *Prog Exp Tumor Res* 1964; 4:207–250.

52. Goldsworthy TL, Hanigan MH, Pitot HC. Models of hepatocarcinogenesis in the rat – contrasts and comparisons. *CRC Crit Rev Toxicol* 1986; 17:61–89.

53. Pitot HC. Stages in neoplastic development, in *Cancer Epidemiology and Prevention* 2nd ed. (Schottenfeld D, Fraumeni JP, eds). Oxford University Press, NY, 1996, pp 65–79.

54. Slaga TJ, Fischer SM, Weeks CE, Klein-Szanto AJP, and Reiners J. Studies on the mechanisms involved in multistage carcinogenesis in mouse skin. *J Cell Biochem* 1982; 18:99–119.

55. Farber E, Sarma DSR. Biology of disease. Hepatocarcinogenesis: a dynamic cellular perspective. *Lab Invest* 1987; 56:4–22.

56. Kakunaga T. The role of cell division in the malignant transformation of mouse cells treated with 3-methylcholanthrene. *Cancer Res* 1975; 35:1637–1642.

57. Columbano A, Rajalakshmi S, Sarma DSR. Requirement of cell proliferation for the initiation of liver carcinogenesis as assayed by three different procedures. *Cancer Res* 1981; 41:2079–2083.

58. Pitot HC, Goldsworthy TL, Moran S, et al. A method to quantitate the relative initiating and promoting potencies of hepatocarcinogenic agents in their dose-response relationship to altered hepatic foci. *Carcinogenesis* 1987; 8:1491–1499.

59. Dragan YP, Hully JR, Nakamura J, et al. Biochemical events during initiation of rat hepatocarcinogenesis. *Carcinogenesis* 1994; 15:1451–1458.

60. Talalay P, De Long MJ, Prochaska HJ. Identification of a common chemical signal regulating the induction of enzymes that protect against chemical carcinogenesis. *Proc Natl Acad Sci USA* 1988; 85:8261–8265.

61. Topal MD. DNA repair, oncogenes and carcinogenesis. *Carcinogenesis* 1988; 9:691–696.

62. Liao D, Porsch-Hällström I, Gustafsson J-A, Blanck A. Sex differences at the initiation stage of rat liver carcinogenesis–influence of growth hormone. *Carcinogenesis* 1993; 14:2045–2049.

63. Grasl-Kraupp B, Bursch W, Ruttkay-Nedecky B, Wagner A, Lauer B, Schulte-Hermann R. Food restriction eliminates preneoplastic cells through apoptosis and antagonizes carcinogenesis in rat liver. *Proc Natl Acad Sci USA* 1994; 91:9995–9999.

64. Maekawa A, Mitsumori K. Spontaneous occurrence and chemical induction of neurogenic tumors in rats–influence of host factors and specificity of chemical structure. *Crit Rev Toxicol* 1990; 20:287–310.

65. Pretlow TP. Alterations associated with early neoplasia in the colon, in *Biochemical and Molecular Aspects of Selected Cancers* vol. 2 (Pretlow TG, Pretlow TP, eds). Academic Press, San Diego, 1994, pp 93–141.

66. Dunham LJ. Cancer in man at site of prior benign lesion of skin or mucous membrane: a review. *Cancer Res* 1972; 32:1359–1374.

67. Pretlow TP, O'Riordan MA, Spancake KM, Pretlow TG. Two types of putative preneoplastic lesions identified by hexosaminidase activity in whole-mounts of colons from F344 rats treated with carcinogen. *Am J Pathol* 1993; 142:1695–1700.

68. Cohen SM, Arai M, Jacobs JB, Friedell GH. Promoting effect of saccharin and DL-tryptophan in urinary bladder carcinogenesis. *Cancer Res* 1979; 39:1207–1217.

69. Dragan YP, Xu X-H, Goldsworthy TL, Campbell HA, Maronpot RR, Pitot HC. Characterization of the promotion of altered hepatic foci by 2,3,7,8-tetrachlorodibenzo-*p*-dioxin in the female rat. *Carcinogenesis* 1992; 13:1389–1395.

70. Beebe LE, Anver MR, Riggs CW, Fornwald LW, Anderson LM. Promotion of *N*-nitrosodimethylamine-initiated mouse lung tumors following single or multiple low dose exposure to 2,3,7,8-tetrachlorodibenzo-*p*-dioxin. *Carcinogenesis* 1995; 16:1345–1349.

71. Poland A, Palen D, Glover E. Tumour promotion by TCDD in skin of HRS/J hairless mice. *Nature* 1982; 30:271–273.

72. Taper HS. The effect of estradiol-17-phenylpropionate and estradiol benzoate on *N*-nitrosomorpholine-induced liver carcinogenesis in ovariectomized female rats. *Cancer* 1978; 42:462–467.

73. Sumi C, Yokoro K, Kajitani T, Ito A. Synergism of diethylstilbestrol and other carcinogens in concurrent development of hepatic, mammary, and pituitary tumors in castrated male rats. *JNCI* 1980; 65:169–175.

74. Kemp CJ, Leary CN, Drinkwater NR. Promotion of murine hepatocarcinogenesis by testosterone is androgen receptor-dependent but not cell autonomous. *Proc Natl Acad Sci USA* 1989; 86:7505–7509.

75. Magnuson BA, Carr I, Bird RP. Ability of aberrant crypt foci characteristics to predict colonic tumor incidence in rats fed cholic acid. *Cancer Res* 1993; 53:4499–4504.

76. Reddy JK, Lalwani ND. Carcinogenesis by hepatic peroxisome proliferators: evaluation of the risk of hypolipidemmic drugs and industrial plasticizers to humans. *CRC Crit Rev Toxicol* 1983; 12:1–58.

77. Pitot HC. Endogenous carcinogenesis: the role of tumor promotion. *Proc Soc Exp Biol Med* 1991; 198:661–666.

78. Hikita H, Vaughan J, Pitot HC. The effect of two periods of short-term fasting during the promotion stage of hepatocarcinogenesis in rats: the role of apoptosis and cell proliferation. *Carcinogenesis* 1997; 18:159–166.

79. Andrews EJ. Evidence of the nonimmune regression of chemically induced papillomas in mouse skin. *JNCI* 1971; 47:653–665.

80. Schulte-Hermann R, Bursch W, Kraupp-Grasl B, et al. Cell proliferation and apoptosis in normal liver and preneoplastic foci. *Environ Health Perspect* 1993; 101:87–90.

81. Wright SC, Zhong J, Larrick JW. Inhibition of apoptosis as a mechanism of tumor promotion. *FASEB J* 1994; 8:654–660.

82. Tatematsu M, Nagamine Y, Farber E. Redifferentiation as a basis for remodeling of carcinogen-induced hepatocyte nodules to normal appearing liver. *Cancer Res* 1983; 43:5049–5058.

83. Hanigan MH, Pitot HC. Growth of carcinogen-altered rat hepatocytes in the liver of syngeneic recipients promoted with phenobarbital. *Cancer Res* 1985; 45:6063–6070.

84. Furth J. A meeting of ways in cancer research: thoughts on the evolution and nature of neoplasms. *Cancer Res* 1959; 19:241–256.

85. Van Duuren BL, Sivak A, Katz C, et al. The effect of aging and interval between primary and secondary treatment in two-stage carcinogenesis on mouse skin. *Cancer Res* 1975; 35:502–505.

86. Sivak A. Cocarcinogenesis. *Biochim Biophys Acta* 1979; 560:67–69.

87. Glauert HP, Schwarz M, Pitot HC. The phenotypic stability of altered hepatic foci: effect of the short-term withdrawal of phenobarbital and of the long-term feeding of purified diets after the withdrawal of phenobarbital. *Carcinogenesis* 1986; 7:117–121.

88. Cohen LA, Kendall ME. et al. Modulation of *N*-nitrosomethylurea-induced mammary tumor promotion by dietary fiber and fat. *JNCI* 1991; 83:496–501.

89. Carter JH, Carter HW, Meade J. Adrenal regulation of mammary tumorigenesis in female Sprague-Dawley rats: incidence, latency, and yield of mammary tumors. *Cancer Res* 1988; 48:3801–3807.

90. Taper HS. The effect of estradiol-17-phenylpropionate and estradiol benzoate on *N*-nitroso-morpholine-induced liver carcinogenesis in ovariectomized female rats. *Cancer* 1978; 42:462–467.

91. Sumi C, Yokoro K, Kajitani T, Ito A. Synergism of diethylstilbestrol and other carcinogens in concurrent development of hepatic, mammary, and pituitary tumors in castrated male rats. *JNCI* 1980; 65:169–175.

92. Kemp CJ, Leary CN, Drinkwater NR. Promotion of murine hepatocarcinogenesis by testosterone is androgen receptor-dependent but not cell autonomous. *Proc Natl Acad Sci USA* 1989; 86:7505–7509.

93. Ashendel CL. The phorbol ester receptor: a phospholipid-regulated protein kinase. *Biochim Biophys Acta* 1985; 822:219–242.

94. Verma AK, Boutwell RK. Effects of dose and duration of treatment with the tumor-promoting agent, 12-O-tetradecanoylphorbol-13-acetate on mouse skin carcinogenesis. *Carcinogenesis* 1980; 1:271–276.

95. Pitot HC. The role of receptors in multistage carcinogenesis. *Mutat Res* 1995; 333:3–14.

96. Dragan YP, Pitot HC. Multistage hepatocarcinogenesis in the rat: insights into risk estimation, in *Relevance of Animal Studies to the Evolution of Human Cancer Risk* (D'Amato R, Slaga T, Farland W, Henry C, eds). Wiley Liss, Inc., New York, 1992, pp 261–279.

97. Foulds L. Multiple etiologic factors in neoplastic development. *Cancer Res* 1965; 25:1339–1347.

98. Pitot HC. Progression: the terminal stage in carcinogenesis. *Jpn J Cancer Res* 1989; 80:599–607.

99. Welch DR, Tomasovic SP. Implications of tumor progression on clinical oncology. *Clin Exp Metastasis* 1985; 3:151–188.

100. Fornace AJ, Jr, Nagasawa H, Little JB. Relationship of DNA repair to chromosome aberrations, sister-chromatid exchanges and survival during liquid-holding recovery in X-irradiated mammalian cells. *Mutat Res* 1980; 70:323–336.

101. Cortés F, Piñero J, Ortiz T. Importance of replication fork progression for the induction of chromosome damage and SCE by inhibitors of DNA topoisomerases. *Mutat Res* 1993; 303:71–76.

102. Ottaggio L, Bonatti S, Cavalieri Z, Abbondandolo A. Chromosomes bearing amplified genes are a preferential target of chemicals inducing chromosome breakage and aneuploidy. *Mutat Res* 1993; 301:149–155.

103. Ledbetter DH. Minireview: cryptic translocations and telomere integrity. *Am J Hum Genet* 1992; 51:451–456.

104. Ames BN, Shigenaga MK, Gold LS. DNA lesions, inducible DNA repair, and cell division: three key factors in mutagenesis and carcinogenesis. *Environ Health Perspect* 1993; 93:35–44.

105. Kitagawa T, Sugano H. Timetable for hepatocarcinogenesis in rat, *in Analytical and Experimental Epidemiology of Cancer.* Proceedings of 3rd International Symposium of Princess Takamatsu Cancer Research Fund, 1973, pp 91–104.

106. Peraino C, Fry R, Staffeldt E. Enhancement of spontaneous hepatic tumorigenesis in C3H mice by dietary phenobarbital. *J Natl Cancer Inst* 1973; 51:1349–1350.

107. Hennings H, Spangler EF, Shores R, Mitchell P, Devor D, Shamsuddin AKM, et al. Malignant conversion and metastasis of mouse skin tumors: a comparison of SENCAR and CD-1 mice. *Environ Health Persp* 1986; 68:69–74.

108. Scherer E. Neoplastic progression in experimental hepatocarcinogenesis. *Biochim Biophys Acta* 1984; 738:219–236.

109. Dragan YP, Sargent L, Xu Y-D, Xu Y-H, Pitot HC. The initiation-promotion-progression model of rat hepatocarcinogenesis. *PSEBM* 1993; 202:16–24.

110. Pitot HC, Dragan YP. The instability of tumor promotion in relation to human cancer risk, in *Growth Factors and Tumor Promotion, Implications for Risk Assessment* (McClain RM, Slaga TJ, Leboeuf R, Pitot H, eds). Wiley-Liss, New York, 1995, pp 21–38.

111. Knudson AG. Genetics and the etiology of childhood cancer. *Pediatr Res* 1976; 10:513–517.

112. Armitage P, Doll R. The age distribution of cancer and a multi-stage theory of carcinogenesis. *Br J Cancer* 1954; 8:1–12.

113. Day NE, Brown CC. Multistage models and primary prevention of cancer. *J Natl Cancer Inst* 1980; 64:977–989.

114. Boice JD Jr, Day NE, Andersen A, et al. Second cancers following radiation treatment for cervical cancer. An international collaboration among cancer registries. *J Natl Cancer Inst* 1985; 74:955–975.

115. Kinlen LJ. Immunosuppressive therapy and cancer. *Cancer Surv* 1982; 1:565–583.

116. Berry CL. Temporal variations in carcinogenic effects. *Hum Toxicol* 1984; 3:3–6.

117. Henson DE, Albores-Saavedra J. (1986) *The Pathology of Incipient Neoplasia* WB, Saunders Company, Philadelphia, PA.

118. Anisimov VN. Carcinogenesis and aging. *Adv Cancer Res* 1983; 40:365–424.

119. Doll R, Peto R. (1981) *The Causes of Cancer.* Oxford University Press, Oxford, UK.

120. Murphree AL, Benedict WF. Retinoblastoma: clues to human oncogenesis. *Science* 1984; 223:1028–1033.

121. Kitamura K, Kuwano H, Yasuda M, Sonoda K, Sumiyoshi K, Tsutsui S-I, et al. What is the earliest malignant lesion in the esophagus? *Cancer Suppl* 1996; 77:1615–1619.

122. Hecker E, Lutz D, Weber J, Goerttler K, Morton JF. *Multistage Tumor Development in the Human Esophagus.* 13th International Cancer Congress, Part B, Biology of Cancer (1), Alan R. Liss, New York, 1983, pp 219–238.

123. Hu J, Nyrén O, Wolk A, Bergström R, Yuen J, Adami H-O, et al. Risk factors for oesophageal cancer in Northeast China. *Int J Cancer* 1994; 57:38–46.

124. Cheng KK, Duffy SW, Day NE, Lam TH, Chung SF, Badrinath P. Stopping drinking and risk of oesophageal cancer. *B Med J* 1995; 310:1094–1097.

125. Antonioli DA. Precursors of gastric carcinoma: a critical review with a brief description of early (curable) gastric cancer. *Hum Pathol* 1994; 25:994–1005.

126. Correa P, Haenszel W, Cuello C, Zavala D, Fontham E, Zarama G, et al. Gastric precancerous process in a high risk population: cross-sectional studies. *Cancer Res* 1990; 50:4731–4736.

127. Rugge M, Farinati F, Di Mario F, Baffa R, Valiante F, Cardin F. Gastric Epithelial Dysplasia: a prospective multicenter follow-up study from the interdisciplinary group on gastric epithelial dysplasia. *Hum Pathol* 1991; 22:1002–1008.

128. Inoue M, Tajima K, Hirose K, Kurioshi T, Gao C-M, Kitoh T. Life-style and subsite of gastric cancer–joint effect of smoking and drinking habits. *Int J Cancer* 1994; 56:494–499.

129. Potter JD. Reconciling the epidemiology, physiology, and molecular biology of colon cancer. *JAMA* 1992; 268:1573–1577.

130. Siu I-M, Pretlow TG, Amini SB, Pretlow TP. Identification of dysplasia in human colonic aberrant crypt foci. *Am J Pathol* 1997; 150:1805–1813.

131. Page DL, Dupont WD, Rogers LW. Ductal involvement by cells of atypical lobular hyperplasia in the breast: a long-term follow-up study of cancer risk. *Hum Pathol* 1988; 19:201–207.

132. Barrett-Connor E, Friedlander NJ. Dietary fat, calories, and the risk of breast cancer in postmenopausal women: a prospective population-based study. *J Am Coll Nutr* 1993; 12:390–399.

133. Hunter DJ, Willett WC. Diet, body build, and breast cancer. *Annu Rev Nutr* 1994; 14:393–418.

134. Longnecker MP, Newcomb PA, Mittendorf R, Greenberg ER, Clapp RW, Bogdan GF, et al. Risk of breast cancer in relation to lifetime alcohol consumption. *J Natl Cancer Inst* 1995; 87:923–929.

135. Nagamoto N, Saito Y, Sato M, Sagawa M, Kanma K, Takahashi S, et al. Lesions preceding squamous cell carcinoma of the bronchus and multicentricity of canceration–serial slicing of minute lung cancers smaller than 1 mm. *Tohoku J Exp Med* 1993; 170:11–23.

136. Zatonski W, Becher H, Lissowska J. Smoking cessation: intermediate nonsmoking periods and reduction of laryngeal cancer risk. *J Natl Cancer Inst* 1990; 82:1427–1428.

137. Samut JM. Health benefits of smoking cessation. *Clin Chest Med* 1991; 12:669–678.

138. Reif AE. Effect of cigarette smoking on susceptibility to lung cancer. *Oncology* 1981; 38:76–85.

139. Sakamoto M, Hirohashi S, Shimosato Y. Early stages of multistep hepatocarcinogenesis: adenomatous hyperplasia and early hepatocellular carcinoma. *Hum Pathol* 1991; 22:172–178.

140. Borzio M, Bruno S, Roncalli M, Mels GC, Ramella G, Borzio F, et al. Liver cell dysplasia is a major risk factor for hepatocellular carcinoma in cirrhosis: a prospective study. *Gastroenterology* 1995; 108:812–817.

141. Longnecker MP, Enger SM. *Clin Chim Acta* 1996; 246:121–141.

142. Edmondson HA, Reynolds TB, Henderson B, Benton B. Regression of liver cell adenomas associated with oral contraceptives. *Ann Intern Med* 1977; 86:180–182.

143. Amin MB, Young RH. Intraepithelial lesions of the urinary bladder with a discussion of the histogenesis of urothelial neoplasia. *Sem Diag Pathol* 1997; 14:84–97.

144. Silverman DT, Hartge P, Morrison AS, Devesa SS. Epidemiology of bladder cancer. *Bladder Cancer* 1992; 6:1–30.

145. Gambrell RD Jr. Pathophysiology and epidemiology of endometrial cancer, in *Treatment of the Postmenopausal Woman: Basic and Clinical Aspects* (Lobo RA, ed). Raven Press, NY, 1994, pp 355–362.

146. Ebeling K, Nischan P, Schindler C. Use of oral contraceptives and risk of invasive cervical cancer in previously screened women. *Int J Cancer* 1987; 39:427–430.

147. Gitsch G, Kainz C, Studnicka M, Reinthaller A, Tatra G, Breitenecker G. Oral contraceptives and human papillomavirus infection in cervical intraepithelial neoplasia. *Arch Gynecol Obstet* 1992; 252:25–30.

148. Pontén J, Adami H-O, Bergström R, Dillner J, Friberg L-G, Gustafsson L, et al. Strategies for global control of cervical cancer. *Intl J Cancer* 1995; 60:1–26.

149. Murthy NS, Sehgal A, Satyanarayana L, Das DK, Singh V, Das BC, et al. Risk factors related to biological behaviour of precancerous lesions of the uterine cervix. *Br J Cancer* 61:732–736.

150. Jones EC, Young RH. The differential diagnosis of prostatic carcinoma, its distinction from premalignant and pseudocarcinomatous lesions of the prostate gland. *Am J Clin Pathol* 1994; 101:48–64.

151. Nomura AMY, Kolonel LN. Prostate cancer: a current perspective. *Am J Epidemiol* 1991; 13:200–227.

152. Gann PH, Hennekens CH, Ma J, Longcope C, Stampfer MJ. Prospective study of sex hormone levels and risk of prostate cancer. *J Natl Cancer Inst* 1996; 88:1118–1126.

153. Beatson GT. On the treatment of inoperable cases of carcinoma of the mamma: suggestions for a new method of treatment with the illustrative cases. *Lancet* 1896; 2:104–107.

154. Allen E, Doisy E. An ovarian hormone: preliminary report on its localization, extraction, and partial purification and action in test animals. *J Am Med Assoc* 1923; 81:819–821.

155. Jensen E, Jacobson H. Basic guides to the mechanism of estrogen action. *Recent Prog Horm Res* 1962; 18:387–414.

156. Jensen E, Block G, Smith S, et al. Estrogen receptors and breast cancer response to adrenalectomy. *Monogr Natl Cancer Inst* 1971; 34:55–70.

157. Furr B, Jordan VC. The pharmacology and clinical uses of tamoxifen. *Pharmacol Ther* 1984; 25:127–205.
158. Cook JW, Dodds EC, Hewett CL. A synthetic oestrus-exciting compound. *Nature (London)* 1933; 131:56.
159. Dodds EC, Lawson W. Synthetic oestrogenic agents without the phenanthrene nucleus. *Nature (London)* 1936; 139:627.
160. Dodds EC, Golberg L, Lawson W, Robinson R. Oestrogenic activity of certain synthetic compounds. *Nature (London)* 1938a; 141:247–248.
161. Robson JM, Schonberg A. Oestrous reactions including mating produced by triphenylethylene. *Nature (London)* 1937; 140:196.
162. Robson JM, Schonberg A, Fahim HA. Duration of action of natural and synthetic estrogens. *Nature (London)* 1938; 142:292–293.
163. Lerner LJ, Holthaus JF, Thompson CR. A non-steroidal estrogen antagonist 1-(p-2-diethylaminoethoxyphenyl)-1-phenyl-2-p-methoxyphenylethanol. *Endocrinology* 1958; 63:295–318.
164. Chang M. Degeneration of the ova in the rat and rabbit following oral administration of 1-(p-2-diethylaminoethoxyphenyl)-1-phenyl-2-p-anisyl-ethanol. *Endocrinology* 1959; 65:339–342.
165. Kistner R, Smith O. Observations on the use of a nonsteroidal estrogen antagonist, MER 25. *Fertil Steril* 1961; 12:121–141.
166. Lerner LJ, Jordan VC. Development of antiestrogens and their use in breast cancer: Eighth Cain Memorial Award Lecture. *Cancer Res* 1990; 50:4177–4189.
167. Jordan VC, Collins MM, Rowsby L, Prestwich G. A monohydroxylated metabolite of tamoxifen with potent antiestrogenic activity. *J Endocrinol* 1977; 75:305–316.
168. Allen KE, Clark ER, Jordan VC. Evidence for the metabolic activation of non-steroidal antiestrogens: a study of structure-activity relationships. *Brit J Pharmacol* 1980; 71:83–91.
169. Lieberman ME, Jordan VC, Fritsch M, Santos MA, Gorski J. Direct and reversible inhibition of estradiol-stimulated prolactin synthesis by antiestrogens in vitro. *J Biol Chem* 1983b; 258:4734–4740.
170. Harper M, Walpole A. Contrasting endocrine activities of cis and trans isomers in a series of substituted triphenylethylenes. *Nature* 1966; 212:87.
171. Harper M, Walpole A. A new derivative of triphenylethylene: effect on implantation and mode of action in rats. *J Reprod Fertil* 1967; 13:101–119.
172. Jordan VC. Biochemical pharmacology of antiestrogen action. *Pharmacol Rev* 1984; 36:245–276.
173. Black LJ, Jones CD, Falcone JF. Antagonism of estrogen action with a new benzothiophene-derived antiestrogen. *Life Sci* 1983; 32:1031–1036.
174. Tonetti DA, Jordan VC. Targeted antiestrogens. *Prog Clin Biol Res* 1997; 396:245–255.
175. Fahey S, Jordan VC, Fritz N, Robinson S, Waters D, Tormey D. Clinical pharmacology and endocrinology of long-term tamoxifen therapy. In: *Long term treatment for breast cancer,* (Jordan VC, ed.), The University of Wisconsin Press, Madison, WI, 1994, pp 27–56.
176. Mani C, Gelboin HV, Park SS, et al. Metabolism of the antimammary cancer antiestrogen agent tamoxifen. I. Cytochrome P-450-catalyzed N-demethylation and 4-hydroxylation. *Drug Metab Dispos* 21:645–656.
177. Lim CK, Yuan Z-X, Lamb JH, et al. A comparative study of tamoxifen metabolism in female rat, mouse and human liver microsomes. *Carcinogenesis* 1994; 15:589–593.
178. Poon GK, Walter B, Lonning PE, et al. Identification of tamoxifen metabolites in human HEP G2 cell line, human liver homogenate, and patients on long-term therapy for breast cancer. *Drug Metab Dispos* 1995; 23:377–382.
179. Tannenbaum S. Comparative metabolism of tamoxifen and DNA adduct formation and in vitro studies on genotoxicity. *Seminars Oncol* 1997; 24:s81–s86.

180. Ruenitz PC, Toledo MM. Inhibition of rabbit liver microsomal oxidative metabolism and substrate binding by tamoxifen and the geometric isomers of clomiphene: *Biochem Pharmacol* 1980; 29:1583–1587.
181. Meltzer NM, Stang P, Sternson LA, Wade A. Influence of tamoxifen and its N-desmethyl and 4-hydroxy metabolites on rat liver microsomal enzymes. *Biochem Pharmacol* 1984; 33:115–123.
182. Ruenitz PC, Bagley JR, Pape CW. Some chemical and biochemical aspects of liver microsomal metabolism of tamoxifen. *Drug Metab Dispos* 1984; 12:478–483.
183. Ruenitz PC, Bagley JR. Comparative fates of clomiphene and tamoxifen in the immature female rat. *Drug Metab Dispos* 1985; 13:582–586.
184. Jacolot F, Simon I, Dreano Y, Beaune P, Riche C, Berthou F. Identification of the cytochrome p450 IIIa family as the enzymes involved in the N-demethylation of tamoxifen in human liver microsomes. *Biochem Pharmacol* 1991; 41:1911–1919.
185. Mani C, Pearce R, Parkinson A, Kupfer D. Involvement of cytochrome P4503A in catalysis of tamoxifen activation and covalent binding to rat and human liver microsomes. *Carcinogenesis* 1994; 15:2715–2720.
186. Mani C, Hodgson E, Kupfer D. Metabolism of the antimammary cancer antiestrogenic agent tamoxifen. II. Flavin-containing monooxygenase-mediated N-oxidation. *Drug Metab Dispos* 1993; 21:657–661.
187. Pathak D, Pangracz K, Bodell W. Activation of 4-hydroxy tamoxifen and the tamoxifen derivative Metabolite E by uterine peroxidases to form DNA adducts: comparison with DNA adducts formed in the uterus of Sprague-Dawley rats treated with tamoxifen. *Carcinogenesis* 1996; 17:1785–1790.
188. Adam HK, Douglas EJ, Kemp JV. The metabolism of tamoxifen in humans. *Biochem Pharmacol* 1979; 27:145–147.
189. Fromson JM, Pearson S, Bramah S. The metabolism of tamoxifen (ICI 46,474) Part I in laboratory animals. *Xenobiotica* 1973; 3:693–709.
190. Foster AB, Griggs LJ, Jarman M, van Maanen JMS, Schulten H-R. Metabolism of tamoxifen by rat liver microsomes: formation of the N-oxide, a new metabolite. *Biochem Pharmacol* 1980; 29:1977–1979.
191. Bates DJ, Foster AB, Griggs LJ, Jarman M, Leclercq G, Devleeschouwer N. Metabolism of tamoxifen by isolated rat hepatocytes: antiestrogenic activity of tamoxifen N-oxide. *Biochem Pharmacol* 1982; 31:2823–2827.
192. Bain RR, Jordan VC. Identification of a new metabolite of tamoxifen in patient serum during breast cancer therapy. *Biochem Pharmacol* 1983; 32:373–375.
193. Jordan VC, Bain RR, Brown RR, Gosden B, Santos MA. Determination and pharmacology of a new hydroxylated metabolite of tamoxifen observed in patient sera during therapy for advanced breast cancer. *Cancer Res* 1983; 43:1446–1450.
194. Kemp JV, Adam HK, Wakeling AE, Slater R. Identification and biological activity of tamoxifen metabolites in human serum. *Biochem Pharmacol* 1983; 32:2045–2052.
195. Lien EA, Solheim E, Ueland PM. Distribution of tamoxifen and its metabolites in rat and human tissues during steady-state treatment. *Cancer Res* 1991; 51:4837–4844.
196. Parr IB, McCague R, Leclercq G, Stoessel S. Metabolism of tamoxifen by isolated rat hepatocytes. *Biochem Pharmacol* 1987; 36:1513–1519.
197. Poon GK, Chui YC, McCague R. Analysis of phase I and phase II metabolites of tamoxifen in breast cancer patients. *Drug Metab Dispos* 1993; 21:1119–1124.
198. Poon G, Walter B, Lonning P, et al. Identification of tamoxifen metabolites in human HEPG2 cell line, human liver homogenates, and patients on long-term therapy for breast cancer. *Drug Metab Dispos* 1995; 23:377–382.
199. Wiseman H, Lewis DFV. The metabolism of tamoxifen by human cytochromes P450 is rationalized by molecular modelling of the enzyme-substrate interactions: potential importance to its proposed anti-carcinogenic/carcinogenic actions. *Carcinogenesis* 1996; 17:1357–1360.

200. Mani C, Kupfer D. Cytochrome P450 mediated activation and irreversible binding of the antiestrogen tamoxifen to proteins in rat and human liver; possible involvement of flavin-containing monooxygenases in tamoxifen activation. *Cancer Res* 1991; 51:6052–6058.
201. Dehal SS, Kupfer D. Evidence that the catechol 3,4-dihydroxy-tamoxifen is a proximate intermediate to the reactive species binding covalently to proteins. *Cancer Res* 1995; 56:1283–1290.
202. White INH, de Matteis F, Gibbs AH, Lim CK, Wolf CR, Henderson C, Smith LL. Species differences in the covalent binding of [^{14}C]tamoxifen to liver microsomes and the forms of cytochrome P450 involved. *Biochem Pharmacol* 1995; 49:1035–1042.
203. Han X, Liehr JG. Induction of covalent DNA adducts in rodents by tamoxifen. *Cancer Res* 1992; 52:1360–1363.
204. Hard G, Iatropoulos M, Jordan K, Radi L, Kaltenberg O, Imondi A, Williams G. Major differences in the hepatocarcinogenicity and DNA adduct forming ability between toremifene and tamoxifen in female CrL:CD(BR) rats. *Cancer Res* 1993; 53:4334–4341.
205. White INH, de Matteis F, Davies A, Smith LL, Crofton-Sleigh C, Venitt S, et al. Genotoxic potential of tamoxifen and analogues in female Fischer F244/n rats, DBA/2 and C57BL/6 mice and human MCL-5 cells. *Carcinogenesis* 1992; 13:2197–2203.
206. Pathak DN, Bodell WJ. DNA adduct formation by tamoxifen with rat and human liver microsomal activation systems. *Carcinogenesis* 1994; 15:529–532.
207. Randerath K, Moorthy B, Mabon N, Sriram P. Tamoxifen: evidence by ^{32}P-postlabeling and use of metabolic inhibitors for two distinct pathways leading to mouse hepatic DNA adduct formation and identification of 4-hydroxytamoxifen as a proximate metabolite. *Carcinogenesis* 1994; 15:2087–2094.
208. Hemminki K, Widlak P, Hou S-M. DNA adducts caused by tamoxifen and toremifene in human microsomal system and lymphocytes in vitro. *Carcinogenesis* 1995; 16:1661–1664.
209. Li D, Dragan Y, Jordan VC, Wang M, Pitot HC. Effects of chronic administration of tamoxifen and toremifene on DNA adducts in rat liver, kidney, and uterus. *Cancer Res* 1997; 57:1438–1441.
210. Blankson EA, Ellis SW, Lennard MS, Tucker GT, Rogers K. The metabolism of tamoxifen by human liver microsomes is not mediated by cytochrome P450IID6. *Biochem. Pharmacol* 1991; 42:S209–S212.
211. Potter GA, McCague R, Jarman M. A mechanistic hypothesis for DNA adduct formation by tamoxifen following hepatic oxidative metabolism. *Carcinogenesis* 1994; 15:439–442.
212. Phillips DH, Potter GA, Horton MN, et al. Reduced genotoxicity of [D$_5$-ethyl]-tamoxifen implicates α-hydroxylation of the ethyl group as a major pathway of tamoxifen activation to a liver carcinogen. *Carcinogenesis* 1994; 15:1487–1492.
213. Phillips D, Carmichael P, Hewer A, Cole K, Poon G. α-Hydroxytamoxifen, a metabolite of tamoxifen with exceptionally high DNA-binding activity in rat hepatocytes. *Cancer Res* 1995; 54:5518–5522.
214. Moorthy B, Sriram P, Pathak DN, Bodell WJ, Randerath K. Tamoxifen metabolic activation: comparison of DNA adducts formed by microsomal and chemical activation of tamoxifen and 4-hydroxytamoxifen with DNA adducts formed in vivo. *Cancer Res* 1996; 56:53–57.
215. Marques MM, Beland FA. Identification of tamoxifen-DNA adducts formed by 4-hydroxy-tamoxifen quinone methide. *Carcinogenesis* 1997; 18:1949–1954.
216. Cunningham A, Klopman G, Rosenkranz H. A study of the structural basis of the carcinogenicity of tamoxifen, toremifene, and their metabolites. *Mutat Res* 1996; 349:85–94.
217. Anttila M, Valavaara R, Kivinen S, Mäenpää J. Pharmacokinetics of toremifene. *J Steroid Biochem* 1990; 36:249–252.
218. Sipilä H, Kangas L, Vuorilehto L, Kalapudas A, Eloranta M, Södervall M, et al. Metabolism of toremifene in the rat. *J Steroid Biochem* 1990; 36:211–215.

219. Kangas L. Introduction to toremifene. *Breast Cancer Res Treat* 1990; 16:S-3–S-7.
220. Kangas L. Biochemical and pharmacological effects of toremifene metabolites. *Cancer Chemother Pharm* 1990; 27:8–12.
221. Kohler PC, Hamm JT, Wiebe VJ, DeGregorio MW, Shemano I, Tormey DC. Phase I study of the tolerance and pharmacokinetics of toremifene in patients with cancer. *Breast Cancer Res Treat* 1990; 16:S-19–S-26.
222. Valavaara R, Pyrhönen S, Heikkinen M, Rissanen P, Blanco G, Thölix E, et al. Toremifene, a new antiestrogenic compound, for treatment of advanced breast cancer. Phase II study. *Eur J Cancer Clin Oncol* 1988; 24:785–790.
223. Wiebe VJ, Benz CC, Shemano I, Cadman TB, DeGregorio MW. Pharmacokinetics of toremifene and its metabolites in patients with advanced breast cancer. *Cancer Chemother Pharmacol* 1990; 25:247–251.
224. Watanabe N, Irie T, Koyama M. Liquid chromatographic-atmospheric pressure ionization mass spectrometric analysis of toremifene metabolites in human urine. *J Chromatogr* 1989; 497:169–180.
225. Robinson SP, Parker CJ, Jordan VC. Preclinical studies with toremifene as an antitumor agent. *Breast Cancer Res Treat* 1990; 16:S-9–S-17.
226. Eppenberger U, Wosikowski K, Küng W. Pharmacologic and biologic properties of droloxifene, a new antiestrogen. *Am J Clin Oncol* 1991; 14:S5–S14.
227. Löser R, Seibel K, Liehn HD, Staab H-J. Pharmacology and toxicology of the antiestrogen droloxifene. *Contr Oncol* 1986; 23:64–72.
228. Hasmann M, Rattel B, Löser R. Preclinical data for droloxifene. *Cancer Lett* 1994; 84:101–116.
229. Coombes RC, Haynes BP, Dowsett M, Quigley M, English J, Judson IR, et al. Idoxifene: report of a phase I study in patients with metastatic breast cancer. *Cancer Res* 1995; 55:1070–1074.
230. Haynes BP, Parr IB, Griggs LJ, Jarman M. Metabolism and pharmacokinetics of pyrrolidino-4-iodotamoxifen in the rat. *Breast Cancer Res Treat* 1991; 19:174.
231. Busch H. Adducts and tamoxifen. *Sem Oncol* 1997; 24:s98–s104.
232. Robinson SP, Langan-Fahey SM, Johnson DA, Jordan VC. Metabolites, pharmacodynamics, and pharmacokinetics of tamoxifen in rats and mice compared to the breast cancer patient. *Drug Metab Dispos* 1991; 19:36–43.
233. Phillips D, Carmichael P, Hewer A, et al. Activation of tamoxifen and its metabolite α-hydroxytamoxifen to DNA binding products: comparisons between human, rat, and mouse hepatocytes. *Carcinogenesis* 1996; 17:89–94.
234. Osborne M, Hewer A, Hardcastle I, Carmichael P, Philips D. Identification of the major tamoxifen-deoxyguanosine adduct formed in the liver DNA of rats treated with tamoxifen. *Cancer Res* 1996; 56:66–71.
235. Carthew P, Martin E, White I, de Matteis F, Edwards R, Dorman B, et al. Tamoxifen induces short-term cumulative DNA damage and liver tumors in rats: promotion by phenobarbital. *Cancer Res* 1995; 55:544–547.
236. Martin E, Rich K, White I, Woods K, Powles T, Smith LL. ^{32}P-postlabeled DNA adducts in liver obtained from women treated with tamoxifen. *Carcinogenesis* 1995; 16:1651–1654.
237. Davies A, Martin E, Jones R, Lim C, Smith L, White I. Peroxidase activation of tamoxifen and toremifene resulting in DNA damage and covalently bound protein adducts. *Carcinogenesis* 1995; 16:539–545.
238. White I, Martin E, Mauthe R, Vogel J, Turtletaub K, Smith LL. Comparisons of the binding of [^{14}C]radiolabeled tamoxifen or toremifene to rat DNA using accelerator mass spectrometry. *Chemico-Biol Interact* 1997; 106:149–160.
239. Hemminki K, Rajaniemi H, Lindahl B, Moberger B. Tamoxifen induced DNA adducts in endometrial samples from breast cancer patients. *Cancer Res* 1996; 56:4374–4377.

240. Vancutsem P, Lazarus P, Williams G. Frequent and specific mutations of the rat p53 gene in hepatocarcinomas induced by tamoxifen. *Cancer Res* 1994; 54:3864–3867.
241. Barakat R, O'Connor B, Banerjee D, Bertino J. Mutation of c-Ki-ras in tamoxifen associated endometrial carcinoma. *Proc. Am. Assoc. Cancer Res* 1995; 36:186(1106A).
242. Davies R, Oreffo V, Martin E, Festing M, White I, Smith LL, Styles JA. Tamoxifen causes gene mutations in the livers of lambda/lacI transgenic rats. *Cancer Res* 1997; 57:1288–1293.
243. Davies R, Oreffo V, Bayliss S, Dinh P, Lilley K, White I, et al. Mutational spectra of tamoxifen-induced mutations in the livers of lacI transgenic rats. *Environ Mol Mutag* 1996; 28:430–433.
244. Randerath K, Bi J, Mabon N, Sriram P, Moorthy B. Strong intensification of mouse hepatic tamoxifen adduct formation by pretreatment with sulfotransferase inhibitor and ubiquitous environmental pollutant pentachlorophenol. *Carcinogenesis* 1994; 15:797–800.
245. Dasaradhi L, Shibutani S. Identification of tamoxifen-DNA adducts formed by α-sulfate tamoxifen and α-acetoxytamoxifen. *Chem Res Toxicol* 1997; 10:189–196.
246. McCague R, Parr IB, Leclercq G, Leung O-T, and Jarman M. Metabolism of tamoxifen by isolated rat hepatocytes. Identification of the glucuronide of 4-hydroxytamoxifen. *Biochem Pharmacol* 1990; 39:1459–1465.
247. Hellriegel ET, Matwyshyn GA, Fei P, Dragnev KH, Nims RW, Lubet RA, Kong A-NT. Regulation of gene expression of various phase I and phase II drug-metabolizing enzymes by tamoxifen in rat liver. *Biochem Pharmacol* 1996; 52:1561–1568.
248. Nuwaysir EF, Daggett DA, Jordan VC, Pitot HC. Phase II enzyme expression in rat liver in response to the antiestrogen tamoxifen. *Cancer Res* 1996; 56:3704–3710.
249. Jarman M, Poon G, Rowlands M, Grimshaw R, Horton M, Potter G, McCague R. The deuterium isotope effect for the α-hydroxylation of tamoxifen by rat liver microsomes accounts for the reduced genotoxicity of [D$_5$-ethyl]-tamoxifen. *Carcinogenesis* 1995; 15:683–688.
250. Phillips D, Potter G, Horton M, Hewer A, Crofton-Sleigh C, Jarman M, Venitt S. Reduced genotoxicity of [D$_5$-ethyl]-tamoxifen implicates α-hydroxylation of the ethyl group as a major pathway of tamoxifen activation to a liver carcinogen. *Carcinogenesis* 1994; 15:1487–1492.
251. McCague R, Seago A. Aspects of tamoxifen metabolism by rat liver microsomes. *Biochem Pharmac* 1986; 35:827–834.
252. Styles J, Davies A, Lim C, DeMatteis F, Stanley L, White I, Yuan Z-X, Smith LL. Genotoxicity of tamoxifen, tamoxifen epoxide, and toremifene in human lymphoblastoid cells containing human cytochrome P450s. *Carcinogenesis* 1994; 15:5–9.
253. Pongracz K, Pathak D, Nakamura T, Burlingame A, Bodell W. Activation of tamoxifen derivative metabolite E to form DNA adducts: comparison with the adducts formed by microsomal activation of tamoxifen. *Cancer Res* 1995; 55:3012–3015.
254. Lim CK, Yuan Z, Jones R, White I, Smith LL. Identification and mechanism of formation of potentially genotoxic metabolites of tamoxifen: study by LC-MS/MS. *J Pharm Biomed Anal* 1997; 15:1335–1342.
255. Shibutani S, Dasaradhi L. Miscoding potential of tamoxifen-derived DNA adducts: α-(N^2-deoxyguanosinyl)tamoxifen. *Biochemistry* 1997; 36:13010–13017.
256. International Agency for Research on Cancer (IARC): Tamoxifen. *IARC Monographs* 1996; 66:274–365.
257. Tucker M, Adam H, Patterson J. Tamoxifen, in *Safety Testing of New Drugs* (Lawrence D, McLean A, Weatherall M, eds). Academic Press, Orlando, FL, 1984, pp 125–161.
258. Montandon F, Williams G. Comparison of DNA reactivity of the polyphenylethylene hormonal agents diethylstilbesterol, tamoxifen, and toremifene in rat and hamster liver. *Arch Toxicol* 1994; 68:272–275.
259. Hemminki K, Widlak P, Hou S-M. DNA adducts caused by tamoxifen and toremifene in human microsomal system and lymphocytes in vitro. *Carcinogenesis* 1995; 16:1661–1664.

260. Tsutsi T, Maizumi H, McLachlan J, Barrett JC. Aneuploidy induction and cell transformation by diethylstilbestrol: a possible chromosomal mechanism in carcinogenesis. *Cancer Res* 1983; 43:3814–3821.

261. Tsutsui T, Degen G, Schiffmann D, Wong A, Maizumi H, McLachlan J, Barrett JC. Dependence on exogenous metabolic activation for induction of unscheduled DNA synthesis in Syrian hamster embryo cells by diethylstilbesterol and related compounds. *Cancer Res* 1984; 44:184–189.

262. Tsutsui T, Suzuki N, Maizumi H, McLachlan J, Barrett JC. Alteration in diethylstilbesterol-induced mutagenicity and cell transformation by exogenous metabolic activation. *Carcinogenesis* 1986; 7:1415–1418.

263. Dragan Y, Xu YD, Pitot HC. Tumor promotion as a target for estrogen/antiestrogen effects in rat hepatocarcinogenesis. *Prev Med* 1991; 20:15–26.

264. Yager J, Roebuck B, Paluszcyk T, Memoli V. Effects of ethinyl estradiol and tamoxifen on liver DNA turnover and new synthesis and appearance of gamma glutamyl transpeptidase positive foci in female rats. *Carcinogenesis* 1986; 7:2007–2014.

265. Ghia M, Mereto E. Induction and promotion of γ-glutamyltranspeptidase-positive foci in the livers of female rats treated with ethinyl estradiol, clomiphene, tamoxifen and their associations. *Cancer Lett* 1989; 46:195–202.

266. Solt D, Farber E. New principle for the analysis of chemical carcinogenesis. *Nature* 1976; 263:701–703.

267. Williams G, Iatropoulos M, Karlsson S. Initiating activity of the anti-estrogen tamoxifen, but not toremifene in rat liver. *Carcinogenesis* 1997; 18:2247–2253.

268. Newberne J, Kuhn W. Elsea J. Toxicologic studies on clomiphene. *Toxic Appl Pharm* 1966; 9:44–56.

269. Gibson J, Newberne J, Kuhn W, Elsea J. Comparative chronic toxicity of three oral estrogens in rats. *Toxic Appl Pharm* 1967; 11:489–510.

270. Juedes MJ, Bulger WH, Kupfer D. Mono-oxygenase mediated activation of chlorotrianisene (TACE) in covalent binding to rat hepatic microsomal proteins. *Drug Metab Dispos* 1987; 15:786–793.

271. Hasmann M, Rattel B, Loser R. Preclinical data for droloxifene. *Cancer Lett* 1994; 84:101–116.

272. Loser R, Seibel K, Liehn H, Staub H-J. Pharmacology and toxicology of the antiestrogen droloxifene. *Contr Oncol* 1986; 23:64–72.

273. Dahme E, Rattel B. Droloxifene induces, in contrast to tamoxifen, no liver tumors in the rat. *Onkologie* 1994; 17(Suppl. 1):6–16.

274. Hirsimaki P, Hirsimaki Y, Nieminen L. The effects of tamoxifen citrate and toremifene citrate on the ultrastructure of the rat liver. *Inst Phys Conf Ser 93:* 1988; 3:235–236.

275. Hirsimaki P, Hirsimaki Y, Nieminen L, Payne BJ. Tamoxifen induces hepatocellular carcinoma in rat liver: a one year study with two antiestrogens. *Arch Toxicol* 1993; 67:49–54.

276. Ahotupa M, Hirsimaki P, Parssinen R, Mantyla E. Alterations of drug metabolizing and antioxidant enzyme activities during tamoxifen-induced hepatocarcinogenesis in the rat. *Carcinogenesis* 1994; 15:863–868.

277. Dragan Y, Vaughan J, Jordan VC, Pitot HC. Comparison of the effects of tamoxifen and toremifene on liver and kidney tumor promotion in female rats. *Carcinogenesis* 1995; 16:2733–2741.

278. Karlsson S, Hirsimaki Y, Mantyla E, Nieminen L, Kangas L, Hirsimaki P, et al. A two year dietary carcinogenicity study of the antiestrogen toremifene in Sprague-Dawley rats. *Drug Chem Toxicol* 1996; 19:245–266.

279. Watanabe M, Tanaka H, Koizumi H, Tanimoto Y, Torii R, Yanagita T. General toxicity studies of tamoxifen in mice and rats. *Jitchuken Zenrinsko Kenkyuko* 1980; 6:1–36.

280. Mishkin SY, Farber E, Ho RK, Mulay S, Mishkin S. Evidence for the hormone dependency of hepatic hyperplastic nodules: inhibition dependency of malignant transformation after endogenous β estradiol and tamoxifen. *Hepatology* 1983; 3:308–316.

281. Kohigashi K, Fukuda Y, Imura H. Inhibitory effect of tamoxifen on DES-promoted hepatic tumorigenesis in male rats and its possible mechanism of action. *Gann* 1988; 79:1335–1339.

282. Francavilla A, Polimeno L, DiLeo A, Barone M, Ove P, Coetzee M, et al. The effect of estrogen and tamoxifen on hepatocyte proliferation in vivo and in vitro. *Hepatology* 1989; 9:614–620.

283. Carthew P, Rich KJ, Martin EA, De Matteis F, Lim C-K, Manson MM, et al. DNA damage as assessed by ^{32}P-postlabeling in three rat strains exposed to dietary tamoxifen: the relationship between cell proliferation and liver tumor formation. *Carcinogenesis* 1995; 16:1299–1304.

284. Kim D, Han S, Ahn B, Lee K, Kang J, Tsuda H. Promotion potential of tamoxifen on hepatocarcinogenesis in female SD or F344 rats initiated with diethylnitrosamine. *Cancer Lett* 1996; 104:13–19.

285. Greaves P, Goonetilleke R, Nunn G, Topham J, Orton T. Two year carcinogenicity study of tamoxifen in Alderley Park Wistar-derived rats. *Cancer Res* 1993; 53:3919–3924.

286. Dragan YP, Fahey S, Street K, Vaughan J, Jordan VC, Pitot HC. Studies of tamoxifen as a promoter of hepatocarcinogenesis in female Fischer F344 rats. *Breast Cancer Res Treat* 1994; 31:11–25.

287. Dragan Y, Fahey S, Nuwaysir E, Sattler C, Babcock K, Vaughan J, et al. The effect of tamoxifen and two of its non-isomerizable fixed ring analogs on multistage rat hepatocarcinogenesis. *Carcinogenesis* 1996; 17:585–594.

288. Williams GM, Iatropoulos MJ, Djordjevic MV, Kaltenberg OP. The triphenylethylene drug tamoxifen is a strong liver carcinogen in the rat. *Carcinogenesis* 1993; 14:315–317.

289. Martin E, Carthew P, White I, Smith LL. A lifetime feeding study of tamoxifen in three strains of mice. The Toxicologist, *Fund Appl Toxiol* 1996; 30:A1026, pg. 201.

290. McLachlan J, Wong A, Degen G, Barrett J. Morphologic and neoplastic transformation of Syrian hamster embryo fibroblasts by diethylstilbesterol and its analogs. *Cancer Res* 1982; 42:3040–3045.

291. Metzler M, Schiffmann D. Structural requirements for the in vitro transformation of Syrian hamster embryo cells by stilbene estrogens and triphenylethylene-type antiestrogens. *Am J Clin Oncol* 1991; 14(Suppl 2):30–35.

292. Styles J, Davies A, Davies R, White I, Smith LL. Clastogenic and aneugenic effects of tamoxifen and some of its analogs in hepatocytes from dosed rats and in human lymphoblastoid cells transfected with human P450 cDNAs (MCL-5 cells). *Carcinogenesis* 1997; 18:303–313.

293. Oshimura M, Barrett JC. Chemically induced aneuploidy in mammalian cells: mechanisms and biological significance in cancer. *Environ Mutag* 1986; 8:129–159.

294. Hayashi N, Hasegawa K, Komine A, Tanaka Y, McLachlan JA, Barrett JC, Tsutsui T. Estrogen-induced cell transformation and DNA adduct formation in cultured Syrian hamster embryo cells. *Mol Carcinog* 1996; 16:149–156.

295. Sargent L, Dragan Y, Bahnub N, Sattler C, Sattler G, Jordan VC, Pitot HC. Tamoxifen induces hepatic aneuploidy and mitotic spindle disruptions after a single in vivo administration to female Sprague-Dawley rats. *Cancer Res* 1994; 54:3357–3360.

296. Sargent L, Dragan Y, Bahnub N, Sattler G, Martin P, Cisneros A, et al. Induction of hepatic aneuploidy in vivo by tamoxifen, toremifene, and idoxifene in female Sprague-Dawley rats. *Carcinogenesis* 1996; 17:1051–1056.

297. Aldaz C, Conti C, Klein-Szanto A, Slaga T. Progressive dysplasia and aneuploidy are hallmarks of mouse skin papillomas: relevance to malignancy. *Proc Natl Acad Sci USA* 1987; 84:2029–2032.

298. Liang J, Brinkley B. Chemical probes and possible targets for the induction of aneuploidy. *Basic Life Sci* 1985; 36:491–505.

299. Osborne C, Boldt D Estrada P. Human breast cancer cell cycle synchronization by estrogens and antiestrogens in culture. *Cancer Res* 1984; 44:1433–1439.

300. Bouhoute A, LeClercq G. Antagonistic effect of triphenylethylenic antiestrogens on the association of estrogen receptor to calmodulin. *Biochem Biophys Res Comm* 1992; 184:1432–1440.

301. Edwards K, Laughton C, Neidle S. A molecular modeling study of the interactions between the antiestrogen drug tamoxifen and several derivatives, and the calcium-binding protein calmodulin. *J Med Chem* 1992; 35:2753–2761.

302. Rowland M, Parr I, McCague R, Jarman M, Goddard P. Variation of the inhibition of calmodulin dependent cyclic AMP phosphodiesterase among analogs of tamoxifen: correlation with cytotoxicity. *Biochem Pharmacol* 1990; 40:283–289.

303. Hardcastle I, Rowlands M, Houghton J, Parr I, Potter G, Jarman M. Rationally designed analogues of tamoxifen with improved calmodulin antagonism. *J Med Chem* 1995; 38:241–248.

304. Musgrove E, Wakeling A, Sutherland R. Points of action of estrogen antagonists and a calmodulin antagonist within the MCF-7 human breast cancer cell cycle. *Cancer Res* 1989; 49:2398–2404.

305. Lam H. Tamoxifen is a calmodulin antagonist in the activation of cAMP-phosphodiesterase. *Biochem Biophys Res Commun* 1984; 118:27–32.

306. Castoria G, Migliaccio A, Nola E, Aurichio F. In vitro interaction of estradiol receptor with Ca^{+2}-calmodulin. *Mol Endocrinol* 1988; 2:167–174.

307. Auricchio F, Migliaccio A, DiDomenico M, Nola E. Estradiol stimulates tyrosine phosphorylation and hormone binding activity of its own receptor in a cell free system. *EMBO J* 1987; 6:2923–2929.

308. Watts C, Sweeney K, Warlters A, Musgrove E, Sutherland R. Antiestrogen regulation of cell cycle progression and cyclin D1 gene expression in MCF-7 human breast cancer cells. *Breast Cancer Res Treat* 1994; 31:95–105.

309. Watts C, Brady A, Sarcevic B, deFaxio A, Musgrove E, Sutherland R. Antiestrogen inhibition of cell cycle progression in breast cancer cells is associated with inhibition of cyclin-dependent kinase activity and decreased retinoblastoma protein phosphorylation. *Mol Endocrinol* 1995; 9:1804–1813.

310. Musgrove E, Hamilton J, Lee C, Sweeney K, Watts C, Sutherland R. Growth factor, steroid, steroid antagonist regulation of cyclin gene expression associated with changes in T-47D human breast cancer cell cycle progression. *Mol Cell Biol* 1993; 13:3577–3587.

311. Pitot HC, Campbell HA. An approach to the determination of the relative potencies of chemical agents during the stages of initiation and promotion in multistage hepatocarcinogenesis in the rat. *Environ Health Persp* 1987; 76:49–56.

312. Pitot HC. Principles of carcinogenesis: chemical, in *Cancer—Principles and Practice of Oncology,* vol. 1, 3rd ed. (DeVita VT, Hellman S, Rosenberg S, eds). J.B. Lippincott Co., Philadelphia, 1989, pp 116–135.

313. Jordan VC. Tamoxifen: toxicities and drug resistance during the treatment and prevention of breast cancer. *Annu Rev Pharmacol Toxicol* 1995; 35:195–211.

314. Tanaka Y, Seiguchi M, Sawamoto T, Hata T, Esumi Y, Sugai S, Ninomiya S. Pharmacokinetics of droloxifene in mice, rats, monkeys, premenopausal and postmenopausal patients. *Eur J Drug Metab Pharmacokinet* 1994; 19:47–58.

315. Pyrhonen S. Phase 3 studies of toremifene in metastatic breast cancer. *Breast Cancer Res Treat* 1990; 16(Suppl):s31–s35.

316. Kallio S, Kangas L, Blanco G, Johansson R, Karalainen A, Perila M, et al. A New triphenylethylene compound Fc-1157a. I. Hormonal effects. *Cancer Chemother Pharmacol* 1986; 17:103–108.

317. McCague R, LeClerq G, Legros N, Goodman J, Blackburn G, Jarman M Foster A. Derivatives of tamoxifen: dependence of antiestrogenicity on the 4-substituent. *J Med Chem* 1989; 32:2527–2533.

318. McCague R, Parr I, Haynes B. Metabolism of the 4-iodo derivative of tamoxifen by isolated rat hepatocytes. *Biochem Pharmacol* 1990; 40:2277–2283.

319. Coombes RC, Haynes B, Dowsxett M, Quigley M, English J, Judson I, et al. Idoxifene: report of a phase I study in patients with metastatic breast cancer. *Cancer Res* 1995; 55:1070–1074.

320. Black L, Jones C, Falcone J. Antagonism of estrogen action with a new benzothiophene-derived antiestrogen. *Life Sci* 1983; 32:1031–1036.

321. Black L, Sato M, Rowley E, Magee D, Bekele A, Williams D, et al. Raloxifene (LY 139481 HCl) prevents bone loss and reduces serum cholesterol without causing uterine hypertrophy in ovariectomized rats. *J Clin Invest* 1994; 93:63–69.

322. Jordan VC, Allen KE, Dix CJ. Pharmacology of tamoxifen in laboratory animals. *Cancer Treat Rep* 1980; 64:745–759.

323. Furr BJA, Jordan VC. The pharmacology and clinical uses of tamoxifen. *Ther Pharm* 1984; 25:127–205.

324. Jordan VC. Long-term adjuvant tamoxifen therapy for breast cancer. *Breast Cancer Res Treat* 1990; 15:125–136.

325. Love R, Weibe D, Newcombe P, Cameron L, Leventhal H, Jordan V, et al. Effects of tamoxifen on cardiovascular risk factors in postmenopausal women with breast cancer. *New Engl J Med* 1992; 326:852–856.

326. Love R, Mazess R, Barden H, Epstein S, Newcomb P, Jordan VC, et al. Effects of tamoxifen on bone mineral density in postmenopausal women with breast cancer. *N Engl J Med* 1992; 326:852–856.

327. Ward RL, Morgan G, Dalley D, Kelley PJ. Tamoxifen reduces bone turnover and prevents lumbar spine and proximal femoral bone loss in early postmenopausal women. *Bone Mineral* 1993; 22:87–94.

328. Gottardis M, Robinson S, Satyaswaroop P, Jordan VC. Contrasting actions of tamoxifen on endometrial and breast tumor growth in the athymic nude mouse. *Cancer Res* 1988; 48:812–815.

329. Jordan VC, Gottardis M, Satyaswaroop P. Tamoxifen-stimulated growth of human endometrial carcinoma. *Ann NY Acad Sci* 1991; 622:439–446.

330. Gottardis M, Ricchio M, Satyaswaroop P. Effect of steroidal and non-steroidal antiestrogens on the growth of a tamoxifen-stimulated human endometrial carcinoma (EnCa101) in athymic mice. *Cancer Res* 1990; 50:3189–3192.

331. Kuiper GG, Gustafsson JA. The novel estrogen receptor-beta subtype: potential role in the cell- and promoter-specific actions of estrogens and anti-estrogens. *FEBS Lett* 1997; 410:87–90.

332. Tremblay GB, Tremblay A, Copeland NG, Gilbert DJ, Jenkins NA, Labrie F, Giguere V. Cloning, chromosomal localization, and functional analysis of the murine estrogen receptor beta. *Mol Endocrinol* 1997; 11:353–365.

333. Mosselman S, Polman J, Dijkema R. ER beta: identification and characterization of a novel human estrogen receptor. *FEBS Lett* 1996; 392:49–53.

334. Carthew P, Edwards RE, Nolan BM. Depletion of hepatocyte nuclear estrogen receptor expression is associated with promotion of tamoxifen induced GST-P foci to tumours in rat liver. *Carcinogenesis* 1997; 18:1109–1112.

335. Paech K, Webb P, Kuiper GG, Nilsson S, Gustafsson J, Kushner PJ, Scanlan TS. Differential ligand activation of estrogen receptors ERα and ERβ at API sites. *Science* 1997; 277:1508–1510.

336. Aaronson SA, Miki T, Meyers K, Chan A. Growth factors and malignant transformation. *Adv Exp Med Biol* 1993; 348:7–22.

337. Ignar-Trowbridge D, Nelson K, Bidwell M, Curtis S, Washburn T, McLachlan J, Korach K. Coupling of dual signaling pathways: epidermal growth factor action involves the estrogen receptor. *Proc Natl Acad Sci USA* 1992; 89:4658–4662.

338. Ignar-Trowbridge D, Teng C, Ross K, Parker M, Korach K, McLachlan J. Peptide growth factors elicit estrogen receptor dependent transcriptional activation of an estrogen-responsive element. *Mol Endocrinol* 1993; 7:992–998.

339. Ignar-Trowbridge D, Pimentel M, Parker M, McLachlan J, Korach K. Peptide growth factor cross-talk with the estrogen receptor requires the A/B domain and occurs independently of protein kinase C or estradiol. *Endocrinology* 1996; 137:1735–1744.

340. Newton C, Buric R, Trapp T, Brockmeier S, Pagotto V, Stella G. The unliganded estrogen receptor (ER) transduces growth factor signals. *J Steroid Biochem* 1994; 48:481–486.

341. Phillips A, Chalbos D, Rochefort H. Estradiol increases and antiestrogens antagonize the growth factor induced activator protein 1 activity in MCF7 breast cancer cells without affecting c-fos and c-jun synthesis. *J Biol Chem* 1993; 268:14103–14108.

342. Sukovich DA, Mukherjee R, Benfield PA. A novel cell-specific mechanism for estrogen receptor mediated gene activation. In the absence of an estrogen-responsive element. *Mol Cell Biol* 1994; 14:7134–7143.

343. Umayahara Y, Kawamori R, Watada H, Iwama E, Morishima T, Yamasaki Y, et al. Estrogen regulation of the insulin-like growth factor 1 gene transcription involves an AP-1 enhancer. *J Biol Chem* 1994; 269:16433–16442.

344. Saeki T, Cristano A, Lynch M, Brattain M, Kim N, Normanno N, et al. Regulation by estrogen through the 5′-flanking region of the transforming growth factor α gene. *Mol Endocrinol* 1991; 5:1955–1963.

345. Webb P, Lopez GN, Uht RM, Kusher PJ. Tamoxifen activation of the estrogen receptor/AP-1 pathway: potential origin for the cell-specific estrogen-like effects of antiestrogens. *Mol Endocrinol* 1995; 9:443–456.

346. Gaub MP, Bellard M, Scheuer I, Chambon P, Sassone-Corsi P. Activation of the ovalbumin gen by the estrogen receptor involves the fos-jun complex. *Cell* 1990; 63:1267–1276.

347. Krishnan V, Wang X, Safe S. Estrogen receptor Sp1 complexes mediate estrogen-induced cathepsin D gene expression in MCF7 human breast cancer cells. *J Biol Chem* 1994; 269:15912–15917.

348. Moulton B. Transforming growth factor-beta stimulates endometrial stromal apoptosis in vitro. *Endocrinology* 1994; 134:1055–1060.

349. Butta A, MacLennan K, Flanders K, Sacks N, Smith I, McKinna A, et al. Induction of transforming growth factor beta in human breast cancer in vivo following tamoxifen treatment. *Cancer Res* 1992; 52:4261–4262.

350. Bentzen S, Skocylas J, Overgaard M, Overgaard J. Radiotherapy-related lung fibrosis enhanced by tamoxifen. *J Natl Cancer Inst* 1996; 88:918–922.

351. Colletta A, Wakefiels L, Howell F, Roozendaal K, Danielpour D, Ebbs S, et al. Anti-estrogens induce the secretion of active transforming growth factor beta from human fetal fibroblasts. *Br J Cancer* 1990; 62:405–409.

6 Preclinical Studies of Raloxifene and Related Compounds

Robin Fuchs-Young

1. HISTORICAL PERSPECTIVE

The development of raloxifene (also know as keoxifene) for clinical use was based on a series of preclinical studies that demonstrated it has a highly desirable tissue-specific activity. Results indicated that the therapeutic effects of raloxifene (LY138481 HCl; LY156758) mimicked some of those of estrogen in ovariectomized animals by reducing bone loss and lowering serum cholesterol levels. Conversely, in mammary and uterine tissue, raloxifene acted as an antiestrogen and inhibited estrogen stimulation without inherent agonist activity (Fig. 1). Raloxifene was originally synthesized by Jones, who was looking for an antiestrogen with strong receptor binding *(1)*. Jones hoped to produce a structure that would combine some features of the estradiol molecule with novel modifications to affect a potent estrogen receptor (ER) antagonist. The product of his efforts, as shown in Fig. 2, was a nonsteroidal benzothiophene derivative with two phenolic hydroxyls, a large basic side chain, and a unique carboxy hinge connecting the side chain to the olefin *(1–3)*. Recent evidence

From: *Hormone Therapy in Breast and Prostate Cancer*
Edited by: V. C. Jordan and B. J. A. Furr © Humana Press Inc., Totowa, NJ

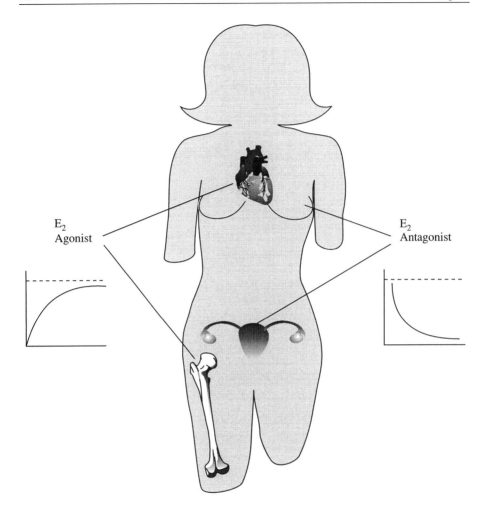

Fig. 1. Tissue specific effects of raloxifene suggest many potential therapeutic applications. This SERM acts as an estrogen agonist on bone and the cardiovascular system but is anti-estrogenic in the uterus and breast.

indicates that the dialkyl amine sidechain is critical for in vivo estrogen antagonism and that the spatial orientation of the side chain and the carbonyl hinge may account for tissue-specific effects, specifically the lack of uterine stimulation *(2,3)*. It is likely that Jones and his colleagues at Eli Lilly and Co. (Indianapolis, IN) have opened a new chapter in medicinal chemistry and that we will see the development of tissue-specific antiestrogens for a number of hormonally dependent disorders ranging from breast and endometrial cancer to uterine leiomyoma and, possibly, Alzheimer's disease (AD).

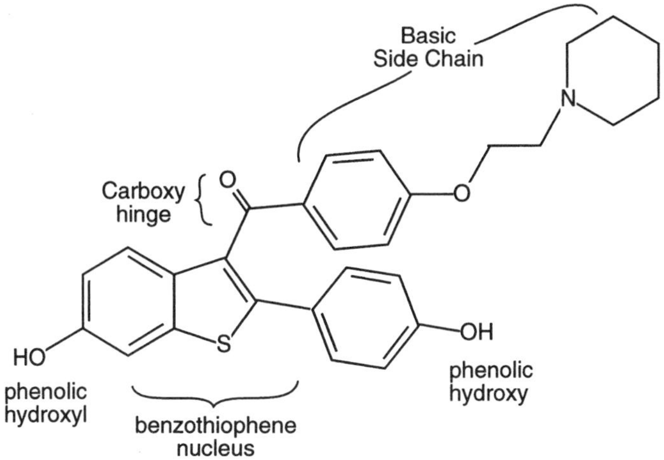

Fig. 2. Raloxifene, formally called keoxifene, is a benzothiophene with two phenolic hydroxyl residues and a large basic sidechain attached to the nucleus through a carboxy hinge. These unique structural aspects mediate the tissue-specific activity. Adapted from ref. *(3)*.

A variety of acronyms have been used to describe compounds like raloxifene that have tissue-specific activity, including SERM (selective estrogen-receptor modulator) and TERM (tissue-specific estrogen-receptor modulator). Generally, SERMs and TERMs are compounds that, like raloxifene, bind to the ER with high affinity (≤ nM) and induce an appropriate receptor conformation that promotes transcriptional regulation of target genes. It has been proposed that a series of distinct receptor conformations may be induced by different SERMs, accounting in part for the spectrum of tissue-specific effects *(4)*. Studies have shown the ability of raloxifene-activated ERs to bind to a unique response element in target-gene promoters, which may mediate the distinctive biological activity *(5)*. During most of the initial studies of raloxifene, the β form of the ER (ERβ) had not been identified. Recent data suggest that raloxifene and tamoxifen, as well as the pure antiestrogen ICI 164,384, bind to ERβ and stimulate transcriptional activation at AP-1 sites, suggesting that tissue-specific activity of some ER ligands may involve this new member of the steroid-receptor superfamily *(6,7)*. However, there is no evidence that raloxifene binds appreciably to other steroid hormone receptors such as those for progesterone or androgen.

2. RALOXIFENE ACTION IN BONE

2.1. Raloxifene In Vitro

The detection of ERs in bone cells, specifically, osteoblasts (which form bone) and osteoclasts (which resolve bone), suggested the possibility that high-affinity ligands act directly on these cells *(8,9)*. Although there were far fewer receptors in these cells than in traditional estrogen-target tissues, measurable effects, such as induction of cellular proliferation and progesterone receptor transcription, indicated that sufficient receptors were present to mediate specific receptor-based cellular responses. Several continuous cell lines have been used in in vitro analyses to predict and analyze the effects of raloxifene in bone. Raloxifene has been shown to act similarly to tamoxifen and 17-β-estradiol in stimulating the upregulation of creatinine kinase expression in cultures of bone cells and tissues. In ROS 17/2.8 rat osteogenic sarcoma cells, female calvaria, and $SaOS_2$ human osteoblast-like cells, nanomolar concentrations of raloxifene increased expression of the marker significantly as compared with no treatment or treatment with ICI 164,384 *(10)*. Both raloxifene and tamoxifen stimulated increases in creatine kinase when added to cultures by themselves, but inhibited E2-stimulated increases when added in combination *(10)*, suggesting the effects of these SERMs are partially agonistic. Further evidence of the estrogenic effects of raloxifene on bone cells or their precursors was reported by Fiorelli et al. *(11)*, who showed that raloxifene bound with high affinity to ERs in the FLG 29.1 human leukemic cell line, which differentiates toward an osteoclastic phenotype in vitro. In addition, raloxifene inhibited cell proliferation, increased progesterone-receptor expression, and induced apoptosis, all of which are expected effects of an estrogen agonist *(11)*.

The effect of raloxifene on osteoclast-mediated resorption has also been assayed in vitro using bone slices. In these analyses, slices were incubated with interleukin-6 (IL-6)-stimulated osteoclast precursors derived from long bones of neonatal rats and increasing doses of raloxifene or 17-β-estradiol *(12,13)*. Both compounds inhibited production of resorption lacunae by differentiating osteoclasts *(12)*. The possibility that an important direct or indirect target of raloxifene action may be the osteoclast or a cellular precursor is also supported by data from Yang et al. *(14)*. Studies have indicated that raloxifene upregulated expression of transforming growth factor-β3 (TGF-β3), which in turn inhibited resorption in a chicken osteoclast-differentiation model *(14)*. Taken together, these results suggest that a similar osteoclast-inhibiting mechanism may be shared by estradiol and raloxifene and that bone protection may occur through the regulation of cytokine activity.

2.2. In Vivo Analyses

A variety of techniques have been used to assess bone density in vivo, including relatively simple measurements of calcium content and dry or ash weight along with more sophisticated imaging approaches, such as peripheral quantitative computed tomography (pQCT) and dual X-ray absorptiometry (DEXA). A recent report by Sato *(15)* suggested that the use of both pQCT and DEXA may be optimal because the two methods are uniquely effective in

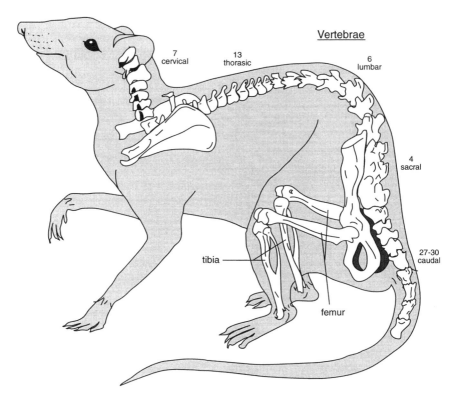

Fig. 3. Most of the preclinical studies involving raloxifene were conducted in rats. Bone-mineral density; labeled perimeters; and breaking force of the femur, tibia and vertebrae were assayed.

assessing appendicular and vertebral bone density, respectively. The in vivo studies have focused on a number of different sites for analysis, including the femur, tibia, and vertebrae, which were chosen primarily for ease of measurement, although two of these sites (femur and vertebrae) are important locations of bone loss in human osteoporosis (Fig. 3) *(16)*.

A challenge to researchers in this field is the application of findings in rodent models that measure osteopenia, or the loss of bone, to the human disease osteoporosis, which becomes clinically relevant when a fracture is diagnosed *(17)*. The fact that the bones of rodents continue to grow longitudinally virtually throughout their life span complicates extrapolation of the data to humans, although this growth is considerably slower in mature animals *(18)*. Osteoporosis involves the loss of both cortical and trabecular (sometimes called cancellous) bone, but a thorough understanding of how these two compartments contribute to bone integrity has not been achieved. While some studies have attempted to improve the applicability of animal experiments by assessing mechanical loading or crush resistance, the determination of true bone strength and susceptibility to fracture in animal models remains controversial. For practical purposes, the rat has proven to be a convenient model for predicting the tendency toward, if not the magnitude of raloxifene-induced bone protection in a hypoovarian milieu.

Early experiments determined that tamoxifen, raloxifene, and estradiol benzoate were all capable of retarding postovariectomy loss of bone density in 9-mo-old rats. The assessment of bone density was done by determining the total ash weight of the rat femurs. Moreover, the increases in total body weight that accompained the loss of bone density after ovariectomy were also inhibited by raloxifene and tamoxifen *(12)*.

Later experiments by Black et al. *(19)* showed that raloxifene inhibited postovariectomy loss of bone-mineral density in the distal metaphysis of the femur and proximal metaphysis of the tibia in 10–11-wk-old Sprague-Dawley rats. In these experiments, raloxifene was given daily by oral gavage at 0.1, 1.0, and 10.0 mg/kg/d for 5 wk, ethynyl estradiol was also given orally, but only at a dose of 0.1 mg/kg/d. The determination of bone density by DEXA showed that the three highest doses (0.1, 1.0, 10 mg/kg/d) of raloxifene were effective at maintaining the density of the femur in treated rats compared to ovariectomized controls. In these studies, the densities of the femurs of animals that received raloxifene and those that received estradiol were not significantly different, but neither treatment was able to maintain bone density at levels observed in intact animals. Results in the tibia were somewhat different; at this site, only the two highest doses of raloxifene were effective in inhibiting bone loss, but the density was indistinguishable from that seen in intact animals. Furthermore, at high doses, raloxifene was more effective at protecting the tibia than was estradiol. These results suggested that raloxifene was efficacious in protecting against bone loss following ovariectomy. However, the studies were criticized because they were conducted in young animals in which longitudinal bone growth was still occurring *(18)*. As explained by Evans et al., osteopenia occurs in immature animals as a result of increased turnover and chrondroclast-mediated resorption *(20)*. While increased turnover can occur in adults, resorption by chondroclasts does not. Because the dosing regimen was short, and the possible contribution of longitudinal bone growth was not considered, the interpretation and relevance of the results were questioned.

Subsequent analysis of the bone-mineral density of the distal femur metaphysis by pQCT showed that raloxifene was also able to inhibit postovariectomy bone loss in older Sprague-Dawley rats (Fig. 4) *(21)*. Bilateral oophorectomy was performed on virgin 6-mo-old animals, which were rested for 4 d and then administered raloxifene, estradiol or tamoxifen for 35 d. Raloxifene was as

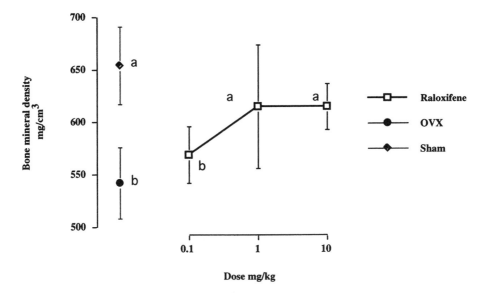

Fig. 4. Raloxifene maintains bone-mineral density of the femur of ovariectomized 6-mo-old rats. The mid-diaphysis of the femur was examined by QCT and volumetric bone-mineral density calculated (mg/cm³) following 35 d of daily dosing of raloxifene or vehicle by oral gavage. a≠b, $p < 0.05$. Adapted from ref. *(22)*.

efficacious as estradiol or tamoxifen in maintaining bone density in these animals, but it proved to be less potent, requiring higher doses to achieve the same effect (calculation of ED_{50}: raloxifene, 0.3 mg/kg/d; tamoxifen, 0.1 mg/kg/d; estradiol, 0.04 mg/kg/d). Interestingly, significant loss of density in the mid-diaphysis of the femur following ovariectomy was not observed during the testing time frame. This suggests that the rate or total amount of bone-mineral density loss may vary at different skeletal sites.

Analysis of the tibia in older animals following ovariectomy detected a significant 14.7–19% decrease in bone-mineral density. Differences in the density of the tibia of sham-operated and ovariectomized rats were first observed 15 d after surgery, with 10% of the loss occurring by d 16 after surgery *(22)*. Images generated by pQCT showed that, compared with the tibiae of sham-operated animals, the tibiae of ovariectomized rats had an increased cross-sectional area, loss of trabecular and cortical bone, and increased marrow space by 38 d after surgery *(22)*. Compared with ovariectomized controls, raloxifene treatment produced significantly higher bone-density levels in the tibia at two of the three doses tested (1 and 10 mg/kg/d at $p < 0.01$ and $p < 0.001$, respectively). Similarly, estradiol protected bone at two of three doses; however, as previously discussed, the effective doses of estradiol were 100-fold less than those of raloxifene.

The effect of raloxifene in animals with established bone loss was also evaluated in a similar model system. Following ovariectomy at 6 mo of age, female rats were rested for 2 mo to allow development of osteopenia. After the resting interval, animals were treated for 4 mo with raloxifene or ethynl estradiol. Analysis of rats 2 mo postovariectomy showed that a significant decrease in bone area had already occurred, and the loss continued in the untreated animals throughout the subsequent 4 mo *(20)*. As compared with their effects in untreated ovariectomized controls, estrogen and raloxifene prevented additional bone loss in treated rats as measured by bone area, trabecular number, and separation between trabeculae. Trabecular thickness was not affected by drugs or surgery.

Neither estrogen nor raloxifene was able to increase cancellous bone area to levels seen in sham-operated animals at any dose. Histomorphometric measurements of fluorochrome labels administered prior to sacrifice indicated that ovariectomy increased several indices of bone turnover. Two mo following ovariectomy, the osteoblast perimeter, osteoclast perimeter, eroded perimeter, labeled perimeter, and bone-formation rate were all elevated. An additional analysis 4 mo later indicated that the indices of bone turnover had fallen significantly, but were still elevated compared with that of sham-operated controls. These results suggested that high turnover rapid bone loss occurred soon after ovariectomy. Raloxifene was able to impact eroded and labeled perimeters most effectively, suggesting that the bone-sparing effects were mediated primarily through action on osteoclasts, as predicted by in vitro bone resorption assays *(5,12,20)*. Neither estradiol nor raloxifene was able to restore density to levels seen in sham-operated animals, indicating a lack of anabolic or bone-forming ability.

Turner et al. *(23)* tested the ability of raloxifene and estradiol to maintain bone strength using either three-point bending or direct force. In these experiments 10–11-wk-old virgin female rats were ovariectomized, rested briefly, and then administered raloxifene, estradiol or vehicle daily for 6 mo. Ovariectomy resulted in a 20% and 22% loss of bone density in the L4 vertebra and proximal tibia, respectively. These studies confirmed the ability of raloxifene and estradiol to inhibit bone density loss at both sites. The protection of bone density achieved by raloxifene was similar to that of estradiol in the vertebral site but raloxifene was less effective in the tibia. Load analyses of the midshaft of the femur, L6 vertebra, and femoral neck were conducted, and the breaking force at each site was determined. Loss of bone strength following ovariectomy was significant at the L6 vertebra and femoral neck but not at the femur midshaft. Although the calculated breaking force of the L6 vertebra was less than that of the femoral neck, raloxifene was more effective at the femoral neck, where post-treatment strength did not differ from that in sham-operated rats (Fig. 5). Both estradiol and raloxifene preserved bone strength at the two weakened sites. These data suggest that maintenance of bone density by estra-

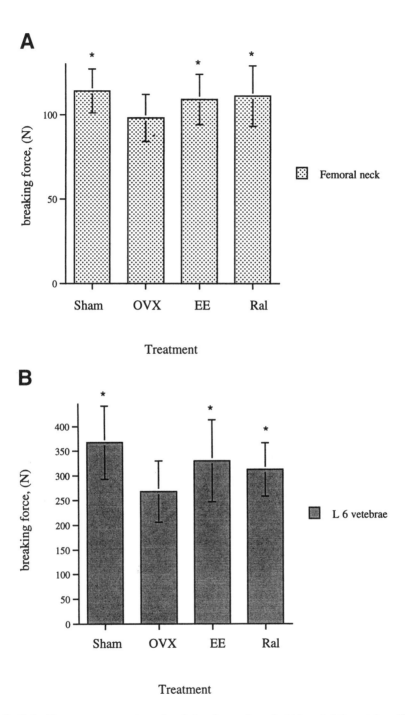

Fig. 5. Raloxifene preserves strength of the femoral neck (**A**) and L6 vertebra (**B**) in ovariectomized rats. Following surgery rats were given raloxifene (Ral) (3 mg/kg/d) or ethynyl estradiol (EE) (0.1mg/kg/d) daily by oral gavage for 6 mo. Breaking force was determined using a materials testing machine. * = $p < 0.05$ vs ovx. OVX = ovariectomized. Adapted from ref. *(24)*.

Table 1
Summary of Bone Effects of Raloxifene

Bone	Measurement	Duration of TX	Preserves bone density	Preserves strength	Anabolic effects	References
Femur	DEXA	5 wk	Yes	NR	NR	(20)
	QCT	5 wk	Yes	NR	NR	(22)
	Ash weight	4 mo	Yes	NR	NR	(19)
Femoral neck	Breaking force	6 mo	NR	Yes	NR	(24)
Tibia	QCT	5 wk	Yes	NR	NR	(23)
	DEXA	5 wk	Yes	NR	NR	(20)
	Histomor-phometry	4 mo*	Yes	NR	no	(21)
	QCT	6 mo	Yes	NR	NR	(24)
	QCT	10 mo	Yes	NR	NR	(50)
L4 vertebrae	QCT	6 mo	Yes	NR	NR	(24)
	QCT	10 mo	Yes	NR	NR	(50)
L6 vertebrae	Breaking force	6 mo	NR	Yes	NR	(24)
	QCT	10 mo	NR	Yes	NR	(50)

* Established osteopenia.

NR, not reported.

diol and raloxifene may result in increased bone strength at some sites in a long-term dosing regimen. These results also help validate the use of surrogate density measurements to assess bone strength and suggest the possible effectiveness of antiresorptives like raloxifene and estradiol in preventing load-induced fracture. The reported effects of raloxifene on bone are summarized in Table 1.

3. RALOXIFENE ACTION IN THE UTERUS

The previous discussion of the effects of raloxifene and estradiol on bone indicates that they act similarly, although with different potency, in protecting bone density and strength. Yet, this is not true in the uterus. In fact, raloxifene has been shown to be far less stimulatory than estrogen or tamoxifen in in vitro and in vivo analyses of uterine tissue. Tamoxifen is a widely used breast-cancer therapeutic with proven efficacy in reducing the risk of relapse and increasing the disease-free interval (24,25), but recent data indicate that long-term tamoxifen therapy may increase the risk of endometrial cancer (26,27). Epidemiologic studies show that an increased incidence of endometrial cancer is strongly associated with several risk factors including obesity, tamoxifen therapy, and unopposed estrogen use. As a result of such studies, hormone-replacement regimens now include progesterone to mitigate the stimulatory effects of estrogen on the endometrium *(28,29)*. At present, the mechanisms by which estradiol and tamoxifen increase the incidence of endometrial lesions, including neoplasia, are not clear, but uterotrophic drugs or hormones that increase proliferation of endometrial cells seem to increase risk.

Meanwhile, some studies have used surrogate measurements of uterine stimulation and cellular proliferation to predict which compounds will more likely increase endometrial risk. For instance, raloxifene is significantly less able than estrogen or tamoxifen to stimulate endometrial cell proliferation, progesterone receptor expression, epithelial hypertrophy, eosinophil-peroxidase activity, and uterine weight. However, there appears to be a significant person-to-person variation in susceptibility to uterine tumorigenesis, and increased proliferation does not necessarily promote cancer *(30)*. Thus, the association of the endpoints just described with endometrial cancer is at present correlative rather than mechanistic, and such analyses are likely to identify mitogenic compounds that impact tumor progression rather than tumor initiation. Therefore, the ability of compounds that stimulate proliferation to affect cellular transformation in the uterus remains controversial.

3.1. In Vitro Analyses

One impediment to in vitro uterine studies has been the lack of continuous cell lines that maintain ER levels and continue to respond predictably to hormones in culture. One cell line that has been reported by several research groups to maintain hormonal responsiveness in vitro is the human endometrial carcinoma line Ishikawa. At least two groups have reported that proliferation of Ishikawa cells was stimulated by tamoxifen (10^{-6} *M*) or estradiol (10^{-8} *M*) *(31,32)*. Raloxifene did not stimulate proliferation of the cells and was able to inhibit estrogen- and tamoxifen-stimulated proliferation as well *(31)*. Raloxifene was also able to inhibit estradiol- and tamoxifen-stimulated phosphorylation of the insulin-like growth factor (IGF-1) receptor β subunit *(31)*. In both analyses, raloxifene was more effective in inhibiting tamoxifen-mediated effects than estradiol-mediated effects. Analyses of alkaline phosphatase activity in Ishikawa cells showed that raloxifene was less stimulatory than estradiol, tamoxifen, droloxifene, or toremifene, but more stimulatory than ICI 182,780 or EM-800 following 5 d of in vitro exposure *(33)*. Raloxifene was also able to block estradiol-induced increases in phosphatase activity.

In related experiments, both estradiol and tamoxifen stimulated creatinine kinase activity in Ishikawa cells in culture *(10,34)*. Raloxifene did not stimulate kinase activity, even at a dose of 1 μM, and was able to inhibit stimulation by estradiol. In contrast to their effects in Ishikawa cells, however, tamoxifen and raloxifene acted as estrogen agonists and stimulated creatinine kinase activity in SaOS$_2$, osteoblast-like cells *(34)*. Thus, differential effects of the SERMs in these two cell types is an in vitro demonstration of tissue-specific

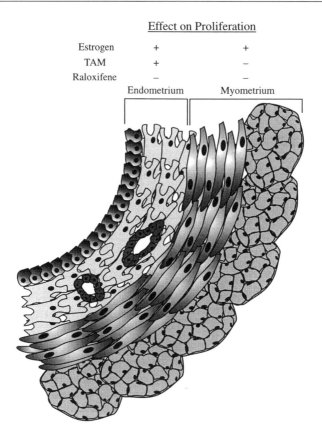

Fig. 6. SERMs have different effects on the endometrial and myometrial compartment of the uterus. Estrogen stimulates proliferation of both endometrial and myometrial cells. Tamoxifen is stimulatory to endometrial cells only, while raloxifene does not stimulate proliferation of either cell type.

activity and further differentiates the activities of raloxifene and tamoxifen in endometrial cells.

Continuous cell lines derived from the uterine myometrium are exceedingly rare, but a series of such lines, designated ELTs (Eker Leiomyoma Tumor-derived), have been derived from leiomyomas in the Eker rat (*35*). Uterine leiomyomas are the most common gynecological tumors in premenopausal women and are the primary reason premenopausal hysterectomies are performed (*36*). These tumors are dependent on ovarian steroids, regress after menopause, and proliferate in cycling women in response to estrogen and perhaps progesterone. Gonadotropin-releasing hormone (GnRH) agonists that create a hypo-ovarian milieu are effective inhibitors of tumor progression in vivo (*37*). An analysis of consecutive hysterectomy specimens revealed that leiomyomas are much more common than previously thought *(38)*. Serial 2-mm sections of the uteri revealed the presence of leiomyomas in 77% of the specimens. Although tumors were smaller in uteri taken from postmenopausal women, incidence was not decreased. These data indicate that while leiomyomas are usually subclinical after menopause, they may not completely regress during the life of the patient *(38)*.

Because leiomyomas are so common, the effect of postmenopausal supplementation therapies on these cells is of interest. Several ELT cell lines have been shown to have ERs and progesterone receptors and to respond proliferatively to estradiol *(35,39)*. Fuchs-Young et al. *(40)* demonstrated that raloxifene did not induce proliferation of ER-positive ELT-3 cells and also inhibited estrogen-stimulated proliferation in vitro. Furthermore, raloxifene inhibited estrogen-stimulated increases in progesterone receptor expression in ELT-3 cells *(40)*. Surprisingly, in contrast to its stimulatory effects in the endometrium, tamoxifen also inhibited the E2-stimulated proliferation and PR expression in ELT cells *(39,40)*, suggesting that an analysis of SERM effects in the uterus must consider both endometrial and myometrial compartments (Fig. 6).

3.2 In Vivo Effects

In vivo analyses of the effects of SERMs on myometrial tumors have been conducted in two different animal models. In the Eker rat, leiomyomas develop in intact females by the age of 12 mo. For these studies, rats were treated for 4 mo starting at 1 yr of age with raloxifene analog, LY326315. This naphthalene compound closely mimics the biologic activity and potency of raloxifene and was utilized during the development of raloxifene for clinical use. Treatment with LY326315 significantly reduced tumor incidence by 50% *(41,42)*. Tamoxifen treatment similarly reduced tumor incidence, as predicted by the in vitro cell-proliferation studies *(41,42)*. In the guinea pig, Porter et al. induced abdominal leiomyomas using chronic estrogen exposure. Raloxifene (10 mg/kg/d) caused a complete regression of all myometrial tumors within 30 days *(43)*.

To evaluate the effects of SERMs on endometrial cancer cells in vivo, Gottardis et al. *(44)* implanted EnCa101 human endometrial cancer cells into athymic, ovariectomized mice. Tamoxifen, raloxifene, and other antiestrogens, including trioxifene, nafoxidine, and enclomiphene, were administered to the mice for 4–6 weeks. Raloxifene stimulated the growth of the endometrial tumors less than any of the other SERMs tested, suggesting a reduced level of inherent agonistic activity. Furthermore, raloxifene was able to inhibit tamoxifen-stimulated tumor progression of the xenografts *(44,45)*. The antiestrogen ICI 164, 384 was similarly able to inhibit tamoxifen-induced growth and was the only compound tested that did not stimulate the tumors.

In short-term studies using ovariectomized rats, raloxifene was far less stimulatory to the uterus than tamoxifen or estradiol. In these analyses, rats were ovariectomized, rested for 2 wk, and then administered drugs daily for 4 d. Compared with tamoxifen and estradiol, raloxifene did not stimulate increases in uterine weight or eosinophil peroxidase activity at the minimally effective dose (2,3,46). When tested at a wide range of doses (0.1–10 mg/kg), raloxifene also displayed a lack of inherent estrogenic activity and did not stimulate increases in luminal epithelial-cell height or infiltration of stromal eosinophils in ovariectomized 5-wk-old rats (19). The results also indicated that raloxifene lacked the ability to induce increases in stromal expansion or myometrial thickness at any dose tested (19). In 3-d assays using immature noncycling rats, raloxifene, but not tamoxifen, was able to inhibit estradiol-stimulated increases in uterine wet weight. At the maximal dose of 10 mg/kg, raloxifene was able to counteract the effects of 0.1 mg estradiol/kg/d and maintain the uterine weight at levels indistinguishable from those of vehicle-treated controls (3). Data also indicate that raloxifene inhibited the stimulatory effects of tamoxifen on uterine weight, eosinophil-peroxidase activity, and epithelial-cell height, further emphasizing the differences in the uterotrophic activity of the two SERMs (47).

Recently, interest in the impact of SERMs on tissues exposed to environmental or xenoestrogens has increased. Although the number of reports on this topic is limited, studies in immature mice treated for 5 consecutive days indicate that raloxifene (5 mg/kg/d) inhibited increases in uterine weight stimulated by DDT (10 mg/kg/d) or methoxychlor (10 mg/kg/d) (48). However, raloxifene was not able to inhibit uterine weight increases stimulated by 17-β estradiol (1 mg/kg) at the dose ratios used in the study.

Some acute studies indicated that raloxifene induced a modest increase in uterine wet weight that was not dose-dependent and was attributed to water imbibition rather than cellular hypertrophy or proliferation (3,22). This contention has been challenged by Ashby et al. (49), whose data demonstrated a small but statistically significant raloxifene-induced increase in both the wet and dry weight of the uterus in immature, ovariectomized rats. Sundstrom et al. (50) also provided evidence that raloxifene could act as an estrogen agonist in the endometrium. Estradiol, tamoxifen, LY117018, and raloxifene all stimulated increased transcription of uterine C3 in luminal epithelial cells of the uteri of immature rats; this effect was inhibited by progesterone.

Claimed by some to be a more appropriate end point, eosinophil peroxidase activity was not stimulated by raloxifene at any dose tested (0.01–10 mg/kg/d) but was stimulated by tamoxifen at all doses tested (0.1, 1.0, and 10 mg/kg/d) (21,47). Photomicrographs of histological uterine sections showed that estrogen- and tamoxifen-treated ovariectomized animals had hypertrophic, columnar luminal epithelium with pseudostratification of the cells. Raloxifene- and vehicle-treated rats had predominantly quiescent cuboidal epithelium, indicating a lack of endometrial stimulation *(3,19,46)*.

In assays in which ovariectomized rats were dosed for a longer period of 5 wk, estradiol, tamoxifen, and nafoxidine stimulated the eosinophil-peroxidase activity level significantly above that in vehicle-treated ovariectomized animals, with estradiol achieving the maximally stimulatory effect *(21)*. Raloxifene, on the other hand, did not stimulate this activity significantly above that in vehicle-treated ovariectomized controls. In assays in which animals were administered drugs for 4–10 mo, ovariectomy resulted in a significant threefold to eightfold reduction in uterine weight. The uterine weights in raloxifene-treated animals were not different from those in ovariectomized animals *(20,51)*.

These data indicate that in acute dosing regimens using ovariectomized animals, raloxifene was significantly less stimulatory than estradiol or tamoxifen. However, in several chronic regimens both raloxifene and tamoxifen reduced the uterine wet weight in intact rats and inhibited estrogen-induced increases in the uterine wet weight in ovariectomized animals following 1–4 mo of dosing administration *(52,53)*. Sourla et al. found that 28 d of tamoxifen administration to intact rats (100 µg/d), reduced uterine weight by 24%, but after 6 mo of tamoxifen exposure, uterine weights were indistinguishable from intact controls. Somewhat surprisingly, these studies and others have shown that in long-term treatment regimens using ovariectomized and intact rats, tamoxifen-treated animals did not have an increased uterine weight at the time of analysis. These data suggest that stimulation of the uterine weight by tamoxifen may be transitory. Studies by Carthew et al. *(54)* showed that continuous treatment with tamoxifen for 24 mo resulted in hyperplasia of the endometrial epithelium for the first 3 mo, followed by atrophy of the endometrium and myometrium for the remaining 21 mo. The lack of a sustained response may be due to the downregulation of ER, suppression of ovarian function, or some other biochemical accomodation of the tissue. Importantly, long-term treatment with tamoxifen (2 yr) was not associated with an increased incidence of uterine tumors in animal studies *(54)*. It is at present unclear how the short-term stimulation of endometrial tissue by tamoxifen in rats is to be reconciled with the increased incidence of uterine carcinoma in women undergoing long-term tamoxifen therapy *(27)*. Although DNA adduct formation in the liver following tamoxifen exposure has been reported, induced adducts have not been detected in the uterus *(55)*. Thus, the long-term effects of SERMs in the uterus require further exploration, and studies of relevant primate models seems appropriate. A summary of the uterine data is shown in Table 2.

Table 2
Summary of Uterine Responses to SERMs and Estradiol

	Endometrium				Myometrium			Whole uterus
	Cell proliferation	Tumor progression	Epithelial cell height	Eosinophil peroxdase activity	C3 expression	Cell proliferation	Tumor progression	Weight
Raloxifene	→	→	→	→	↑	→	→	+/—
(Ref)	(32)	(42)	(3,22,45,46,47)	(3,22,45,46,47)	(48)	(40,41)	(42,43,44)	(3,6,20,45)
TAM	↑	↑	↑	↑	↑	→	→	↑
(Ref)	(32,33)	(33,42,43)	(3,22,45,46)	(3,22,46)	(48)	(40)	(42,43,44)	(3,45)
Estradiol	↑	↑	↑	↑	↑	↑	↑	
(Ref)	(32)	(33,42,44)	(3,22,45,46,47)	(3,22,45,46,47)	(48)(36,40,41)	(42,43,44)	(3,20,45)	

Table 3
Summary of Mammary Effect of Raloxifene and Tamoxifen

	Breast-cancer cell proliferation	Tumor progression	Chemoprevention
Ral	↓	↓	Yes
TAM	↓	↓	Yes
Ref	*(2,3,44,54,56)*	*(59,61)*	*(62,63)*

4. RALOXIFENE EFFECTS IN MAMMARY TISSUE

4.1. In Vitro Analyses

Unlike uterine cells, many estrogen-responsive breast-cancer cell lines are available for analysis of antiestrogens. Raloxifene and 4-OH tamoxifen have been shown to inhibit estrogen-induced proliferation of MCF-7 breast-cancer cells in vitro with IC_{50}s of 0.2 nM and 0.5 nM, respectively *(2,3,46)*. As Thomas and Kiang *(56)* have reported, raloxifene is highly effective at inhibiting MCF-7 cell growth, achieving a 54% inhibition of proliferation, compared with a 33% inhibition by 4-OH tamoxifen. In addition to inhibiting proliferation, benzothiophene antiestrogens also inhibit the transcription of estrogen-regulated genes in breast-cancer cells. The raloxifene analog LY117018, which shares the tissue-specific profile of raloxifene, inhibited the estrogen induction of four mRNA transcripts in the ER containing cell line EMF-19 *(57)*. Moreover, as Poulin and Labrie *(58)* have shown, raloxifene competitively inhibited estrogen stimulation of ZR-75-1 human breast-carcinoma cells, a line that proliferates in response to the adrenal steroids androst-5-ene-3b,7b-diol (C_{19}-d^5-diol[3]), dehydroepiandrosterone (DHEA), and dehydroepiandrosterone sulfate (DHEAS). Raloxifene was highly effective at inhibiting proliferation promoted by any of these adrenal steroids and 17-β estradiol, and in the case of DHEA and DHEAS, raloxifene completely abolished all stimulatory effects.

4.2. In Vivo Effects of Raloxifene

Raloxifene has been tested in a number of in vivo models of mammary development and carcinogenesis. A summary of these data is shown in Table 3. In a study of 7,12-dimethylbenz{a}anthracene (DMBA)-induced carcinomas in Sprague-Dawley rats, raloxifene and tamoxifen significantly inhibited tumor growth, although tamoxifen was more effective *(59)*. Both compounds were also tested for their ability to inhibit mammary-gland development in intact rats and estrogen-induced increases in uterine weight in ovariectomized rats; raloxifene was more inhibitory than tamoxifen in both organs *(59)*. The inhibitory effect of raloxifene on mammary morphogenesis was confirmed in subsequent studies showing that raloxifene inhibited estrogen stimulation of mammary end-bud formation but tamoxifen did not *(60)*. Taken together, these studies suggest that raloxifene is a potent antiestrogen in the mammary gland.

Because DMBA-induced tumors are dependent on prolactin and estradiol for growth, N-nitrosomethylurea (NMU)-induced tumors are preferred by some investigators for evaluating the efficacy of antiestrogens. For example, in studies by Gottardis and Jordan *(61)*, animals received antiestrogens starting 7 wk after the NMU injections; raloxifene and tamoxifen reduced tumor incidence to 46 and 13%, respectively *(61)*. In assays in which antiestrogens were administered 2 wk after the NMU and continued for 7 wk, the final tumor incidence at 25 wk was 29% for raloxifene-treated animals and 28% for tamoxifen-treated animals *(61)*. Refractory tumors appeared earlier in raloxifene-treated animals, even though it was used at a fivefold higher dose. Raloxifene (500 µg) and tamoxifen (100 µg) were similarly effective in reducing the average number of tumors per animal. These data suggest that while tamoxifen is more effective and potent at inhibiting tumor growth and incidence, raloxifene is highly antiestrogenic in mammary tissue, has some ability to prevent tumor development and thus may be a useful tumor preventative. This possibility is intriguing, especially in light of the reduced stimulation of uterine tissues by raloxifene as compared with tamoxifen.

The possibility that raloxifene and tamoxifen prevent mammary tumors was specifically addressed in studies by Anzano et al. *(62,63)*. In these studies, 55-d-old rats were injected with a single 50-mg NMU/kg dose. Starting 1 wk later and continuing for 4.5–5 mo, animals were given either 60 or 20 mg of raloxifene per kg of food. Raloxifene exposure significantly increased the number of tumor-free rats and decreased the average number of tumors per rat and the average tumor burden. There was little difference in effect between the two doses, so no lower efficacy limit could be determined. The results obtained with raloxifene were comparable with those obtained with tamoxifen, although tamoxifen was effective at substantially lower doses (1.0 or 0.5 mg/kg food).

5. THE EFFECT OF RALOXIFENE ON SERUM CHOLESTEROL

In contrast to its effects in uterine and mammary tissue, raloxifene acts as an estrogen agonist on cholesterol metabolism. Multiple studies have shown that raloxifene, like estrogen, can lower serum lipid levels in ovariectomized rats *(2,19–22)*. Postmenopausal women are at increased risk of cardiovascular disease, including atherosclerosis, primarily because of a reduction in circulating estrogen, but this risk may be lowered by hormone-replacement therapy *(64–66)*. Although the exact mechanism by which estrogen protects against cardiovascular disease is unknown, it has been shown that estrogen lowers serum lipid levels and directly affects vascular smooth-muscle cells *(67,68)*.

However, these proven cardiovascular benefits are partially offset by the association between estrogen-replacement therapy and increased risk of endometrial and breast cancer *(69–71)*. The addition of progesterone to estrogen-replacement therapy protected the endometrium, but combined hormonal therapy was still associated with an increased risk of breast cancer *(69)*. Thus, the potential therapeutic benefit of a tissue-specific antiestrogen is substantial if the cardiovascular benefits can be realized without increased risk of breast and uterine cancer.

When evaluating the role of estradiol or tissue-specific antiestrogens on serum lipid levels in rat models, it is important to recognize that the predominant form of cholesterol in rat is high-density lipoprotein (HDL) *(72)*. In humans, estrogens lower low-density lipoprotein (LDL) and raise HDL levels, both changes probably contribute to the decrease in cardiovascular disease *(72–75)*. In rats, however, estrogens lower both LDL and HDL levels, making an evaluation of the potentially beneficial increases in HDL levels impossible *(72)*. The use of the rat model to study the effects of estrogen on serum lipid levels is considered by most to be valid, but extrapolation of results must be tempered by differences between the lipid profile of humans and rodents.

In 35- and 75-d-old rats, raloxifene, tamoxifen, and estradiol were able to significantly lower serum cholesterol levels below those in ovariectomized controls after only 4 d of dosing *(19,45,76)*. Over a 7-d course, raloxifene began lowering serum cholesterol levels on d 1 and was maximally effective by d 2 *(77)*. In 3-wk assays, serum cholesterol levels in the raloxifene, tamoxifen, and estradiol treatment groups remained below those in ovariectomized and sham-operated throughout the 21 d of dosing *(76)*. Unfortunately, the cholesterol levels in the sham-operated and ovariectomized groups were the same at all times. Both estradiol and raloxifene were able to lower total and HDL cholesterol levels significantly compared with those in ovariectomized controls starting at a dose of 0.03 mg/kg/d and 0.3 mg/kg/d, respectively. However, cholesterol levels were significantly lower in estrogen-treated animals than in raloxifene-treated animals. Lundeen et al. *(72)* found that raloxifene and tamoxifen lowered the total cholesterol level after 4 d but found reduced efficacy of both compounds compared to other reports. Raloxifene lowered cholesterol at all doses tested (0.005–5.0 mg/kg) but tamoxifen was effective only at the two highest doses, 1.0 and 10.0 mg/kg.

Longer-term studies may be more informative because, in some, ovariectomized animals have significantly higher cholesterol levels than do sham-operated animals. When serum levels were analyzed 39 d after surgery, ovariectomy increased the serum cholesterol level by 8–38%. Compared with ovariectomy, estradiol (0.1 mg/kg), tamoxifen (10 mg/kg), and raloxifene (10 mg/kg) reduced the cholesterol level by 70, 50, and 62%, respectively *(21,22)*. In these analyses, estradiol was more potent than raloxifene or tamoxifen. In 4- and 10-mo treatment protocols, raloxifene significantly reduced serum choles-

Table 4
Summary of Effects on the Cardiovascular System

	Serum cholesterol	LDL oxidation	Aortic cholesterol
Ral	↓	↓	↓
TAM	↓	NR	NR
Estradiol	↓	↓	↓
References	(20,22,23,40,74)	(77)	(76)

NR, not reported.

terol levels below those in ovariectomized or sham-operated rats (22,51). Data from the 10-mo study indicated that raloxifene was more efficacious than estradiol in reducing serum cholesterol levels.

In studies in which ovariectomized rabbits received treatment for 45 wk, estradiol and raloxifene lowered serum levels of very low-density lipoprotein (VLDL) cholesterol and triglycerides compared with those in placebo-treated controls (78). Neither compound significantly lowered the serum LDL level, and estrogen alone lowered the serum HDL level. In addition to their effects on serum lipids, estradiol and raloxifene also reduced the cholesterol content of the inner layer of the thoracic aorta. Both compounds were able to induce this antiatherosclerotic effect, but aortic cholesterol levels as well as serum triglycerides were lower in estradiol-treated rabbits than in raloxifene-treated rabbits (78).

Analysis of coronary arteries harvested from normal New Zealand white rabbits showed that both estradiol and raloxifene were able to cause relaxation of pre-contracted arterial rings (79). This effect was demonstrated in rings obtained from both male and female rabbits, however, higher levels of raloxifene than estradiol were needed to achieve similar relaxation. Additional evidence of the antiatherosclerotic activity of raloxifene was reported by Zuckerman and Bryan (80). They reported their assessment of LDL oxidation and myeloperoxidase-dependent radical formation in murine peritoneal macrophages, noting that inflammatory processes are an important component of the tissue damage associated with plaque formation. In these analyses, raloxifene was a more potent inhibitor of in vitro LDL oxidation than was estradiol. Raloxifene was also effective at inhibiting myeloperoxidase-induced dityrosine radical formation and neutrophil-mediated myeloperoxidase activity.

Taken together, the studies discussed in this section suggest that, in addition to lowering serum lipid levels, raloxifene may have specific antiatherosclerotic activities in the vessel wall. In addition, most studies indicate that estrogen is more potent and effective than raloxifene at lowering lipids, but that raloxifene may have other important attributes that contribute to its protection against cardiovascular disease. A summary of the effects of raloxifene, tamoxifen and estradiol on the cardiovascular system is shown in Table 4.

6. MECHANISM OF ACTION

The mechanism of action of raloxifene and other SERMs is the subject of research in a number of laboratories. From all available data, it appears that raloxifene acts primarily through interaction with the ERs, which act as regulators of transcription and that the unique target-specific profiles of raloxifene result from a combination of factors involving the ER itself and its interaction with cofactors and specific DNA sequences. McDonnell et al. *(4)* have proposed that ER ligands be classified as types I–IV based on their activity in a number of in vitro analyses. In brief, protease digestion revealed that ligands like raloxifene, that can act as estrogen agonists or antagonists, induce distinct ER conformations. In reporter assays, estrogen and 4-OH tamoxifen acted as agonists when a chimeric receptor was cotransfected into cells along with an estrogen response element (ERE), but only estrogen was agonistic when the wild-type receptor was present. ICI 164,384 was antagonistic in both settings. Raloxifene acted as an estrogen antagonist when the wild-type receptor was cotransfected with a C3 reporter, but was agonistic when the AF-1 receptor mutant (mutated AF-2 domain) was included. Using these types of analyses, the specific profile of ER ligands was determined, allowing their classification into four groups represented by estradiol, tamoxifen, raloxifene, and ICI 164,384. The proposed basis for the differing biological activity is partly structural and centers around the ability of a ligand to promote productive interaction of the AF-1 or AF-2 domain of the receptor with DNA. The ability of some promoters to discriminate between ligands is also considered pivotal to achieving tissue-specific activity.

In one report, this discriminatory ability was dependent on a transferable *cis* element about 90 bp upstream of the promoter *(81)*. The distal and proximal promoters of the progesterone-receptor gene controlled expression of the two receptor forms and were found to be differentially responsive to transcriptional repression by antiestrogens. Transcriptional activity from the distal promoter (PRD) was stimulated by estrogen but only partially antagonized when ICI 164,384 or the raloxifene analog LY117018 was added. The proximal promoter (PRP) was completely inhibited when antiestrogens were added. The difference in ligand responsiveness was found to reside in a transferable element 5′ of the distal promoter. This fragment was found to be both positionally independent and transferable, satisfying the criteria for a *cis* element. These data suggest that the tissue-specific activity of SERMs is in part promoter-specific and is in this case mediated by a *cis*-acting element that is probably acted on in turn by soluble *trans* factors whose expression may also be tissue-specific.

Yang et al. *(5)* have shown that one possible mechanism of the estrogen-agonist activity of raloxifene in bone is the interaction of a receptor with a unique response element. A unique polypurine sequence that preferentially mediated raloxifene-induced transcription of TGF-β3 in osteosarcoma cells was identified. Importantly, the DNA binding domain of the receptor was not required for the induction of reporter activity, suggesting an indirect association of the receptor with DNA, perhaps through tissue-specific cofactors. The estrogen metabolites 17-epiestriol and 16-keto-17β-estradiol were more effective activators of transcription through the response element than was estradiol, indicating that the endogenous ligand could be a steroid metabolite. Although some of these data have been subsequently qualified, it seems likely that this unique interaction plays a role in the agonistic activity of raloxifene in bone.

Recent data showing that ER-β was highly expressed in bone (RNA) and moderately expressed in the uterus suggest the possible involvement of this alternate receptor in mediating tissue-specific activity by raloxifene and other SERMs *(82,83)*. As mentioned earlier, raloxifene binds to ER-β and activates transcription through the AP-1 site. ER-β is also capable of activating transcription of ERE containing reporters in a ligand-dependent manner *(84)*. It has also been demonstrated that ER-α and ER-β form heterodimers that can activate transcription of some ERE-containing promoters *(84,85)*. Together, these results suggest new mechanisms by which the β receptor may participate in the tissue-specific activity of raloxifene and other SERMs. Relative levels of ER-β expression or the ERα:ERβ ratio could determine the activity of tissue-specific ligands. The discovery of this new receptor, along with promoter-specific responses, tissue-specific cofactors, and unique ligand-induced receptor structures, continues to increase the number and complexity of possible mechanisms responsible for tissue-specific activity.

In summary, the preponderance of available data indicates that raloxifene is a high-affinity ER ligand that acts as an estrogen agonist in bone and the cardiovascular system but is antiestrogenic in the mammary gland and uterus. The data also suggest that raloxifene inhibits postovariectomy loss of bone density and bone strength but is significantly less potent than estradiol. Although there is still some debate about the level and importance of uterine-weight stimulation, raloxifene is clearly less uterotrophic than tamoxifen or estradiol, at least in terms of the eosinophil-peroxidase activity and epithelial-cell height. Moreover, raloxifene is highly antiestrogenic in the developing mammary gland and in mammary cancer cells. The mechanism of this tissue-specific activity has not been elucidated but is likely to involve unique receptor structure, specialized promoter usage, and possibly the newly discovered ER-β.

ACKNOWLEDGMENTS

The author would like to thank C.L. Walker for her review of the manuscript and her artistic contribution to Fig. 6. The author would also like to thank D. Swafford for reviewing the manuscript, C. Yone for the figures, and M. Gardiner and B. Brooks for typing and editing.

REFERENCES

1. Jones CD, Suarez T, Massey EH, Black LJ, Tinsley FC. Synthesis and antiestrogenic activity of [3,4-dihydro-2-(4-methoxyphenyl)-1-naphthalenyl][4-[2-(1-pyrrolidinyl)ethoxy]-phenyl]methanone, methanesulfonic acid salt. *J Med Chem* 1979; 22:962–966.
2. Grese TA, Cho S, Finley DR, Godfrey AG, Jones CD, Lugar CW, III, et al. Structure-Activity Relationships of selective estrogen receptor modulators: modifications to the 2-arylbenzothiophene core of raloxifene. *J Med Chem* 1997; 40:146–167.
3. Grese TA, Sluka JP, Bryant HU, Cullinan GJ, Glasebrook AL, Jones CD, et al. Molecular determinants of tissue selectivity in estrogen receptor modulators. *Proc Natl Acad Sci USA* 1997; 94:14105–14110.
4. McDonnell DP, Clemm DL, Hermann T, Goldman ME, Pike JW. Analysis of estrogen receptor function in vitro reveals three distinct classes of antiestrogens. *Molec Endocrinol* 1995; 9:659–669.
5. Yang NN, Venugopalan M, Hardikar S, Glasebrook A. Identification of an estrogen response element activated by metabolites of 17 beta-estradiol and raloxifene. *Science* 1996; 273:1222–1225.
6. Kuiper G, Enmark E, Pelto-Huikko M, Nilsson S, Gustafsson J. Cloning of a novel estrogen receptor expressed in rat prostate and ovary. *Proc Natl Acad Sci USA* 1996; 93:5925–2930.
7. Paech K, Webb P, Kuiper GGJM, Nilsson S, Gustafsson J-A, Kushner PJ, Scanlan TS. Differential ligand activation of estrogen receptors ERα and ERβ at AP1 Sites. *Science* 1997; 277:1508–1510.
8. Eriksen EF, Colvard DS, Berg NJ, Graham ML, Mann KG, Spelsberg TC, Riggs BL. Evidence of estrogen receptors in normal human osteoblast-like cells. *Science* 1988; 24:84–86.
9. Pensler JM, Radosevich JA, Higbee R, Langman CB. Osteoclasts isolated from membranous bone in children exhibit nuclear estrogen and progesterone receptors. *J Bone Min Res* 1990; 5:797–802.
10. Somjen D, Waisman A, Kaye AM. Tissue selective action of tamoxifen methiodide, raloxifene and tamoxifen on creatine kinase B activity in vitro and in vivo. *J Ster Biochem Mol Biol* 1996; 59:389–396.
11. Fiorelli G, Martineti V, Gori F, Benvenuti S, Frediani U, Formigli L, et al. Heterogeneity of binding sites and bioeffects of raloxifene on the human leukemic cell line FLG 29.1. *Biochem Biophys Res Commun* 1997; 240:573–579.
12. Sato M, Bryant HU. Raloxifene efficacy in nonreproductive and reproductive tissues in rat models in vivo and in vitro. In vitro *Biol Sex Ster Horm Act* 1996; 406–421.
13. Sato M, Kim J, Bryant H. Estrogen, tamoxifen, raloxifene, and nafoxidine have different effects on ovariectomized rats and on rat osteoclasts. *J Bone Min Res* 1994; 9:A272.
14. Yang NN, Bryant HU, Hardikar S, Sato M, Galvin RJS, Glasebrook AL, Termine JD. Estrogen and raloxifene stimulate transforming growth factor-β3 gene expression in rat bone: a

potential mechanism for estrogen- or raloxifene-mediated bone maintenance. *Endocrinology* 1996; 137:2075–2084.

15. Sato M. Comparative X-ray densitometry of bones from ovariectomized rats. *Bone* 1995; 17:157S–162S.

16. Lindsay R. Prevention and treatment of osteoporosis. *Lancet* 1993; 341:801–805.

17. Dempster DW, Lindsay R. Pathogenesis of osteoporosis. *Lancet* 1993; 351:797–801.

18. Kimmel DB. Quantitative histologic changes in the proximal tibial growth cartilage of aged female rats. *Cell Mater* 1991; S1:11–18.

19. Black L, Sato M, Rowley E, Magee D, Bekele A, Williams D, et al. Raloxifene (LY139481 HCI) prevents bone loss and reduces serum cholesterol without causing uterine hypertrophy in ovariectomized rats. *J Clin Invest* 1994; 93:63–69.

20. Evans GL, Bryant HU, Magee DE, Turner RT. Raloxifene inhibits bone turnover and prevents further cancellous bone loss in adult ovariectomized rats with established osteopenia. *Endocrinology* 1996; 137:4139–4144.

21. Sato M, Rippy MK, Bryant HU. Raloxifene, tamoxifen, nafoxidine, or estrogen effects on reproductive and nonreproductive tissues in ovariectomized rats. *FASEB J* 1996; 10:905–912.

22. Sato M, Kim J, Short LL, Slemenda CW, Bryant HU. Longitudinal and cross-sectional analysis of raloxifene effects on tibiae from ovariectomized aged rats. *J Pharmacol Exp Ther* 1995; 272:1252–1259.

23. Turner CH, Sato M, Bryant HU. Raloxifene preserves bone strength and bone mass in ovariectomized rats. *Endocrinology* 1994; 135:2001–2005.

24. Fisher B, Costantino J, Remond C. A randomized clinical trial evaluating tamoxifen in the treatment of patients with node-negative breast cancer who have estrogen-receptor-positive tumors. *N Engl J Med* 1989; 320:479–484.

25. Fisher B, Redmond C, Wickerham L. Systemic therapy in patients with node-negative breast cancer. A commentary based on two National Surgical Adjuvant Breast and Bowel Project (NSABP) clinical trials. *Ann Intern Med* 1989; 111:703–712.

26. Kedar RP, Bourne TH, Powles TJ, Collins WP, Ashley SE, Cosgrove DO, Campbell S. Effects of tamoxifen on uterus and ovaries of postmenopausal women in a randomised breast cancer prevention trial. *Lancet* 1994; 343:1318–1321.

27. Fisher B, Costantino JP, Redmond CK, Fisher ER, Wickerham DL, Cronin WM. Endometrial cancer in tamoxifen-treated breast cancer patients: findings from the National Surgical Adjuvant Breast and Bowel Project (NSABP) B-14. *J Natl Cancer Inst* 1994; 86:527–537.

28. Hulka BS. Epidemiologic analysis of breast and gynecologic cancers. *Prog Clin Biol Res* 1997; 396:17–29.

29. Greven KM, Corn BW. Endometrial cancer. *Curr Probl Cancer* 1997; 21:65–127.

30. Farber E. Cell proliferation as a major risk factor for cancer: a concept of doubtful validity. *Cancer Res* 1995; 55:3759–3762.

31. Kleinman D, Karas M, Danilenko M, Arbell A, Roberts CT, LeRoith D, et al. Stimulation of endometrial cancer cell growth by tamoxifen is associated with increased insulin-like growth factor (IGF)-I induced tyrosine phosphorylation and reduction in IGF binding proteins. *Endocrinology* 1996; 137:1089–1095.

32. Anzai Y, Holinka CF, Kuramoto H, Gurpide E. Stimulatory effects of 4-hydroxytamoxifen on proliferation of human endometrial adenocarcinoma cells (Ishikawa line). *Cancer Res* 1989; 49:2362–2365.

33. Simard J, Sanchez R, Poirier D, Gauthier S, Singh SM, Merand Y, et al. Blockade of the stimulatory effect of estrogens, OH-tamoxifen, OH-toremifene, droloxifene, and raloxifene on alkaline phosphatase activity by the antiestrogen EM-800 in human endometrial adenocarcinoma Ishikawa cells. *Cancer Res* 1997; 57:3494–3497.

34. Fournier B, Haring S, Kaye AM, Somjen D. Stimulation of creatine kinase specific activity in human osteoblast and endometrial cells by estrogens and antiestrogens and its modulation by calciotropic hormones. *J Endocrinol* 1996; 150:275–285.
35. Howe SR, Gottardis MM, Everitt JI, Goldsworthy TL, Wolf DC, Walker C. Rodent model of reproductive tract leiomyomata: establishment and characterization of tumor-derived cell lines. *Am J Pathol* 1995; 146:1568–1579.
36. ACOG. Uterine Leiomyomata. *ACOG Tech Bul* 1994; 192:1–9.
37. Friedman AJ, Hoffman DI, Comite F, Browneller RW, Miller JD. Treatment of leiomyomata uteri with leuprolide acetate depot: a double-blind, placebo-controlled, multicenter study. The Leuprolide Study Group. *Obstet Gynecol* 1991; 77:720–725.
38. Cramer SF, Patel A. The frequency of uterine leiomyomas. *Am J Clin Pathol* 1990; 94:435–438.
39. Howe SR, Gottardis MM, Everitt JI, Walker C. Estrogen stimulation and tamoxifen inhibition of leiomyoma cell growth in vitro and in vivo. *Endocrinology* 1995; 136:4996–5003.
40. Fuchs-Young R, Howe S, Hale L, Miles R, Walker C. Inhibition of estrogen-stimulated growth of uterine leiomyomas by selective estrogen receptor modulators. *Mol Carcinog* 1996; 17:151–159.
41. Fuchs-Young R, Burroughs KD, Everitt J, Davis B, Walker C (1998) Discrimination of the tissue-specific biologic activity of therapeutic antiestrogens in vivo. Keystone Symposia – Molecular & Cellular Biology, pp 425.
42. Walker CL, Burroughs KD, Davis B, Sowell K, Everitt JI, Fuchs-Young R. Preclinical evidence for therapeutic efficacy of selective estrogen receptor modulators for uterine leiomyoma. *J Soc Gynecol Invest* 2000; 7:249–256.
43. Porter KB, Tsibris JC, Porter GW, Fuchs-Young R, Nicosia SV, O'Brien WF, Spellacy WN. Effects of raloxifene in a guinea pig model for leiomyomas. *Am J Obstet Gynecol* 1998; 179:1283–1287.
44. Gottardis MM, Ricchio ME, Satyaswaroop PG, Jordam VC. Effect of steroidal and non-steroidal antiestrogens on the growth of a tamoxifen-stimulated human endometrial carcinoma (EnCa101) in athymic mice. *Cancer Res* 1990; 50:3189–3192.
45. Jordan VC, Gottardis MM, Satyaswaroop PG. Tamoxifen-stimulated growth of human endometrial carcinoma. *Ann NY Acad Sci* 1991; 622:439–446.
46. Fuchs-Young R, Glasebrook AL, Short LL, Draper MW, Rippy MK, Cole HW, et al. Raloxifene is a tissue-selective agonist/antagonist that functions through the estrogen receptor. *Ann NY Acad Sci* 1995; 355–360.
47. Fuchs-Young R, Magee DE, Cole HW. (1995) Raloxifene is a tissue-specific antiestrogen that blocks tamoxifen or estrogen-stimulated uterotrophic effects. Program of the 77th Annual Meeting of The Endocrine Society, Washington, DC.
48. Al-Jamal JH, Dubin NH. The effect of raloxifene on the uterine weight response in immature mice exposed to 17beta-estradiol, 1,1,1-trichloro-2, 2-bis(p-chlorophenyl)ethane, and methoxychlor. *Am J Obstet Gynecol* 2000; 182:1099–1102.
49. Ashby J, Odum J, Foster JR. Activity of raloxifene in immature and ovariectomized rat uterotrophic assays. *Regul Toxicol Pharmacol* 1997; 25:226–231.
50. Sundstrom SA, Komm BS, Xu Q, Boundy V, Lyttle R. The stimulation of uterine complement component C3 gene expression by antiestrogens. *Endocrinology* 1990; 126:1449–1456.
51. Sato M, Bryant HU, Iversen P, Helterbrand J, Smietana F, Bemis K, et al. Advantages of raloxifene over alendronate or estrogen on nonreproductive and reproductive tissues in the long-term dosing of ovariectomized rats. *J Pharmacol Exp Ther* 1996; 279:298–305.
52. Jordan C, Phelps E, Lindgren U. Effects of anti-estrogens on bone in castrated and intact female rats. *Br Cancer Res Treat* 1987; 10:31–35.

53. Sourla A, Luo S, Labrie C, Belanger A, Labrie F. Morphological changes induced by 6-month treatment of intact and ovariectomized mice with tamoxifen and the pure antiestrogen EM-800. *Endocrinology* 1997; 138:5605–5617.

54. Carthew P, Edwards RE, Nolan BM, Martin EA, Smith LL. Tamoxifen associated uterine pathology in rodents: relevance to women. *Carcinogenesis* 1996; 17:1577–1582.

55. Li D, Dragan Y, Jordan VC, Wang M, Pitot HC. Effects of chronic administration of tamoxifen and toremifene on DNA adducts in rat liver, kidney, and uterus. *Cancer Res* 1997; 57:1438–1441.

56. Thomas T, Kiang DT. Additive growth-inhibitory effects of Dl-alpha-difluoromethylornithine and antiestrogens on MCF-7 breast cancer cell line. *Biochem Biophys Res Comm* 1987; 148:1338–1345.

57. Westley B, May FEB, Brown AMC, Krust A, Chambon P, Lippmann ME, Rochefort H. Effects of antiestrogens on the estrogen-regulated pS2 RNA and the 52- and 160-kilodalton proteins in MCF7 cells and two tamoxifen-resistant sublines. *J Biol Chem* 1984; 259:10030–10035.

58. Poulin R, Labrie F. Stimulation of cell proliferation and estrogenic response by Adrenal C_{19}-!delta^5-steroids in the ZR-75-1 human breast cancer cell line. *Cancer Res* 1986; 46:4933–4937.

59. Clemens J, Bennett D, Black L, Jones C. Effects of a new antiestrogen, keoxifene (LY156759), on growth of carcinogen-induced mammary tumors and on LH and prolactin levels. *Life Sci* 1983; 32:2869–2875.

60. Daniel CW, Silberstein GB, Strickland P. Direct action of 17B-estradiol on mouse mammary ducts analyzed by sustained release implants and steroid autoradiography. *Cancer Res* 1987; 47:6052–6057.

61. Gottardis MM, Jordan VC. Antitumor actions of keoxifene and tamoxifen in the N-Nitrosomethylurea-induced rat mammary carcinoma model. *Cancer Res* 1987; 47:4020–4024.

62. Anzano MA, Byers SW, Smith JM, Peer CW, Mullen LT, Brown CC, et al. Prevention of breast cancer in the rat with 9-cis-retinoic acid as a single agent and in combination with tamoxifen. *Cancer Res* 1994; 54:4614–4617.

63. Anzano MA, Peer CW, Smith JM, Mullen LT, Shrader MW, Logsdon DL, et al. Chemoprevention of mammary carcinogenesis in the rat: combined use of raloxifene and 9-cis-retinoic acid. *J Natl Cancer Inst* 1996; 88:123–125.

64. Barrett-Connor E, Bush TL. Estrogen and coronary heart disease in women. *J Am Med Assn* 1991; 265:1861–1867.

65. Levy H, Boas EP. Coronary artery disease in women. *J Am Med Assn* 1936; 107:97.

66. Stampfer MJ, Colditz GA. Estrogen replacement therapy and coronary heart disease: a quantitative assessment of the epidemiologic evidence. *Prev Med* 1991; 20:47–63.

67. Baysal K, Losordo DW. Estrogen receptors and cardiovascular disease. *Clin Exp Pharmacol Physiol* 1996; 23:537–548.

68. Nabulsi A, Folsom A, White A, Patsch W, Heiss G, Wu K, Szklo M. Association of hormone-replacement therapy with various cardiovascular risk factors in postmenopausal women. *N Engl J Med* 1993; 15:1069–1075.

69. Colditz GA, Hankinson SE, Hunter DJ, Willett WC, Manson JE, Stampfer MJ, et al. The use of estrogens and progestins and the risk of breast cancer in postmenopausal women. *N Engl J Med* 1995; 332:1589–1593.

70. Smith DC, Prentice R, Thompson DJ, Herrmann WL. Association of exogenous estrogen and endometrial carcinoma. *N Engl J Med* 1975; 293:1164–1167.

71. Jick H, Watkins RN, Hunter JR, Dinan BJ, Madsen S, Rothman KJ, Walker AM. Replacement estrogens and endometrial cancer. *N Engl J Med* 1979; 300:218–222.

72. Lundeen SG, Carver JM, McKean ML, Winneker RC. Characterization of the ovariectomized rat model for the evaluation of estrogen effects on plasma cholesterol levels. *Endocrinology* 1997; 138:1552–1558.

73. Sullivan JM, Fowlkes LP. Estrogens, menopause, and coronary artery disease. *Cardiol Clin* 1996; 14:105–116.

74. Yla-Herttuala S, Luoma J, Kallionpaa H, Laukkanen M, Lehtolainen P, Viita H. Pathogenesis of atherosclerosis. *Maturitas* 1996; 23(Suppl):S47–49.
75. Schwartz J, Freeman R, Frishman W. Clinical pharmacology of estrogens: cardiovascular actions and cardioprotective benefits of replacement therapy in postmenopausal women. *J Clin Pharmacol* 1995; 35:314–329.
76. Frolik CA, Bryant HU, Black EC, Magee DE, Chandrasekhar S. Time-dependent changes in biochemical bone markers and serum cholesterol in ovariectomized rats: effects of raloxifene HC1, tamoxifen, estrogen, and alendronate. *Bone* 1996; 18:621–627.
77. Kauffman RF, Bensch WR, Roudebush RE, Cole HW, Bean JS, Phillips DL, et al. Hypocholesterolemic activity of raloxifene (LY139481): pharmacological characterization as a selective estrogen receptor modulator. *J Pharmacol Exp Ther* 1997; 280:146–153.
78. Bjarnason NH, Haarbo J, Byrjalsen I, Kauffman RF, Christiansen C. Raloxifene inhibits aortic accumulation of cholesterol in ovariectomized, cholesterol-fed rabbits. *Circulation* 1997; 96:1964–1969.
79. Figtree GA, Lu Y, Webb CM, Collins P. Raloxifene acutely relaxes rabbit coronary arteries in vitro by an estrogen receptor-dependent and nitric oxide-dependent mechanism. *Circulation* 1999; 100:1095–1101.
80. Zuckerman SH, Bryan N. Inhibition of LDL oxidation and myeloperoxidase dependent tyrosyl radical formation by the selective estrogen receptor modulator raloxifene (LY139481 HCL). *Atherosclerosis* 1996; 126:65–75.
81. Montano MM, Kraus WL, Katzenellenbogen BS. Identification of a novel transferable cis element in the promoter of an estrogen-responsive gene that modulates sensitivity to hormone and antihormone. *Mol Endocrinol* 1997; 11:330–341.
82. Onoe Y, Miyaura C, Ohta H, Nozawa S, Suda T. Expression of estrogen receptor beta in rat bone. *Endocrinology* 1997; 138:4509–4512.
83. Couse JF, Lindzey J, Grandien K, Gustafsson JA, Korach KS. Tissue distribution and quantitative analysis of estrogen receptor- alpha (ERalpha) and estrogen receptor-beta (ERbeta) messenger ribonucleic acid in the wild-type and ERalpha-knockout mouse. *Endocrinology* 1997; 138:4613–4621.
84. Pace P, Taylor J, Suntharalingam S, Coombes RC, Ali S. Human estrogen receptor beta binds DNA in a manner similar to and dimerizes with estrogen receptor alpha. *J Biol Chem* 1997; 272:25832–25838.
85. Cowley SM, Hoare S, Mosselman S, Parker MG. Estrogen receptors alpha and beta form heterodimers on DNA. *J Biol Chem* 1997; 272:19858–19862.

7 Pure Antiestrogens

Alan E. Wakeling

1. INTRODUCTION

The first antiestrogen, MER 25, described by Lerner et al. *(1)* 40 years ago was discovered in the course of a drug-hunting program seeking new lipid-lowering agents. In the process of evaluating the pharmacologic activity of new chemical entities, it became clear that MER 25 blocked the action of estradiol on the vagina. Further studies confirmed that MER 25 has the primary characteristic of an antiestrogen, that is, it blocks the trophic actions of endogenous or exogenous estradiol on the uterus and vagina. When administered to ovariectomized mice, MER 25 had little effect on the vagina and minimally stimulated the uterus; thus, MER 25 alone was only a weak agonist on estrogen target organs and can be thought of as the first "pure" antiestrogen. The term "pure" is used in the pharmacological sense, meaning an antagonist capable of complete blockade of the actions of the natural ligand (estradiol) and, as a corollary of this, being devoid of agonist (trophic) activity. The distinction between the properties of pure antiestrogens and the large number of other partial-agonist antiestrogens that have been described since the original work of Lerner et al. *(1,2),* and that are exemplified by tamoxifen is the subject of this chapter.

From: *Hormone Therapy in Breast and Prostate Cancer*
Edited by: V. C. Jordan and B. J. A. Furr © Humana Press Inc., Totowa, NJ

A high level of interest in antiestrogens has been sustained by their therapeutic potential; original pharmaceutical research was driven primarily by their potential utility in fertility regulation and although this expectation has proven largely unjustified, their application to the treatment of breast cancer has amply rewarded this interest. The discovery and subsequent clinical application of tamoxifen (2,3) provides the historical perspective for development of novel pure antiestrogens. Tamoxifen was discovered in an antifertility research program where synthetic homologues of the nonsteroidal estrogen chloro-triphenylethylene were tested for their capacity to block implantation of the fertilized ovum in rats (4,5). Tamoxifen emerged as the perfect contraceptive in rats—unfortunately this did not extend to humans—but tamoxifen has subsequently been established as the endocrine treatment of choice for breast cancer. From its first successful application in the therapy of advanced breast cancer (6), the use of tamoxifen was extended to first-line treatment of advanced disease and then to adjuvant treatment of primary breast cancer until today, tamoxifen is being evaluated in large-scale clinical trials to test whether it can prevent the development of breast cancer in women at high risk of developing the disease (7). The recent report of over 45% reduction in breast-cancer occurrence in women at high risk of development of the disease in a large NCI trial, amply justifies consideration of prophylactic therapy with tamoxifen in spite of potential increased risk of endometrial cancer.

The clinical and commercial success of tamoxifen is based on the beneficial combination of therapeutic efficacy and modest level of side-effects, together with the ease of treatment offered by once or twice daily oral administration. Until very recently when chloro-tamoxifen (toremiphene) was registered for clinical use (8), no other antiestrogen had reached the U.S. market. This may be surprising in view of the very large number of other nonsteroidal antiestrogens that have been described in the literature in the past 40 years, including other triphenylethylene analogues (droloxifene [9], idoxifene [10]), substituted tetrahydronaphthalenes (nafoxidene [11], trioxifene [12]), indole derivatives (zindoxifene [13]) and benzothiophenes (keoxifene [14]), but none of these has yet proved to offer a sufficient combination of advantages over tamoxifen in respect of efficacy and tolerance to merit drug registration. All of these antiestrogens share with tamoxifen the pharmacologic characteristic of partial-agonist activity; while they antagonize estrogen action, this activity is incomplete for the reason that each compound has intrinsic estrogen-like stimulatory (agonist) activity. Thus, the net effect of drug treatment is a balance between agonist and antagonist activity. In the original studies of tamoxifen reported by Harper and Walpole (4,5), it was clear that the balance between agonism and antagonism varied depending on the test endpoint used and the species in which the assay(s) were performed. The term "partial-agonist" accurately conveys the the idea that all of these antiestrogens have some estrogenic

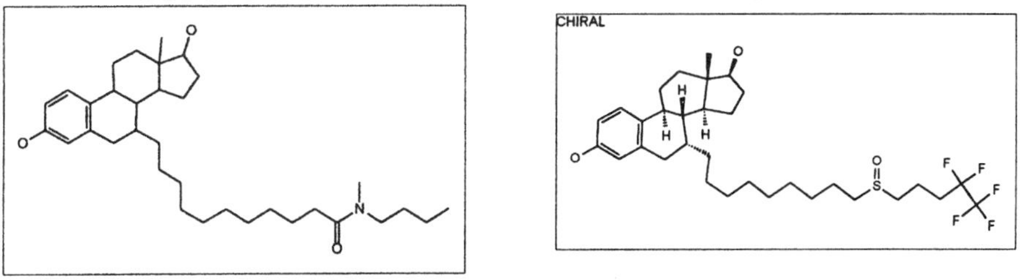

Fig. 1. Structures of pure antiestrogens.

activity but it does not adequately describe their complex organ, cell and gene-specific actions *(2,15,16)*.

In clinical use it is not clear to what extent, if any, the partial agonism of the current generation of antiestrogens affects either efficacy, side-effect profile, or toxicity. In the case of tamoxifen, although estrogen-like effects on the uterus, on bone density, and on serum lipid profiles are observed in patients *(17)*, there is no evidence for tumor-stimulatory effects in patients other than a transient effect at the start of treatment in a minority of patients *(18)*. Among newer partial agonist antiestrogens, the potential to target tissue-specific agonist actions, for example on the bone, while avoiding stimulation of the uterus has lead to renewed clinical interest *(19)*. Agents of this kind have been termed selective estrogen-receptor modulators (SERMs; *20*) and raloxifene (previously known as keoxifene) has recently been approved by the Food and Drug Administration (FDA) for the treatment of osteoporosis *(19)*. Despite this imaginitive exploitation of the selective agonist pharmacology of nonsteroidal antiestrogens, the major thrust of most research in the field has been the desire to eliminate partial agonism. This objective was pursued in Zeneca (formerly ICI) Pharmaceuticals and produced the first of a new series of antiestrogens, ICI 164384 (Fig. 1), which most closely conform to the pharmacologic definition of pure antiestrogens *(21,22)*. The remainder of this chapter compares and contrasts the pharmacology and mode of action of pure and partial-agonist antiestrogens.

2. DISCOVERY OF PURE ANTIESTROGENS

Although the primary pharmacological property of pure antiestrogens is clearly defined and the *potential* clinical advantage(s) of more rapid, more complete or longer-lasting remissions in breast cancer may be readily understood, it was less clear how such compounds might be realized. At the end of the second decade of antiestrogen research (late 1970s) the accumulated experience in Zeneca and many other industrial and academic laboratories pro-

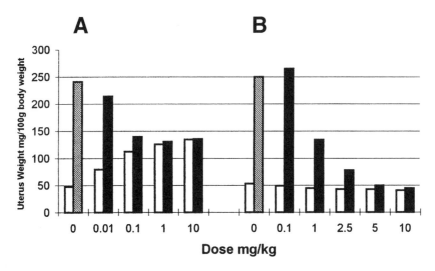

Fig. 2. Effects of tamoxifen and ICI 164384 on the immature rat uterus. Groups of 5 immature female rats received the indicated doses of tamoxifen **(A)** or ICI 164384 **(B)** alone (open bars) or together with 0.5 μg 17β-estradiol benzoate (filled bars) s.c.once daily for 3 d. The vehicle alone (open bar) and estradiol alone (hatched bar) controls are shown (0 dose) for each experiment. The weight of the uterus was recorded 24 h after the 3rd dose.

duced one clear conclusion: further synthetic chemistry based on existing nonsteroidal lead structures was unlikely to be productive. Attention thus turned to the potential for modifying the structure of the natural hormone estradiol while retaining the capacity of target molecules to bind tightly to the cognate receptor. A high affinity for the estrogen receptor was thought likely to improve the chance of achieving potency and selectivity. A starting point for chemistry emerged from collaborative studies between the laboratories of Roussel-Uclaf Pharmaceuticals and Etienne Baulieu in Paris *(23),* which had the objective of preparing an affinity matrix to facilitate purification of the estrogen receptor (ER). These studies reported that the carbon atom at position 7 in estradiol provided the optimum site for attachment of an alkylene bridge structure between the ligand and the matrix material. Our initial chemistry exploited this observation by synthesizing a series of 7-alkyl analogues of estradiol *(22).* The second requirement, that for a facile and efficient means of testing for activity, was satisfied by the rat-uterus assay *(24,* and *see* Fig. 2). This assay, as well as providing a reliable means to distinguish between pure and partial agonist antiestrogens in vivo, has the additional advantage of requiring modest quantities of compound, a particularly important consideration when the complexity of chemical synthesis may have a major impact on the length of each cycle of synthesis and testing in the drug-discovery

Table 1
Effects of 7-Substituted Estradiol Analogues on the Immature Rat Uterus

Compound	R	Dose mg/kg sc	Uterotrophic activity	
			% Agonism	% Antagonism
Tamoxifen	–	1	40	60
18	$-CO_2H$	25	23	30
19	$-CH_2OH$	25	28	33
20	$-CH_2NEt_2$	10	33	62
21	$-CONH(CH_2)_5CO_2H$	25	19	33
22	$-CONHC_4H_9$	10	–3	92

process. Additional in vitro tests, for example relative binding affinity (RBA) assays using ER *(25)* and inhibition of the growth of human breast-cancer cells *(26),* were available to monitor intrinsic potency that may not parallel in vivo data because of variations in absorption and metabolism. Although RBA assays are quicker to perform than the rat assay, and in vitro temperature-shift assays had been proposed at this time to distinguish between agonists and antagonists *(27),* this was rejected as the primary screen because the latter claim proved to be incorrect *(25).* We also had a clear concept of what mode of action might underlie pure antagonism. At this time (late 1970s), it was thought that ligand binding to ER initiated translocation of ER from the cyto-plasm to the cell nucleus to initiate DNA binding and transcription activation. A simple concept of how pure antiestrogens might act was to find ligands which, while binding ER, did not stimulate nuclear transfer. Although one could measure ER translocation and there was an established precedent for the existance of such ER ligands *(28),* the complexity of the assay mitigated against its routine use. As we shall see later this conceptualization of the mol-ecular basis for pure antagonism was not entirely unfounded.

Synthesis of 7-alkyl analogues of estradiol where a C10 side chain, together with a variety of end groups, initially produced partial agonists (Table 1) but an early breakthrough to the desired profile in the rat-uterus assay emerged with compound 22, (ICI 163964; ref. *21*), which incorporates a secondary amide in

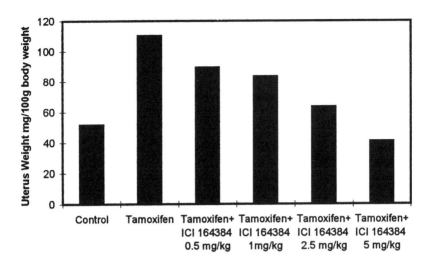

Fig. 3. Inhibition of the uterotrophic effect of tamoxifen by ICI 164384. Groups of 5 immature female rats were treated with veicle alone (control), tamoxifen 1 mg/kg alone, or tamoxifen plus the indicated doses of ICI 164384 s.c. once daily for 3 d. The weight of the uterus was recorded 24 h after the 3rd dose.

the side-chain. This compound was devoid of agonism when administered parenterally but had some uterotrophic activity when given orally *(21)*.

Comparison of the activity of the 7α- and 7β-isomers (ICI 163964 and ICI 164275 *(21)* showed that biological activity resides in the 7α-isomer. Conversion to the tertiary amide produced ICI 164384 (Fig. 1) which is a pure antiestrogen via both routes; that is it antagonized the uterotrophic action of estradiol in a dose-dependent and complete manner and, when administered in the absence of estradiol, had no uterotrophic activity *(21)*. The contrast between the old and new antiestrogens in the rat-uterus assay is illustrated in Fig. 2, where tamoxifen (A) or ICI 164384 (B) were administered alone (open bars) or together with estradiol (filled bars).

The trophic, estrogenic action of tamoxifen limits its capacity to antagonize estrogen stimulation of the uterus when co-administered with estradiol, whereas ICI 164384 does not stimulate the uterus and is able to inhibit estrogen action in a dose-dependent and complete manner. The difference between pure and partial agonist antiestrogens is further illustrated in Fig. 3 where co-administration to immature rats showed that ICI 164384 also blocked the uterotrophic action of tamoxifen in a dose-dependent and complete manner *(21)*. This experiment provides cogent support for the view that each ligand class—that is, full agonists (estradiol), partial agonists (tamoxifen), and pure antagonists (ICI 164384—

share a common mechanism of action mediated exclusively through the ER and that the antiestrogen-specific binding sites (AEBS) to which tamoxifen also binds *(29)* play no role in mediating tamoxifen partial agonism, since the pure antiestrogens do not bind to AEBS *(30)* and would therefore not block AEBS-mediated effects of tamoxifen. Consistent with this interpretation of the data is the demonstration that both tamoxifen and ICI 164384 compete with [^{3}H]-estradiol for binding to the ER in a concentration-dependent manner parallel to that of estradiol *(21)*. ICI 164384 has an RBA of 19, significantly greater than that of tamoxifen (RBA = 2.5) and as desired in our drug profile, more like that of estradiol (RBA = 100). Comparing oral and parenteral routes of administration, ICI 164384 was approx 10-fold less potent orally suggesting either modest absorption and/or metabolism in the gut.

Enhanced potency was sought by further modifications of the side-chain *(22)* to produce ICI 182780 (Fig. 1) in which the alkyl bridge is 9 rather than 10 carbon atoms long, the amide is replaced by sulphoxide and the terminal chain is fluorinated to reduce metabolic susceptibility *(31)*. ICI 182780, now named Faslodex®, has entered drug develoment and has successfully completed a Phase II clinical trial *(32)*.

Subsequent to the description of ICI 164384 several other laboratories have reported pure antiestrogens that encompass further synthetic modifications of the steroidal 7α-alkyl amides *(33)*, alternative positioning of the side chain on the steroid nucleus as in the 11β-amidoalkoxyphenyl derivatives *(34)*, as well as nonsteroidal pure antiestrogens from Zeneca *(35)* and elsewhere *(36,37)*.

3. PHARMACOLOGY OF PURE ANTIESTROGENS

3.1. Reproductive Tract

As we have seen the pure antiestrogens, unlike tamoxifen, do not stimulate the uterus. This difference is likely to be of clinical significance for two reasons. First, lack of uterotrophic activity should eliminate the concerns that have arisen from the reports of an increased incidence of endometrial cancer in patients treated with tamoxifen *(38)* and second, the possibility is opened up that pure antiestrogens could treat proliferative disorders of the uterus such as endometriosis and fibroids, conditions where treatment with partial agonists is inappropriate.

That there is a mechanistic connection between tamoxifen partial agonism and endometrial carcinoma is founded on the well-known association between unopposed estrogen replacement therapy in postmenopausal women and an increased incidence of the disease. However, this connection remains unproven for tamoxifen in women and caution is indicated by the fact that the predominant action of tamoxifen on the rodent uterus is to cause hypertrophy rather than hyperplasia of the luminal epithelium *(39)*. The risk-benefit equation remains strongly in favor of continuing tamoxifen therapy in women with breast cancer *(40)*. Comparative studies of tamoxifen and pure antiestrogens in two animal models serve to illustrate further potential advantages in use of the new agents. Studies by Gottardis et al. *(41)* with a human endometrial carcinoma grown in nude mice, which is stimulated by tamoxifen *(42)*, showed that pure antiestrogens inhibit both estrogen- and tamoxifen-stimulated tumor growth *(41)*. Again direct extrapolation to the clinical setting should be moderated by the apparent paradox that tamoxifen has been used with some success to treat endometrial cancer *(43)*. The estrogenic activity of tamoxifen and other partial agonists causes developmental abnormalities of the reproductive tract in neonatal rodents *(44–46)*. As might be anticipated, pure antiestrogens did not cause such effects and, when co-administered with tamoxifen, blocked these "toxicological" consequences *(46)*. The absence of effects on reproductive-tract development could be particularly relevent to the anticipated use of pure antiestrogens to treat gynecologic conditions in premenopausal women.

The effects of pure antiestrogens on reproductive function in cycling rats and in menstruating primates have also been studied to investigate likely outcomes in women. In adult female rats, comparison of the effects of treatment with ICI 182780 with that of ovariectomy showed a similar rate of uterine involution *(31)* and in ovariectomized, estrogen-treated primates, ICI 182780 treatment achieved a similar rate and extent of endometrial involution as estrogen withdrawal *(47)*. In rats, pure antiestrogens block ovulation and cyclical vaginal cornification *(35,48)*. In menstruating monkeys, ICI 182780 completely blocked cyclical endometrial proliferation in the majority where plasma steroid measurements indicated that ovulation was also blocked *(49)*. In those monkeys where ovulation occurred during ICI 182780 treatment (approx 25%), endometrial proliferation was still reduced but was not blocked completely *(49)*. The reasons for differential responses to the same dose of drug between individuals is not known but differences between individuals may simply be an extension of the well-established differential thresholds for response between different reproductive-tract endpoints *(35)*. A complicating factor in interpreting antiestrogen effects on the uterus is their concurrent action on the hypothalamic-pituitary-ovarian axis and consequent effects on estrogen secretion. In rats, ICI 182780 at doses which proved effective in reducing the weight of the uterus, had no effect on plasma gonadotrophin concentrations *(31)* suggesting that pituitary function was unaffected. In monkeys treated with ICI 182780, no postcastration-like increase of plasma gonadotrophins was detected (Fig. 4) but plasma estradiol concentrations did increase (Fig. 5; Dukes and Wakeling, unpublished studies). A similar increase of plasma estradiol without a concurrent change in gonadotrophins was noted in premenopausal women treated with ICI 182780 for 7 d prior to hysterectomy; in these women endometrial proliferation was blocked by ICI 182780 *(50)*. This increased estrogen secretion following pure antiestrogen treatment

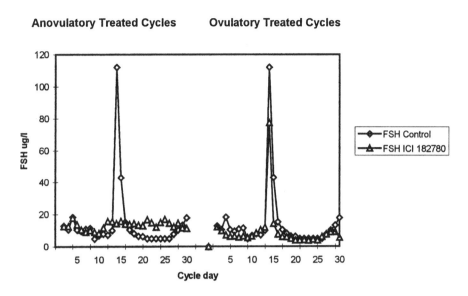

Fig. 4. Plasma FSH in ICI 182780-treated monkeys.

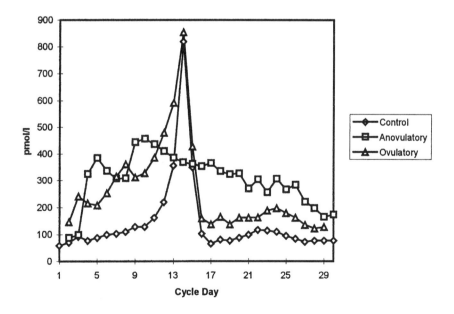

Fig. 5. Plasma estradiol in c ntrol and ICI 182780-treated menstrual cycles in monkeys.

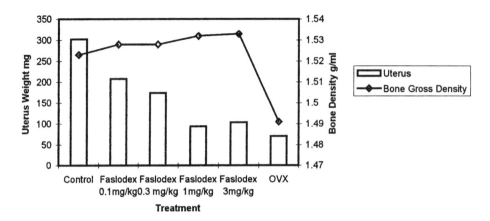

Fig. 6. Effect of ICI 182780 on uterus weight and bone density in adult rats.

remains to be explained. Further analysis of the central effects of pure antie-strogens is presented later.

The therapeutic efficacy of pure antiestrogens in benign gynecologic condi-tions remains to be explored further in clinical trials but the successful clinical pharmacology study of Thomas et al. *(50)*, together with the effective treat-ment with ICI 182780 of a monkey with uterine adenomyosis *(51)*, provide preliminary evidence that such studies are worth pursuing.

3.2. Bone

An important potential consequence of the therapeutic use of pure antiestro-gens is the anticipated loss of bone by analogy with that seen in women treated with GnRH analogues *(52)*, which reflects that seen as a natural consequence of the cessation of ovarian function at the menopause. Model studies in rats have provided conflicting evidence. Experiments with ICI 182780 did not reveal any gross loss of bone or reduction of mineral density at doses which caused an ovariectomy-like involution of the uterus (Fig. 6; *53)*. Similarly, EM-800 did not reduce bone density at effective antiuterotrophic doses *(54)* and ICI 164384 did not affect bone turnover or trabecular bone volume *(55)*. However other investigators have reported bone loss in rats treated with ICI 182780 *(56,57)*. It is probable that there is a differential threshold for antiestro-gen action between the bone and uterus and direct evidence for this is reported in studies with the nonsteroidal pure antiestrogen, ICI 189154 *(35)*. In the case of ICI 182780, a Phase II trial currently in progress is designed to test whether a dose of drug can be chosen that is effective on the uterus but which is also bone-sparing. The outcome of this study will have important implications because if pure antiestrogens do not cause bone loss, it will open up for the first time the prospect of effective, well-targeted, long-term medical treatment of endometriosis and fibroids.

3.3. Brain

The balance between positive and negative feedback of estrogens on the hypothalamus and pituitary controls ovarian function and the menstrual cycle. In general, negative feedback through ERs in the hypothalamus controls luteinizing hormone-releasing hormone (LH-RH) secretion which in turn determines pituitary output of follicle-stimulating hormone (FSH) and LH. Direct effects of estrogen on ER in the pituitary gonadotrophs can also affect gonadotrophin secretion. Thus, blockade by pure antiestrogens of ER action in either or both tissues is likely to cause significant disruption of the menstrual cycle. An anticipated outcome is an inappropriate stimulation of the ovary. Studies with EM-800 in mice have reported this effect; a significant increase in ovarian size *(58)*. Studies with another nonsteroidal antiestrogen, ICI 189154 showed ovarian hyperstimulation at a dose >15-fold that required to inhibit ovulation *(35)*. Although as previously noted, ICI 182780 also caused increased estrogen secretion in monkeys and women, there was no evidence of ovarian hyperstimulation or changes in gonadotrophin secretion in rats *(31,48)* or monkeys (Zeneca, unpublished studies). The difference between ICI 182780 and the two nonsteroidal antiestrogens might be explained by the apparent inability of ICI 182780 to penetrate the blood-brain barrier (BBB) first proposed to explain the lack of an effect of ICI 182780 on plasma gonadotrophins and body-weight gain in rats *(31,48)*. Whole-body autoradiographs of rats treated with ^{14}C-ICI 182780 showed the lack of penetration of the drug into the brain and cerebrospinal fluid (CSF) (Zeneca, unpublished studies), a result confirmed independently by the studies of the capacity of tamoxifen or ICI 182780 to block the uptake of [^{3}H]estradiol by rat tissues *(59)*. Tamoxifen blocked uptake in all tissues including the uterus, pituitary, and hypothalamus but ICI 182780 blocked uptake in all tissues including the uterus and pituitary *except* the hypothalamus (note: the pituitary is outside the BBB). The limited data available in humans from the clinical pharmacology studies that show that ICI 182780 did not alter gonadotrophin concentrations *(32,50)*, is consistent with a failure of ICI 182780 to penetrate the BBB in women.

Estrogens in the brain have important physiological effects other than those associated with reproductive function as well as profound psychological effects on mood, sleep patterns, and cognitive ability *(60)*. One of the most common debilitating symptoms of the menopause is the onset of frequent and sometimes severe hot flashes associated with estrogen withdrawal-induced vasomotor instability. Not surprisingly, the most common side effect of tamoxifen treatment is hot flushes *(61)*, an effect also reported in women treated with the SERM, raloxifene *(62)*. Since ICI 182780 does not enter the brain, it can be anticipated that the drug will not cause central estrogen withdrawal-like effects in patients. This is supported by the limited clinical data available to date, which noted no increase in the severity of hot flushes in patients where symptoms were already apparent and no onset of flushes in women free of flushes before treatment began *(32)*. Longer-term studies, particularly in premenopausal patients, are necessary to establish whether drug treatment with ICI 182780 will avoid the psychological effects of estrogen withdrawal from the brain. The profound importance of this is clear and further emphasized by recent data that indicate the role estrogen withdrawal might play in the onset or progression of Alzheimer's disease (AD) *(60)*.

3.4. Normal and Cancerous Breast

The effect of pure antiestrogens on the normal breast has been studied in the rat and mouse. In both species, the mammary gland develops postpubertally by outgrowth from the nipple of an extensively branched structure to fill the mammary fat pads. In the rat ovariectomized at 30 d of age, hormone replacement with either estradiol, tamoxifen, or other partial agonists mimicked the normal developmental process, whereas ICI 164384 had no effect and, when co-administered with estradiol or tamoxifen, completely blocked ductal extension *(63)*. Similarly, local implantation of either ICI 164384 or ICI 182780 into the developing mouse mammary gland caused ductal regression and inhibited DNA synthesis in terminal end buds *(64)*. Thus, ICI 164384 and ICI 182780 are pure antiestrogens in the normal breast.

In breast-cancer models, the pure antiestrogens also inhibit tumor growth. This activity was demonstrated in carcinogen-induced rat and mouse mammary tumors *(65,66)* as well as in two different human breast tumors grown as xenografts in nude mice *(31,67)*. Although tamoxifen also inhibits the growth of human breast-tumor xenografts in nude mice, its activity in these model systems appears to be short-lived since all of these tumors resume growth after about 3 mo *(68,69)*. The development of resistance to continued tamoxifen treatment in this model system reflects the clinical situation where most patients whose tumors respond initially, experience relapse of the disease. In nude mice, the growth of these tamoxifen-resistant tumors can be attenuated by treatment with pure antiestrogens *(67,70,71)*, clearly demonstrating the absence of cross-resistance between the two classes of antiestrogen, and strongly implying that a major cause of relapse in patients is related to the estrogenic activity of tamoxifen. Direct comparison of the efficacy and duration of antitumor activity of tamoxifen and ICI 182780 in xenografts of human MCF-7 breast-cancer cells showed that the pure antiestrogen prevents tumor growth for at least twice as long as tamoxifen and may also provide a greater degree of tumor regression *(71)*. In the latter studies, although resistance to the antitumor action of ICI

182780 developed, tumors did not grow in all of the animals, suggesting an indefinite and potentially "curative" effect in some. This would be consistent with studies with MCF-7 cells in vitro, which showed that ICI 182780 blocked cell growth in more than 90% of cells, whereas tamoxifen effected growth blockade in only 60% of cells *(31)*. This difference in efficacy could be sufficient in some tumors to lead to effective cure of the disease.

In patients with breast cancer, a Phase I trial in which tumors were biopsied before and after 7 d treatment with ICI 182780, showed that the drug caused significant reductions of ER, of progesterone receptor (an estrogen-regulated protein), of Ki67 an indicator of proliferative activity *(72)* and an increase in the number of apoptotic cells *(73)*. Following this study, a Phase II trial of ICI 182780 was conducted in patients who had relapsed on tamoxifen treatment (analogous to the nude mouse studies referred to earlier). Drug treatment produced responses in two-thirds of patients *(32)*. The mean duration of response of 26 mo was significantly longer than that achieved previously in such a group of patients using the standard high-dose progestin therapy *(74)*. These clinical results are consistent with what was predicted from the animal-model studies. Faslodex is now being assessed in Phase III trials in patients with advanced disease treated previously with tamoxifen.

4. MODE OF ACTION

Target-cell response to estrogens is dictated by the presence or absence of ER; estradiol binding to ER initiates a sequence of events that includes dissociation of heat-shock proteins, dimerization, and binding to discrete DNA sequences termed estrogen-response elements (EREs) in the regulatory regions of target genes *(75)*. The ligand-receptor complex regulates gene activity by recruiting other proteins to the transcriptional complex; these proteins may act with ER as coactivators or corepressors of transcription *(76)*. There is no precise molecular description of these events but ligand-induced conformational changes in the ER dimer, which differ for estradiol and antiestrogens *(77)*, are likely to influence strongly protein-protein interactions in the transcriptional complex since such changes will alter the relative orientation of the two major independent transcriptional activation domains (AF1/AF2) of the ER *(78)*. Partial agonism of tamoxifen has been attributed to the fact that one of the activation domains (N-terminal AF1) of ER remains active in the tamoxifen-ER complex *(78)*, but more complex schemes involving the efficiency of coactivator or corepressor coupling in the transcriptional complex are necessary to account for the gene-specific actions of antiestrogens *(79)*. Thus, among partial agonists that show varying degrees of agonism depending on which response is measured, agonism is cell-, promotor-, and effector-sensitive *(79,80)*. Further complexity is added by the recent description of a third activation domain

(AF2a) in ER, which may function when AF1 and AF2 are inactive and might thus account for how certain ligands act as full agonists in the bone and cardio-vascular system *(81)*, and of a novel form of ER designated ERβ *(82,83)*. Furthermore, the ER can be activated in a ligand-independent manner by other signaling molecules, for example dopamine *(84)*, epidermal growth factor (EGF) *(85)*, cAMP *(86)*, and insulin-like growth factor (IGF-1) *(86,87)* and so antiestrogen effects, for example on IGF-1 synthesis *(88)*, could indirectly affect ER activity. Recently, it has been shown that growth factor-induced phosphorylation of ER can amplify the partial agonist effect of tamoxifen *(89)*.

In contrast to the partial agonists, studies examining the mode of action of the pure antiestrogens have produced a uniform conclusion; that is that the ability of the ER to activate or inhibit transcription in a ligand-dependent or independent manner in vivo is completely attenuated by ICI 164384 and ICI 182780 *(16)*. Multiple changes in ER function following pure antiestrogen treatment appear to contribute to the blockade of estrogen action. These include impaired dimerization *(90)*, increased turnover *(91)* and disrupted nuclear localization *(92)*. The rapid loss of ER following ICI 164384-treatment of cells in culture *(91,93)*, or from the uterus after in vivo treatment *(94)* is likely to play a major role in abrogating estrogen action and would account for the efficacy of pure antiestrogens in blocking ER activation induced by other mediators like dopamine, cAMP, and growth factors *(84–87,95)*. This could have important therapeutic implications in breast cancer since no other treatment option leads to removal of the ER. In women with breast cancer treated with ICI 182780, the median tumor ER index was reduced from a pre-treatment median of 0.72 to 0.02 *(72)* suggesting that the pure antiestrogen also leads to rapid loss of ER in humans.

As a consequence of the "downregulation" of ER by ICI 164384 and ICI 182780, the transcription of ER-regulated genes should be inhibited. This has been studied both in animal models and in humans. In the rat uterus, estradiol and tamoxifen stimulate the expression of a number of genes, including complement component C3 *(96)*, calbindin-D *(97)*, IGF-I *(88)*, vascular endothelial-cell growth factor and c-*fos* *(98)*. In each case ICI 164384 or ICI 182780 showed no induction of transcription and, when adminstered prior to estradiol or tamoxifen, completely blocked estrogen or tamoxifen induction of these genes *(88,96–98)*. Similarly, these two compounds act as pure antiestrogens on the transcription of estrogen-inducible genes in human breast-cancer cells in vitro *(93,99,100)*, in vivo *(71)*, and in patients with breast cancer *(72)*.

The contrasting actions of tamoxifen and the pure antiestrogens also extend to effects on genes that are downregulated by estrogens. For example, expression of the IGF-binding protein 3 (IGFBP3), is suppressed by estradiol and tamoxifen, whereas ICI 182780 significantly stimulated expression *(101)*. Similarly, blockade by ICI 182780 of estrogen-suppressed transcription of several other genes, pMGT1 *(102)*, IGFBP5 *(103)*, and quinone reductase *(104)*, allows these genes to be expressed. ICI 164384 and ICI 182780 also effectively inhibit cell growth and the transcription of estrogen-regulated genes in human breast-cancer cells resistant to growth inhibition by tamoxifen *(105,106)* consistent with the absence of cross-resistance in vivo between the two classes of antiestrogen *(32,71)*. It is not known whether ERβ functions in vivo in the control of transcription of specific target genes but in vitro transfection studies have demonstrated this potential. The pure antiestrogens are fully effective in blocking ERβ-induced transcription in vitro *(83,107)*.

5. CONCLUSIONS

Clinical experience with tamoxifen has established unequivocally the tremendous value of antiestrogen therapy in the treatment of breast cancer and has illustrated the potential of antiestrogen treatment to reduce the incidence of the disease in women at high risk. The development of new agents, termed "pure" antiestrogens and exemplified by Faslodex, was based on the understanding that tamoxifen-like drugs are not devoid of estrogen-like actions and that their intrinsic partial-agonist effects may have undesired consequences. The potential therapeutic advantage of the pure antiestrogens, which have no partial agonist activity, has been demonstrated in disease models where Faslodex blocked breast-tumor growth for twice as long as tamoxifen, more effectively reduced the development of the disease, and was effective against tamoxifen-resistant breast and endometrial tumors. Based on successful Phase II clinical trials that demonstrated efficacy in women experiencing disease progression following tamoxifen treatment, Faslodex is currently in Phase III trials in advanced breast cancer. The mode of action of Faslodex is unique; the downregulation of ER following drug exposure implies that all cell-growth signals operating through the receptor will be attenuated. This novel action may provide greater efficacy than can be achieved with conventional antiestrogens or other drugs like aromatase inhibitors, which reduce estrogen synthesis.

Complete blockade of estrogen action by Faslodex could potentially have adverse effects in patients, for example unfavorable changes of serum lipid profile, increased rates of bone loss, and adverse effects in the brain. Only clinical trials will determine the extent or significance of these, but data available to date have indicated no change in serum lipids in patients and that the drug dose required to achieve a full antagonist effect on the uterus in the rat had no effect on bone density. Also, in rats there is evidence that Faslodex does not cross the BBB. The possible adverse effects of pure antiestrogens may assume greater significance for drug treatment of benign gynecological conditions such as endometriosis, where effects on bone could limit utility. Phase II clinical trials are currently addressing these important questions.

REFERENCES

1. Lerner LJ, Holthaus JF, Thompson A nonsteroidal estrogen antagonist (1-(p-2-diethy-laminoethoxyphenyl)-1-phenyl-2-p-methoxyphenyl\ ethanol. *Endocrinology* 1958; 63:295–318.
2. Jordan VC, Murphy CS. Endocrine pharmacology of antiestrogens as antitumor agents. *Endocr Rev* 1990; 11:578–610.
3. Jordan VC. The development of tamoxifen for breast cancer therapy: a tribute to the late Arthur L Walpole. *Breast Cancer Res Treat* 1988; 11:197–209.
4. Harper MJK, Walpole AL. A new derivative of triphenylethylene: effect on implantation and mode of action in rats. *J Reprod Fert* 1967a; 13:101–119.
5. Harper MJK, Walpole AL. Mode of action of ICI 46,474 in preventing implantation in rats. *J Endocr* 1967b; 37:83–92.
6. Cole MP, Jones CTA, Todd IDH. A new antiestrogenic agent in late breast cancer. An early clinical appraisal of ICI 46474. *Br J Cancer* 1971; 25:270–275.
7. Jordan VC. Tamoxifen: the herald of a new era of preventive therapeutics. *J Natl Cancer Inst* 1997; 89:747–749.
8. Wiseman LR, Goa KL. Toremifene. A review of its pharmacological properties and clinical efficacy in the management of advanced breast cancer. *Drugs* 1997; 54:141–160.
9. Bruning PF. Droloxifene, a new anti-estrogen in postmenopausal advanced breast cancer; preliminary results of a double-blind dose-finding Phase II trial. *Eur J Cancer* 1992; 28A:1404–1407.
10. Johnson SRD, Riddler S, Haynes BP, A'Hern R, Smith IE, Jarman M, Dowsett M. The novel anti-estrogen idoxifene inhibits the growth of human MCF-7 breast cancer xenografts and reduces the frequency of acquired anti-estrogen resistance. *Br J Cancer* 1997; 75:804–809.
11. Duncan GW, Lyster SC, Clark JJ, Lednicer D. Antifertility activities of two diphenyl-dihy-dronaphthalene derivatives. *Proc Soc Exp Biol Med* 1963; 112:439–442.
12. Jones CD, Suarez T, Massey EH, Black LJ, Tinsley J. Synthesis and antiestrogenic activity of [3,4-dihydro-2-(4-methoxyphenyl)-1-naphthalenyl](4-(1-pyrolidinyl) ethoxyphenyl methanone, methanesulphonic acid salt. *J Med Chem* 1979; 22:962–966.
13. Stein RC, Dowsett M, Cunningham DC, Davenport J, Ford HT, Gazet J-C, von Angerer E, Coombes RC. Phase I/II study of the anti-estrogen zindoxifene (D 16726) in the treatment of advanced breast cancer. A Cancer Research Campaign PhaseI/II clinical trials committee study. *Br J Cancer* 1990; 61:451–453.
14. Clemens JA, Bennett DR, Black LJ, Jones CD. Effects of a new antiestrogen, keoxifene (LY 156758), on growth of carcinogen-induced mammary tumors and on LH and prolactin levels. *Life Sci* 1983; 32:2869–2875.
15. Furr BJA, Jordan VC. The pharmacology and clinical uses of tamoxifen. *Pharmacol Ther* 1984; 25:127–205.
16. Wakeling AE. Use of pure antiestrogens to elucidate the mode of action of estrogens. *Biochem Pharmacol* 1995; 49:1545–1549.
17. Fornander T, Rutqvist LE, Wilking N, Carlstrom K, von Schoultz B. Oestrogenic effects of adjuvant tamoxifen in postmenopausal breast cancer. *Eur J Cancer* 1993; 29A:497–500.
18. Plotkin D, Lechner JJ, Jung WE, Rosen PJ. Tamoxifen flare in advanced breast cancer. *J Am Med Assoc* 1978; 240:2644–2646.
19. Mitlak BH, Cohen FJ. In search of optimal long-term female hormone replacement: the potential of selective estrogen receptor modulators. *Hormone Res* 1997; 48:155–163.
20. Kauffman RF, Bryant HU. Selective estrogen receptor modulators. *Drug News Perspect* 1995; 8:531–539.
21. Wakeling AE, Bowler J. Steroidal pure antiestrogens. *J Endocr* 1987; 112:R7–R10.

22. Bowler J, Lilley TJ, Pittam JD, Wakeling AE. Novel steroidal pure antiestrogens. *Steroids* 1989; 54:71–99.

23. Bucort R, Vignau M, Torelli V, Richard-Foy H, Geynet C, Secco-Millet C, Redeuilh G, Baulieu EE. New biospecific adsorbents for the purification of estradiol receptor. *J Biol Chem* 1978; 253:8221–8228.

24. Wakeling AE, Valcaccia B. Antioestrogenic and antitumour activities of a series of non-steroidal antiestrogens. *J Endocr* 1983; 99:455–464.

25. Wakeling AE. Anti-hormones and other steroid analogues, in *Steroid Hormones: A practical Approach* (Green B, Leake RE, eds). IRL Press, Oxford, 1987, pp 219–236.

26. Wakeling AE, Valcaccia B, Newboult E, Green LR. Non-steroidal antiestrogens – receptor binding and biological response in rat uterus, rat mammary carcinoma and human breast cancer cells. *J Steroid Biochem* 1984; 20:111–120.

27. Raynaud JP, Bouton MM, Ojasoo T. The use of interaction kinetics to distinguish potential antagonists from agonists. *Trends Pharmacol Sci* 1980; 1:324–327.

28. Muldoon TG. Characterization of steroid binding sites by affinity labelling: further studies of the interaction between 4-mercuri-17β-estradiol and specific estrogen-binding proteins. *Biochemistry* 1971; 10:3780–3784.

29. Sutherland RL, Murphy LC, Foo MS, Green MD, Whybourne AM. High-affinity anti-estrogen binding site distinct from the estrogen receptor. *Nature* 1980; 288:273–275.

30. van den Koedijk CDMA, van Heemst CV, Elsendoorn GM, Thijssen JHH, Blankenstein MA. Comparative affinity of steroidal and non-steroidal antiestrogens, cholesterol derivatives and compounds with dialkylamino side chain for the rat liver antiestrogen binding site. *Biochem Pharmacol* 1992; 34:2511–2518.

31. Wakeling AE, Dukes M, Bowler J. A potent specific pure antiestrogen with clinical potential. *Cancer Res* 1991; 51:3867–3873.

32. Howell A, DeFriend D, Robertson J, Blamey R, Walton P. Response to a specific antiestrogen (ICI 182780) in tamoxifen-resistant breast cancer. *Lancet* 1995; 345:29–30.

33. Levesque C, Merand Y, Dufour JM, Labrie C, Labrie F. Synthesis and biological activity of new halo-steroidal anti-estrogens. *J Med Chem* 1991; 34:1624–1630.

34. Nique F, Van de Velde P, Bremaud J, Hardy M, Philibert D, Teutsch G. 11β-amidoalkoxyphenyl estradiols, a new series of pure antiestrogens. *J Steroid Biochem Mol Biol* 1994; 50:21–29.

35. Dukes M, Chester R, Yarwood L, Wakeling AE. Effects of a non-steroidal pure antiestrogen, ZM 189,154, on estrogen target organs of the rat including bones. *J Endocr* 1994; 41:335–341.

36. Gauthier S, Caron B, Cloutier J, Dory YL, Favre A, Larouche D, et al. (S)-(+)-4-[7-(2,2-dimethyl-1-oxopropoxy)-4-methyl-2[4-[2-(1-piperidinyl)-ethoxy] phenyl]-2*H*-1-benzopyran-3-yl]-phenyl 2,2-dimethylpropanoate (EM800): a highly potent, specific, and orally active nonsteroidal antiestrogen. *J Med Chem* 1997; 40:2117–2122.

37. Day BW, Magarian RA, Jain PT, Pento JT, Mousissian GK, Meyer KL. Synthesis and biological evaluation of a series of 1, 1-dichloro-2,2,3-triarylcyclopropanes as pure antiestrogens. *J Med Chem* 1991; 34:842–851.

38. Fisher B, Costantino JP, Redmond CK, Fisher ER, Wickerham DL, Cronin WM, Other NSABP contributors. Endometrial cancer in tamoxifen-treated breast cancer patients: findings from the National Surgical Adjuvant Breast and Bowel project (NSABP) B-14. *J Natl Cancer Inst* 1994; 86:527–537.

39. Martin L. Effects of antiestrogens on cell proliferation in the rodent reproductive tract, in *Non-Steroidal antiestrogens. Molecular Pharmacology and Antitumour Activity* (Sutherland RL, Jordan VC, eds). Academic Press, Sydney, 1981, pp 143–163.

40. Assikis VJ, Neven P, Jordan VC, Vergote I. A realistic clinical perspective of tamoxifen and endometrial carcinogenesis. *Eur J Cancer* 1996; 32:1464–1476.

41. Gottardis MM, Ricchio ME, Satyaswaroop PG, Jordan VC. Effect of steroidal and nonsteroidal antiestrogens on the growth of tamoxifen-stimulated human endometrial carcinoma (EnCa101) in athymic mice. *Cancer Res* 1990; 50:3189–3192.

42. Gottardis MM, Robinson SP, Satyaswaroop PG, Jordan VC. Contrasting actions of tamoxifen on endometrial and breast tumor growth in the athymic mouse. *Cancer Res* 1988; 48:812–815.

43. White JO, Owen GI, De Clerq NAM, Soutter WP. Antiestrogens in the treatment of endometrial carcinoma. *Rev Endocr Rel Cancer* 1993; 44:47–57.

44. Chamness GC, Bannayan GA, Landry LA Jr, Sheridan PJ, McGuire WL. Abnormal reproductive development in rats neonatally administered antiestrogen (tamoxifen). *Biol Reprod* 1979; 21:1087–1090.

45. Clark JF, Guthrie SC. The estrogenic effects of clomiphene during neonatal period in the rat. *J Steroid Biochem* 1983; 18:513–517.

46. Branham WS, Fishman R, Streck RD, Medlock KL, DeGeorge JJ, Sheehan DM. ICI 182,780 inhibits estrogen-dependent rat uterine growth and tamoxifen-induced developmental toxicity. *Biol Reprod* 1996; 54:160–167.

47. Dukes M, Miller D, Wakeling AE, Waterton JC. Antiuterotrophic effects of a pure antiestrogen, ICI 182,780: magnetic resonance imaging of the uterus in ovariectomized monkeys. *J Endocr* 1992; 135:239–247.

48. Wakeling AE, Bowler J. Novel antiestrogens without partial agonist activity. *J Ster Biochem* 1988; 31:645–653.

49. Dukes M, Waterton JC, Wakeling AE. Antiuterotrophic effects of the pure antiestrogen ICI 182,780 in adult female monkeys *(Macaca nemestrina):* quantitative magnetic resonance imaging. *J Endocrinol* 1993; 138:203–209.

50. Thomas EJ, Walton PL, Thomas NM, Dowsett M. The effects of ICI 182,780, a pure antiestrogen, on the hypothalamic-pituitary-ovarian axis and on endometrial proliferation in pre-menopausal women. *Human Reprod* 1994; 9:1991–1996.

51. Waterton JC, Breen SA, Dukes M, Horrocks M, Wadsworth PF. A case of adenomyosis in a pigtailed monkey diagnosed by magnetic resonance imaging and treated with the novel pure antiestrogen, ICI 182,780. *Lab Animal Sci* 1993; 43:247–251.

52. Perry CM, Brogden RN, Goserelin. A review of its pharmacodynamic and pharmacokinetic properties, and therapeutic use in benign gynaecological disorders. *Drugs* 1996; 51:319–346.

53. Wakeling AE. The future of new pure antiestrogens in clinical breast cancer. *Breast Cancer Res Treat* 1993; 25:1–9.

54. Luo S, Sourla A, Labrie C, Belanger A, Labrie F. Combined effects of dehydroepiandrosterone and EM-800 on bone mass, serum lipids, and the development of dimethylbenz(a)anthracene(DMBA)-induced mammary carcinoma in the rat. *Endocrinology* 1997; 138:4435–4444.

55. Baer PG, Willson TM, Morris DC. Lack of effect on bone of 28-days treatment of OVX and intact rats with a pure anti-estrogen (ICI 164384). *Cal Tissue Int* 1994; 54:338 (Abstract).

56. Gallagher A, Chambers TJ, Tobias JH. The estrogen antagonist ICI 182, 780 reduces cancellous bone volume in female rats. *Endocrinology* 1993; 133:2787–2791.

57. Sibonga JD, Dobnig H, Harden RM, Turner RT. ICI 182,780 has complex effects on the rat skeleton. *Endocrinology* 1998; 139:3736–3742.

58. Luo S, Martel C, Sourla A, Gauthier S, Merand Y, Belanger A, Labrie C, Labrie F. Comparative effects of 28-day treatment with the new antiestrogen EM-800 and tamoxifen on estrogen-sensitive parameters in the intact mouse. *Intl J Cancer* 1997; 73:381–391.

59. Wade GN, Blaustein JD, Gray JM, Meredith JM. ICI 182,780: a pure antiestrogen that affects behaviours and energy balance in rats without acting in the brain. *Am J Physiol* 1993; 43:R1392–R1398.

60. Sherwin BB. Estrogenic effects on the central nervous system: clinical effects, in *Estrogens and Antiestrogens: Basic and Clinical Aspects* (Lindsay R, Dempster DW, Jordan VC, eds). Lippincott-Raven, Philadelphia, 1997, pp 75–87.

61. Pritchard K. Effects on breast cancer. Clinical aspects, in *Estrogens and Antiestrogens: Basic and Clinical Aspects* (Lindsay R, Dempster DW, Jordan VC, eds). Lippincott-Raven, Philadelphia, 1997, pp 75–210.

62. Draper MW, Flowers DE, Huster WJ, Nield JA, Harper KD, Arnaud C. A controlled trial of raloxifene (LY139481)HC1: impact on bone turnover and serum lipid profile in healthy postmenopausal women. *J Bone Min Res* 1996; 11:835–842.

63. Nicholson RI, Gotting KE, Gee J, Walker KJ. Actions of estrogens and antiestrogens on rat mammary gland development: relevance to breast cancer prevention. *J Steroid Biochem* 1988; 30:95–103.

64. Silberstein GB, Van Horn K, Shyamala G, Daniel CW. Essential role of endogenous estrogen in directly stimulating mammary growth demonstrated by implants containing pure antiestrogens. *Endocrinology* 1994; 134:84–90.

65. Wakeling AE, Bowler J. Biology and mode of action of pure antiestrogens. *J Steroid Biochem* 1988; 30:141–147.

66. Parczyk K, Schneider M. The future of antihormone therapy: innovations based on an established principle. *J Cancer Res Clin Oncol* 1996; 122:383–396.

67. Nique F, Van de Velde P, Bremaud J, Hardy M, Philibert D, Teutsch G. 11β-amidoalkoxyphenyl estradiols, a new series of pure antiestrogens. *J Steroid Biochem Mol Biol* 1994; 50:21–29.

68. Gottardis MM, Jordan VC. Development of tamoxifen-stimulated growth of MCF-7 tumors in athymic mice after long-term antiestrogen administration. *Cancer Res* 1988; 48:5183–5187.

69. Osborne CK, Coronado E, Allred DC, Wiebe V, DeGregorio M. Acquired tamoxifen resistance: correlation with reduced breast tumor levels of tamoxifen and isomerization of *trans*-4-hydroxytamoxifen. *J Natl Cancer Inst* 1991; 83:1477–1482.

70. Gottardis MM, Jiang S-Y, Jeng M-H, Jordan VC. Inhibition of tamoxifen-stimulated growth of an MCF-7 tumor variant in athymic mice by novel steroidal antiestrogens. *Cancer Res* 1989; 49:4090–4093.

71. Osborne CK, Coronado-Heinsohn EB, Hilsenbeck SG, McCue BL, Wakeling AE, McClelland RA, et al. Comparison of the effects of a pure steroidal antiestrogen with those of tamoxifen in a model of human breast cancer. *J Natl Cancer Inst* 1995; 87:746–750.

72. DeFriend DJ, Howell A, Nicholson RI, Anderson E, Dowsett M, Mansel RE, et al. Investigation of a new pure antiestrogen (ICI 182780) in women with primary breast cancer. *Cancer Res* 1995; 54:408–414.

73. Ellis PA, Saccani-Jotti G, Clarke R, Johnson SRD, Anderson E, Howell A, et al. Induction of apoptosis by tamoxifen and ICI 182780 in primary breast cancer. *Intl J Cancer* 1997; 72:608–613.

74. Robertson JFR, Howell A, DeFriend DJ, Blamey R, Walton P. Duration of remission to ICI 182,780 compared to megestrol acetate in tamoxifen resistant breast cancer. *Breast* 1997; 6:186–189.

75. Beato M. Gene regulation by steroid hormones. *Cell* 1989; 56:335–344.

76. Horwitz KB, Jackson TA, Bain DL, Richer JK, Takimoto GS, Tung L. Nuclear receptor coactivators and corepressors. *Mol Endocrinol* 1996; 10:1167–1177.

77. Bzozowski AM, Pike ACW, Dauter Z, Hubbard RE, Bonn T, Engström O, et al. Molecular basis of agonism and antagonism in the estrogen receptor. *Nature* 1997; 389:753–758.

78. Tzukerman MT, Esty A, Santiso-Mere D, Danielian P, Parker M, Stein RB, et al. Human estrogen receptor transactivational capacity is determined by both cellular and promotor context and mediated by two functionally distinct intramolecular regions. *Mol Endocrinol* 1994; 8:21–30.

79. Katzenellenbogen JA, O'Malley BW, Katzenellenbogen BS. Tripartite steroid hormone receptor pharmacology: interaction with multiple effector sites as a basis for the cell- and promotor-specific action of these hormones. *Mol Endocrinol* 1996; 10:119.

80. McDonnell DP, Clemm DL, Hermann T, Goldman ME, Pike JW. Analysis of estrogen receptor function in vitro reveals three distinct classes of antiestrogens. *Mol Endocrinol* 1995; 9:659–669.

81. Norris JD, Fan d, Kerner SA, McDonnell DP. Identification of a third autonomous activation domain within the human estrogen receptor. *Mol Endocrinol* 1997; 11:747–754.

82. Kuiper GGJM, Enmark E, Pelto-Huikko M, Nilsson BS, Gustafsson J-A. Cloning of a novel estrogen receptor expressed in rat prostate and ovary. *Proc Natl Acad Sci USA* 1996; 93:5925–5930.

83. Mosselman S, Polman J, Dijkema R. ERβ: identification and characterization of a novel human estrogen receptor. *FEBS Lett* 1996; 392:49–53.

84. Smith CL, Conneely OM, O'Malley BW. Modulation of the ligand-independent activation of the human estrogen receptor by hormone and antihormone. *Proc Nat Acad Sci USA* 1993; 90:6120–6124.

85. Ignar-Trowbridge DM, Teng CT, Ross KA, Parker MG, Korach KS, McLachlan JA. Peptide growth factors elicit estrogen receptor-dependent transcriptional activation of an estrogen-responsive element. *Mol Endocrinol* 1993; 7:992–998.

86. Aronica SM, Katzenellenbogen BS. Stimulation of estrogen receptor-mediated transcription and alteration in the phosphorylation state of the rat uterine estrogen receptor by estrogen, cyclic adenosine monophosphate, and insulin-like growth factor-1. *Mol Endocrinol* 1993; 7:743–752.

87. Newton CJ, Buric R, Trapp T, Brockmeier S, Pagatto U, Stalla G. The unliganded estrogen receptor (ER) transduces growth factor signals. *J Steroid Biochem Mol Biol* 1994; 48:481–486.

88. Huynh HT, Pollack M. Insulin-like growth factor I gene expression in the uterus is stimulated by tamoxifen and inhibited by the pure antiestrogen ICI 182780. *Cancer Res* 1993; 53:5585–5588.

89. Kato S, Endoh H, Masuhiro Y, Kitamoto T, Uchiyama S, Sasaki H, et al. Activation of the estrogen receptor through phosphorylation by mitogen-activated protein kinase. *Science* 1995; 270:1491–1494.

90. Fawell SE, White R, Hoare S, Sydenham M, Page M, Parker MG. Inhibition of estrogen-receptor-DNA binding by the "pure" antiestrogen ICI 164,384 appears to be mediated by impaired receptor dimerization. *Proc Natl Acad Sci USA* 1990; 87:6883–6887.

91. Dauvois S, Danielian PS, White R, Parker MG. Antiestrogen ICI 164,384 reduces cellular estrogen receptor content by increasing its turnover. *Proc Natl Acad Sci USA* 1992; 89:4037–4041.

92. Dauvois S, White R, Parker MG. The antiestrogen ICI 182780 disrupts estrogen receptor nucleocytoplasmic shuttling. *J Cell Sci* 1993; 106:1377–1388.

93. Nicholson RI, Gee JMW, Manning DL, Wakeling AE, Montano MM, Katzenellenbogen BS. Responses to pure antiestrogens (ICI 164384, ICI 182780) in estrogen-sensitive and -resistant experimental and clinical breast cancer. *Ann NY Acad Sci* 1995; 761:148–162.

94. Gibson MK, Nemmers LA, Beckman WC Jr, Davis VL, Curtis SW, Korach KS. The mechanism of ICI 164,384 antiestrogenicity involves rapid loss of estrogen receptor in uterine tissue. *Endocrinology* 1991; 129:2000–2010.

95. EI-Tanani MK, Green CD. Two independent mechanisms for ligand-independent activation of the estrogen receptor. *Mol Endocrinol* 1997; 11:928–937.

96. Galman MS, Sundstrom SA, Lyttle CR. Antagonism of estrogen- and antiestrogen-induced uterine complement component C3 expression by ICI 164,384. *J Steroid Biochem* 1990; 36:281–286.

97. Blin C, L'Horset F, Leclerc T, Lambert M, Colnot S, Thomasset M, Perret C. Contrasting effects of tamoxifen and ICI 182780 on estrogen-induced calbindin-D 9k gene expression in the uterus and in primary culture of myometrial cells. *J Steroid Biochem* 1995; 55:1–7.

98. Hyder SM, Chieppetta C, Murthy L, Stancel GM. Selective inhibition of estrogen-regulated gene expression in vivo by the pure antiestrogen ICI 182,780. *Cancer Res* 1997; 57:2547–2549.

99. May FEB, Johnson MD, Wiseman LR, Wakeling AE, Kastner P, Westley BR. Regulation of progesterone receptor mRNA by estradiol and antiestrogens in breast cancer cell lines. *J Steroid Biochem* 1989; 33:1035–1041.

100. Wiseman LR, Wakeling AE, May FEB, Westley BR. Effects of the antiestrogen, ICI 164,84, on estrogen induced RNAs in MCF-7 cells. *J Steroid Biochem* 1989; 33:1–6.

101. Huynh H, Pollack M. Uterotropic actions of estradiol and tamoxifen are associated with inhibition of uterine insulin-like growth factor binding protein 3 gene expression. *Cancer Res* 1994; 54:3115–3119.

102. Manning DL, Nicholson RI. Isolation of pMGT1: a gene that is repressed by estrogen and increased by antiestrogens and antiprogestins. *Eur J Cancer* 1993; 29(A):759–762.

103. Huynh H, Yang X-F, Pollak M. A role for insulin-like growth factor binding protein 5 in the antiproliferative action of the antiestrogen ICI 182780. *Cell Growth Diff* 1996; 7:1501–1506.

104. Montano MM, Katzenellenbogen BS. The quinone reductase gene: a unique estrogen receptor-regulated gene that is activated by antiestrogens. *Proc Natl Acad Sci USA* 1997; 94:2581–2586.

105. Coopman P, Garcia M, Brunner N, Derocq D, Clarke R, Rochefort H. Anti-proliferative and anti-estrogenic effects of ICI 164,384 and ICI 182,780 in 4-OH-tamoxifen resistant human breast cancer cells. *Intl J Cancer* 1994; 56:295–300.

106. Lykkesfeldt AE, Madsen MW, Briand P. Altered expression of estrogen-regulated genes in a tamoxifen-resistant and ICI 164,384 and ICI 182,780 sensitive human breast cancer cell line, MCF-7TAM^R-1. *Cancer Res* 1994; 54:1587–1595.

107. Tremblay GB, Tremblay A, Copeland NG, Gilbert DJ, Jenkins NA, Labrie F, Giguere V. Cloning, chromosomal localization, and functional analysis of the murine estrogen receptor β. *Mol Endocrinol* 1997; 11:353–365.

II   ANTIESTROGENS: CLINICAL

8 Tamoxifen for the Treatment of Breast Cancer

V. Craig Jordan

CONTENTS

INTRODUCTION
OVERVIEW OF CLINICAL TRIALS
CONCLUSIONS
REFERENCES

1. INTRODUCTION

During the 1960s, many pharmaceutical companies around the world were involved in the study of the structure-activity relationships of the antiestrogens. Each compound was an effective antifertility agent in the laboratory rat, but it was clear that the properties scientists were observing in animals did not translate into a clinically useful contraceptive. A number of preliminary clinical trials in breast cancer were conducted with several new antiestrogens because of the recognized link between estrogen and the growth of some breast cancers *(1,2)*. It had also been found in the laboratory that antiestrogens could block the binding of radioactive estradiol in its target tissues, so the rationale for clinical studies in the 1970s was strong.

The Upjohn Company in Kalamazoo, MI conducted extensive tests on their new antiestrogen, nafoxidine; but in the 1970s, after numerous clinical studies around the world, development was abandoned because all patients suffered severe toxic side effects *(3)*. Similarly, clomiphene, an impure mixture of geometric isomers, was tested, but concerns about potential side effects or toxicities, particularly cataracts, prevented further clinical development for long-term treatment. Clinical studies were abandoned in the early 1970s *(4)*.

From: *Hormone Therapy in Breast and Prostate Cancer*
Edited by: V. C. Jordan and B. J. A. Furr © Humana Press Inc., Totowa, NJ

Table 1
Comparison of Earlier Clinical Experience with Antiestrogens as a Treatment
for Advanced Breast Cancer

Antiestrogen	Daily dose (mg)	Year	Response rate (%)	Toxicity
Ethamoxytriphetol	500–4500	1960	25	Acute psychotic episodes
Clomiphene	100–300	1964–1974	34	Fear of cataracts
Nafoxidine	180–240	1976	31	Cataracts, ichthyosis, photophobia
Tamoxifen	20–40	1971–1973	31	Transient thrombocytopenia

The late Dr. Arthur Walpole deserves the credit for pursuing the application of tamoxifen as a potential palliative treatment for advanced breast cancer in postmenopausal women *(5)*. Tamoxifen, however, was only one of numerous compounds being tested by pharmaceutical companies during the 1960s. Table 1 compares and contrasts the different compounds that underwent evaluation.

Dr. Mary Cole and coworkers at the Christie Hospital in Manchester, UK, conducted the first preliminary evaluation of ICI 46, 474 for the palliative treatment of breast cancer. Initially, 46 postmenopausal patients with late-stage disease were treated with the drug; 10 patients responded *(6)*. These results were subsequently confirmed in a small dose-response study by Dr. Harold Ward in Birmingham, UK *(7)*. Over the past 20 years, tamoxifen has become the endocrine treatment of choice for all stages of breast cancer *(8)*. However, the results of the adjuvant clinical trials have been evaluated rigorously, so it is possible to draw some conclusions about the actions of tamoxifen.

2. OVERVIEW OF CLINICAL TRIALS

The 1998 Oxford Overview Analysis *(9)* involved any randomized trial that was started before 1990. The analysis included 55 trials of adjuvant tamoxifen vs no tamoxifen before recurrence. The study population was 37,000 women with node-positive and node-negative breast cancer, thus comprising 87% of world evidence of known randomized clinical trials. Of these women, fewer than 8000 had a very low or zero level of estrogen receptor (ER) and 18,000 were classified as ER-positive. The remaining nearly 12,000 women were unknown for ER but the authors estimated that two-thirds would be ER-positive based on the normal distribution of ER in random populations.

This clinical-trial database *(9)* can now be used to answer the questions raised over the past two decades by laboratory results and hypotheses. In the 1970s, three laboratory observations emerged that merited evaluation in clinical trial: 1) tamoxifen blocks estrogen binding to the ER so patients with ER-positive disease would be more likely to respond than those with ER-negative disease *(10);* 2) tamoxifen prevents mammary cancer in rats *(11,12)* so the drug could reduce the incidence of primary breast cancer; and 3) long-term treatment was better than short-term treatment to prevent rat mammary carcinogenesis, so longer adjuvant therapy with tamoxifen should be superior to short-term adjuvant therapy *(13–15,),* i.e., five yr of tamoxifen should be superior to 1 yr of tamoxifen. By the late 1980s, tamoxifen had been shown in the laboratory to block estrogen-stimulated breast-tumor growth but to encourage the growth of human endometrial cancer implanted in the same athymic mouse *(16,17).* The clinical question, therefore, became "are patients, who are receiving long term adjuvant tamoxifen therapy, at risk for an increased incidence of endometrial cancer?" *(17).*

In the process of evaluating the impact of translational research, it is important to establish what works, and achieves clinical progress, and what does not. A clinical trial should not be started without a strong hypothesis and the incorporation of the relevant scientific results. For convenience, the discussion in this section will be subdivided, but the end points of duration of tamoxifen usage, menopausal status, and ER status interact, so the size of a pharmacologic effect can change.

2.1. ER Status and the Duration of Tamoxifen

The ER status of the patient is highly predictive of a treatment response to long-term tamoxifen therapy. The treatment effect, based on receptor status, is summarized in Table 1. The recurrence reductions produced by tamoxifen in ER-positive patients are all highly significant ($2p < 0.00001$) and the trend between the different devation of tamoxifen is also highly significant ($\chi^2 = 45.5$, $2p < 0.00001$). By contrast, the therapeutic effect of tamoxifen on ER-negative patients is minimal. Additionally, the questions could be asked, "Does more ER give a better response to tamoxifen?" and "Does an additional progesterone receptor (PgR) assay help to improve the results with tamoxifen?" In the trials of about 5 yr of tamoxifen, the proportional reductions of recurrence were $43 \pm 5\%$ and $60 \pm 6\%$ for patients with below or above 100-femtomoles/mg cytosol ER protein. This translated to a reduction in mortality of $23 \pm 6\%$ and $36 \pm 7\%$, respectively. Clearly, one can conclude the ER is a powerful predictor of tamoxifen response; a conclusion consistent with tamoxifen's proven mechanism of action as an estrogen antagonist in breast cancer *(18).* Although PgR positive status might be thought to be of benefit, these data show that there was little additional value if the tumor was already ER-positive. A comparison of interactions is shown in Table 2. Comparing the 2,000 women who had ER-positive and PgR-negative tumors and the 7,000 women who had ER-positive and PgR-positive tumors shows there was no apparent difference in the effect of tamoxifen on either the recurrence rates or mortality rates. Additionally, the numbers were too few (602 women) in the Overview

Table 2
A Comparison of the Proportional Risk Reduction of Adjuvant Tamoxifen Therapy
Based on ER Status[a]

Patient Response	Duration of tamoxifen (yr)		
	1	2	5
Estrogen receptor-poor			
Percent reduction in recurrence rates (± SD)	6 ± 8	13 ± 5	6 ± 11
Percent reduction in death rates (± SD)	6 ± 8	7 ± 5	−3 ± 11
Estrogen receptor-positive			
Percent reduction in recurrence rates (± SD)	21 ± 5	28 ± 3	50 ± 4
Percent reduction in death rates (± SD)	14 ± 5	18 ± 4	28 ± 5

[a] Nearly 8000 patients are ER-poor and 18,000 patients are ER-positive.

Adapted with permission from ref. *(9)*.

Analysis *(9)* to allow a meaningful prediction of the benefits of tamoxifen in-patients who had an ER-negative but PgR-positive tumor.

The Overview Analysis also provides unequivocal proof of the laboratory principle *(13–15)* that longer adjuvant tamoxifen therapy was predicted to provide more benefit. The duration of therapy is extremely important for the ER-positive premenopausal woman with large amounts of circulating estrogen that can rapidly reverse the effect of short-term tamoxifen treatment. The effect of the duration of tamoxifen treatment on the reduction of recurrence rates and the reduction of death rates is shown in Fig. 1. The duration of tamoxifen is critical for the premenopausal patient, as an effect is virtually nonexistent with 1 yr of treatment compared with the benefit of 5 yr of treatment. It is also important to point out that the reduction of death rates in women under 50 yr of age and over 60 yr of age treated with 5 yr of tamoxifen is identical, at around 33% (Table 3). By contrast, the effect of tamoxifen duration on women over the age of 60 is less dramatic because 1 yr of tamoxifen is much more effective in post-menopausal women. These data are illustrated in Table 4, which shows a two- to threefold increase in the effectiveness of tamoxifen by increasing the duration from 1 to 5 yr, whereas there is a 20-fold increase in tamoxifen's effectiveness for premenopausal women with an increased duration of 1 to 5 yr (Fig. 1).

2.2. Contralateral Breast Cancer

Tamoxifen consistently reduces the risk of contralateral breast cancer (i.e., a second primary breast cancer in the other breast) independent of age *(9)*. Women have a proportional risk reduction that is 27 ± 11% or 31 ± 7% if they are below or above the age of 50, respectively. The principle "longer is better" is also true for the reduction of risk for contralateral breast cancer with adjuvant tamoxifen ther-

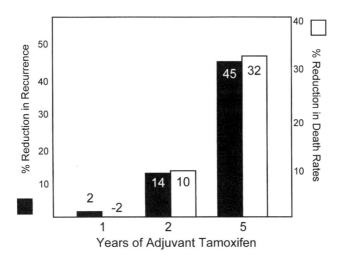

Fig. 1. The relationship between the duration of adjuvant tamoxifen therapy in ER-positive premenopausal patients and the reduction in recurrence and death rate. A longer duration of treatment has a dramatic effective on patient survival. Adapted from ref. *(9)*.

Table 3
A Comparison of the Proportional Risk Reduction of Adjuvant Tamoxifen Therapy
Based on PgR Status in Populations of ER-Positive Patients.

Patient Response	ER + PgR– (n = 2000)	ER + PgR+ (n = 7000)
Percent reduction in recurrence rates (± SD)	32 ± 6	37 ± 3
Percent reduction in death rates (± SD)	18 ± 7	16 ± 4

Adapted from ref. *(9)*.

Table 4
Proportional Risk reductions in 60–69-yr-old breast-cancer patients when the known
ER-poor Patients are Excluded[a].

Patient Response	Duration of tamoxifen (yr)		
	1	2	5
Percent reduction in recurrence rates (± SD)	26 ± 6	33 ± 4	54 ± 5
Percent reduction in death rates (± SD)	12 ± 6	12 ± 5	33 ± 6

[a] The duration of adjuvant tamoxifen is 1, 2, or 5 yr.

Adapted with permission from ref. *(9)*.

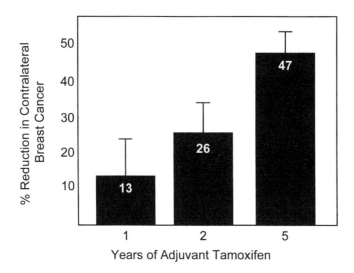

Fig. 2. The relationship between the duration of adjuvant tamoxifen and the reduction in contralateral breast cancer. A longer duration is clearly superior and the 5-yr result that produces a 47% reduction in contralateral breast cancer is equivalent to the result observed in the tamoxifen-prevention trial. Adapted from ref. *(9)*.

apy. Five years is better then 2 yr or 1 yr of adjuvant therapy with tamoxifen (Fig. 2). In fact, 1 yr of adjuvant tamoxifen does not significantly reduce the incidence of contralateral breast cancer compared to control because the standard deviation (SD) is so large (13 ± 13% reduction compared to control).

It is interesting to note that a quarter of the women allocated to the known adjuvant trials in the Overview Analysis *(9)* were Japanese, who have an annual incidence of contralateral breast cancer in patients not receiving tamoxifen of 2 per 1000 compared with 6 per 1000 elsewhere in the world. Therefore, if 5 yr of tamoxifen can halve contralateral breast cancer, then the absolute benefit for Japanese women would be 1 per 1000 and 3 per 1000 elsewhere for both young and old women. Finally, the proportional reduction in contralateral breast cancer appears to be similar in women whose initial tumor being treated with tamoxifen was ER-poor (29 ± 15%) compared with the rest of the study population (30 ± 6%). This is an important result for the potential application of tamoxifen for the reduction of contralateral breast cancer in the woman with a primary breast cancer that is unequivocally ER-negative.

2.3. Endometrial Cancer

The overall increase in the incidence of endometrial cancer in the Overview Analysis was two- to threefold *(9)*. There was no association with dose, i.e., 20 mg and 30–40 mg daily produced relative risk ratios of 2.7 and 2.4, respectively. However, there was a suggestion that 1 and 2 yr of tamoxifen doubled the incidence of endometrial cancer and 5 yr quadrupled incidence. However, the side effect is so rare (i.e., the numbers are too small) that the risk ratios are not significantly different from one another for each duration of tamoxifen. It is, however, important to state that the absolute increase in endometrial cancer was only half as big as the absolute decrease in contralateral breast cancer.

The Overview Analysis was able to identify 3,673 women who took 5 yr of adjuvant tamoxifen. With 26,400 woman-years of follow-up before breast-cancer recurrence in this group, there were seven endometrial-cancer deaths. It is estimated that during the whole first decade, the cumulative risk was 2 deaths per 1,000 women. It is important to state that the current knowledge about the association of tamoxifen with endometrial cancer will improve these statistics. In general, the reported trials were conducted without awareness of the endometrial side effects of tamoxifen. This is no longer the situation and early detection will improve mortality figures associated with tamoxifen.

3. CONCLUSIONS

Tamoxifen has been extensively tested in clinical trials of adjuvant therapy for 20 years. The Overview shows that the proportional mortality reductions were similar for women with node-positive or node-negative disease *(9)*. However, the absolute reductions in mortality were much greater in node-positive than node-negative disease. Additionally, patients with ER-positive disease have an increased reduction in death rate with longer duration of tamoxifen treatment, whereas patients who are ER-negative do not benefit from tamoxifen, regardless of the duration of therapy. The value of a long duration of treatment is most important for the premenopausal patient (Fig. 1). This latter finding is new, as the results for premenopausal women could not be ascertained with certainty in earlier Overviews *(19)*. The Oxford Overview Analysis has established the veracity of the laboratory concepts that tamoxifen would be most effective in ER-positive disease, longer duration would be more beneficial, and tamoxifen would prevent primary breast cancer, in this case contralateral disease *(9–15)*.

Overall, the absolute improvement in recurrence was greater during the first 5 yr following surgery but improvement in survival increased steadily throughout the first 10 yr. This is an important finding because the patient is clearly benefiting from tamoxifen despite stopping therapy. There is an accumulation of the tumoristatic/tumoricidal actions of tamoxifen for at least the first 5 yr of treatment, but the benefit continues after therapy stops. This is also true for the reduction in contralateral breast cancer; the breast seems to be protected so the value remains after therapy stops. This observation is extremely important for the application of tamoxifen as a preventive because a 5-yr course of tamoxifen would be expected to protect a woman from breast cancer for many years afterwards.

Finally, the risk/benefit ratio of tamoxifen therapy can be stated to be strongly in the benefit category. The risk of endometrial cancer, a concept derived from laboratory studies *(17)*, is of concern, but the benefits clearly outweigh the risks. In contrast, early concerns about the carcinogenic effects of tamoxifen in the rat liver do not translate to the clinic as there is no evidence from the Overview Analysis of an increase in either liver or colorectal cancer in-patients who take tamoxifen *(9)*.

REFERENCES

1. Beatson GT. On the treatment of inoperable cases of carcinoma of the mamma: suggestions for a new method of treatment with illustrative cases. *Lancet* 1896; ii:104–107.
2. Boyd S. On oophorectomy in cancer of the breast. *BMJ* 1900; 2:1161–1167.
3. Bloom HJG, Biesen E. Antiestrogens in the treatment of breast cancer. Value of raloxidine in 52 advanced cases. *BMJ* 1974; 2:7–14.
4. Legha SS, Carter SK. Antiestrogen in the treatment of breast cancer. *Cancer Treat Rev* 1976; 3:205–216.
5. Jordan VC. The development of tamoxifen for breast cancer therapy: a tribute to the late Arthur Walpole. *Breast Cancer Res Treat* 1988; 11:197–209.
6. Cole MP, Jones CTA, Todd IDH. A new antioestrogenic agent in late breast cancer. An early appraisal of ICI 46, 474. *Br J Cancer* 1971; 25:270–275.
7. Ward HWC. Antioestrogenic therapy for breast cancer: a trial of tamoxifen at two dose levels. *BMJ* 1973; 1:13–14.
8. Osborne CK. Tamoxifen in the treatment of breast cancer. *N Engl J Med* 1998; 339:1609–1618.
9. Early Breast Cancer Trialists' Collaborative Group Tamoxifen for early breast cancer: an overview of the randomized trials. *Lancet* 1998; 351:1451–1467.
10. Jordan VC, Jaspan T. Tamoxifen as an antitumour agent: estrogen binding as a predictive test for tumour response. *J Endocrinol* 1976; 68:453–460.
11. Jordan VC. Antitumour activity of the antiestrogen ICI 46, 474 (tamoxifen) in the dimethyl-benzanthracene (DMBA)-induced rat mammary carcinoma model. *J Steroid Biochem* 1974; 5:354.
12. Jordan VC. Effect of tamoxifen (ICI 46,474) on initiation and growth of DMBA-induced rat mammary carcinomata. *Eur J Cancer* 1976; 12:419–424.
13. Jordan VC, Dix CJ, Allen KE. The effectiveness of long term tamoxifen treatment in a laboratory model for adjuvant hormone therapy of breast cancer, in *Adjuvant Therapy of Cancer II* (Salmon SE, Jones SE, eds). Grune & Stratton New York, NY Inc., 1979, pp 19–26.
14. Jordan VC, Allen KE. Evaluation of the antitumour activity of the nonsteroidal antiestrogen monohydroxytamoxifen in the DMBA-induced rat mammary carcinoma model. *Eur J Cancer* 1980; 16:239–251.
15. Jordan VC. Laboratory studies to develop general principles for the adjuvant treatment of breast cancer with antiestrogens: problems and potential for future clinical applications. *Breast Cancer Res Treat* 1983; 3, pp 73–86.
16. Satyaswaroop PG, Zaino RJ, Mortel R. Estrogen-like effects of tamoxifen on endometrial carcinoma transplanted in nude mice. *Cancer Res* 1984; 44:4006–4010.

17. Gottardis MM, Robinson SP, Satyaswaroop PG, Jordan VC. Contrasting actions of tamoxifen on endometrial and breast tumor growth in the athymic mouse. *Cancer Res* 1988; 48:812–815.

18. MacGregor JI, Jordan VC. Basic guide to the mechanisms of antiestrogen action. *Pharm Rev* 1998; 50:151–196.

19. Early Breast Cancer Trialists' Collaborative Group. The effects of adjuvant tamoxifen and of cytotoxic chemotherapy on mortality in early breast cancer: an overview of 61 randomized trials among 28,896 women. *N Engl J Med* 1988; 319:1681–1692.

9 Clinical Utility of New Antiestrogens

Ruth M. O'Regan and William J. Gradishar

CONTENTS

INTRODUCTION
TAMOXIFEN-LIKE ANTIESTROGENS
RALOXIFENE-LIKE ANTIESTROGENS
REFERENCES

1. INTRODUCTION

Tamoxifen (Fig. 1) is the endocrine treatment of choice for all stages of hormone-responsive breast cancer. Additionally tamoxifen has been shown to reduce the incidence of cancer of the opposite breast *(1)* and has recently been demonstrated to prevent breast cancer *(2)*. Although most women with hormone-responsive advanced breast cancer respond to tamoxifen, their disease eventually becomes refractory to tamoxifen. These patients are known to respond to second-line hormonal therapies. In this chapter, we will focus on new antiestrogens that are currently available or are being developed for use following tamoxifen failure. We have divided these new agents into three groups according to their target-site specificity and molecular properties *(3);* tamoxifen-like agents, raloxifene-like agents, and pure antiestrogens.

2. TAMOXIFEN-LIKE ANTIESTROGENS

2.1. Toremifene

Toremifene (Fig. 1) is a chlorinated derivative of tamoxifen, which is currently approved in the US for the treatment of advanced breast cancer in postmenopausal women. Toremifene was initially developed in Finland and is marketed in the US under the name Farnesdon®. The recommended daily dose is 60 mg administered orally.

From: *Hormone Therapy in Breast and Prostate Cancer*
Edited by: V. C. Jordan and B. J. A. Furr © Humana Press Inc., Totowa, NJ

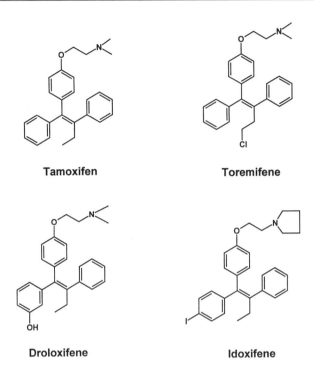

Fig. 1. Structures of tamoxifen-like antiestrogens, toremifene, droloxifene, and idoxifene, compared with tamoxifen.

2.1.1. PRECLINICAL STUDIES

At low concentrations (10^{-7} to 10^{-6}), toremifene has an estrogen antagonistic effect on the growth of ER-positive, MCF-7 cell lines, while at higher doses ($>10^{-6}$), it is oncolytic and its effects can not be reversed by estrogen *(4–7)*. Toremifene controls the growth of DMBA-induced rat mammary carcinomas *(8–11)* but appears to be three times less potent than tamoxifen *(12)*, which correlates with clinical observations.

Toremifene blocks the growth of ER-positive, MCF-7 tumors implanted in athymic mice but does not inhibit the growth of ER-negative, MDA-MB-231 tumors or mixed tumors containing both ER-positive and ER-negative cells *(13)*. Interestingly, however, toremifene has been shown to have a cytolytic effect, in vivo, on an ER-negative, glucocorticoid-sensitive mouse uterine sarcoma *(4)*. Like tamoxifen, acquired resistance to toremifene has been reported in mice implanted with MCF-7 tumors, in the form of toremifene-stimulated tumors *(14)*.

Toremifene acts as a partial estrogen antagonist on the rat uterus and results in modest increases in uterine weight when administered alone

(8,15,16). Toremifene, like tamoxifen, stimulates the growth of human endometrial tumors implanted in athymic mice *(17).* To date, there has been no increase in the incidence of liver or uterine cancers associated with toremifene use, but the drug has only been used in patients with advanced breast cancer and has not yet been evaluated in the adjuvant setting, where long-term toxicity can be assessed.

2.1.2. TOXICOLOGY

Large doses of toremifene do not produce DNA adducts in rat liver and long-term therapy does not result in liver cancers in rats *(18,19).* Large doses of toremifene can, however, promote rat liver and kidney carcinogenesis *(20).*

2.1.3. PHARMACOLOGY

Toremifene is extensively metabolized in animals and humans *(16,21).* Toremifene is metabolized in a similar manner to tamoxifen, with demethylation, deamination, and production of a more potent 4-hydroxylated derivative being the predominant pathways *(22).* The time to steady state and terminal half-life of toremifene, as measured by high-performance liquid chromatography (HPLC), are 2 wk and 5 d, respectively *(21,23–27).*

2.1.4. CLINICAL STUDIES

2.1.4.1. Phase I and II. Phase I studies demonstrated that toremifene is well-tolerated with minimal toxicity and has activity against breast cancer *(23,28,29).*

Phase II studies of toremifene in postmenopausal women with advanced breast cancer demonstrated response rates of 21–68%, at doses of 20–240 mg daily, used as a first-line therapy (Table 1) *(30–35).* Toxicity was mild, with approx 50% of patients reporting hot flashes *(33).* Responses were seen in soft tissue and visceral sites and did not appear to be related to level of ER concentrations *(30).* Median duration of response was approx 14 mo *(33).*

2.1.5. DOSE-RESPONSE TRIALS

In one clinical trial, patients with advanced breast cancer were treated with toremifene at a dose of 240 mg daily *(34).* An objective response rate of 68%, with 26% complete response (CR) rate, was reported suggesting that high doses of toremifene may improve outcome *(34).* However, a recent clinical trial, which randomized patients with untreated, advanced breast cancer to tamoxifen (20 mg/d) or toremifene (60 mg or 200 mg/d), reported no statistically significant difference in response rate between the toremifene arms *(36).* In addition, another small randomized trial reported a worse response rate with 240 mg daily compared with 60 mg daily of toremifene *(37).*

Table 1

Phase II Trials of Toremifene in Postmenopausal Women with Advanced,
Previously Untreated Breast Cancer

Dose of toremifene (mg qd)	Response rate (%)			References
	CR	PR	SD	
20	21	0	26	Valavaara (31)
60	54	17	26	Valavaara (30)
	48	26	26	Gunderson (33)
	50	25	42	Modig (35)
	45	15	35	Valavaara (32)
240	68	26		Hietenen (34)

CR, complete response; PR, partial response; SD, stable disease.

Table 2

Clinical Trials Comapring Toremifene with Tamoxifen in Postmenopausal Women with Advanced Breast Cancer

Dose/schedule (mg qd)	Response rate (%)		References
	RR	CR	
TOR 60	50	0	Konstantinova (37)
TOR 240	35	6	
TAM 40	36	1	
TOR 40	26	14	Nomura (38)
TAM 20	28	5	
TOR 240	29	3	Stenbygaard (39)
TAM 40	42	16	
TAM 20	19	5.8	Hayes (36)
TOR 60	21	5.6	
TOR 200	23	5.6	

TOR, toremifene; TAM, tamoxifen; RR, response rate; CR, complete response; qd, daily.

2.1.6. TOREMIFENE VS TAMOXIFEN

Three small, randomized trials have compared tamoxifen to toremifene as
first-line treatment for advanced breast cancer (Table 2) (37–39). One trial noted
similar response rates for tamoxifen (20 mg/d) compared with toremifene (40
mg/d) (38). A comparison of tamoxifen (40 mg/d) with toremifene (60 mg or 240
mg/d), reported superior response rates for toremifene 60 mg daily compared
with the other treatment arms (37). In contrast, another trial reported inferior

Table 3
Clinical Trials of Toremifene in Patients with Advanced,
Tamoxifen-Refractory Breast Cancer

Dose/schedule (mg qd)	Response rate (%)		References
	RR	CR	
200	33	0	Ebbs (40)
60	25	0	Hindy (41)
300	33	0	
240	0		Jonsson (42)
120	14	0	Asaishi (43)
120	4	2	Pyrhonen (44)
200	5	2	Vogel (45)

RR, response rate; CR, complete response; qd, daily.

response rates for toremifene, 240 mg daily, compared with tamoxifen, 40 mg daily (39). However, these trials were too small to be statistically significant and, therefore, no firm conclusions can be drawn.

An international trial randomized 648 previously untreated patients with advanced breast cancer to tamoxifen 20 mg daily or toremifene 60 mg or 200 mg daily (36). There was no statisically significant difference between the three arms with respect to response rate, median survival, or time to disease progression (36). In addition, quality-of-life assessments were similar between the three arms, although less nausea was observed in the toremifene-treated patients (36). Therefore, it appears that toremifene is a suitable alternative to tamoxifen as first-line treatment of hormone-responsive, advanced breast cancer.

2.1.7. TOREMIFENE AFTER TAMOXIFEN

Response rates to toremifene following tamoxifen failure in Phase II trials are generally low, suggesting that toremifene exhibits cross-resistance to tamoxifen (Table 3) (40–45). In the largest of these trials, patients who had been heavily pretreated for advanced breast cancer received toremifene 200 mg daily following tamoxifen failure (45). A response rate of 5%, with a 2% CR rate was reported, suggesting cross-resistance between the two agents (45).

2.1.8. TOREMIFENE AND ER-NEGATIVE TUMORS

Toremifene has been reported to have a cytolytic effect on the growth of an ER-negative mouse uterine sarcoma (4) and therefore, a mechanism of action independent of the ER has been postulated. In one small trial of nine patients with ER-unknown, tamoxifen-resistant advanced breast cancer, a 33%

response rate was reported for toremifene at a dose of 200 mg daily *(40)*. However, the Cancer and Leukemia Group B (CALGB), reported a 0% response rate in 20 patients with ER-negative, moderately pretreated advanced breast cancer treated with toremifene 400 mg daily *(46)*. This suggests that the predominant mode of action of toremifene is through the ER.

2.1.9. EFFECTS ON BONES AND LIPIDS

Similar to tamoxifen, toremifene does not appear to increase bone loss in postmenopausal women *(47)*. A recent study suggests that the beneficial effects of toremifene on bones can be augmented by concurrent bisphosphonate treatment *(47)*.

Toremifene has similar effects to tamoxifen on the lipid profile, resulting in a reduction of low-density lipoprotein (LDL) and total cholesterol *(47)*. In contrast to tamoxifen, however, toremifene appears to increase high-density lipoprotein (HDL) cholesterol *(47)*.

2.2. Droloxifene

Droloxifene (Fig. 1) or 3-hydroxytamoxifen was originally developed in Germany and later in Japan. Despite being previously tested in metastatic breast cancer, is currently being developed as an osteoporosis agent.

2.2.1. PRECLINICAL STUDIES

Compared with tamoxifen, both droloxifene and N-desmethyldroloxifene bind to MCF-7 cells with 10 times greater avidity *(48,49)*. Droloxifene arrests estrogen-induced cell replication *(50–52)* in G_0/G_1 *(53)*. Droloxifene does not inhibit the growth of ER-negative breast-cell lines and therefore, its mode of action appears to be predominantly through the ER *(52)*.

Although droloxifene has antiestrogenic effects in the immature rat uterine-weight test, it causes a partial increase in uterine wet weight when administered alone *(50,54)*. The partial estrogen agonist effects of droloxifene are slightly less potent than those of tamoxifen *(51,54)* but result in maintenance of bone density in the ovariectomized rat *(55)*. Droloxifene inhibits the growth of the rat mammary tumor-DMBA-*(50,56)* and NMU-*(57)* induced rat mammary tumors. Droloxifene inhibits only the growth of ER-positive tumors in athymic mice *(52,54)*.

2.2.2. TOXICOLOGY

Droloxifene, does not produce DNA adducts or hepatocellular carcinomas in rats. In comparison, tamoxifen, administered at a similar dose for 2 yr, resulted in 100% incidence of hepatocellular carcinomas *(53)*. There was a 2% incidence of hepatocellular carcinomas in rats administered droloxifene at very high doses for 2 yr *(53)*.

Table 4
Clinical Trials Utilizing Different Doses
of Droloxifene in Advanced Breast Cancer[a]

Dose of droloxifene (mg)	Response rate (%)	References
20	30	Raushning (59)
	17	Bellmunt (60)
	14	Abe (62)
40	47	Raushning (59)
	30	Bellmunt (60)
	5	Abe (62)
100	44	Raushning (59)
	31	Bellmunt (60)
	17	Abe (62)
	15	Haarstad (64)
	60/80	Ahlemann (61)
120	15	Abe (63)

[a] Patients received droloxifene at 100 mg
every 2 or 3 d.

2.2.3. PHARMACOLOGY

Unlike tamoxifen, droloxifene is rapidly absorbed and excreted and does not seem to accumulate. Steady-state levels are achieved within 5 h (58). Droloxifene is metabolized to N-desmethyldroloxifene and 4-methoxydroloxifene and both free and glucuronide conjugates of the parent drug and metabolites can be detected in the blood (58).

2.2.4. CLINICAL STUDIES

Droloxifene has been primarily tested in patients with advanced, pretreated breast cancer. Results of phase II trials are shown in Table 4 (59–65).

In the largest study, 369 postmenopausal patients, with metastatic, inoperable recurrent or primary locoregional breast cancer, were randomized to receive 20, 40, or 100 mg daily, with response rates of 30, 47, and 44%, respectively (59). In a similar study, in which 68% of patients were pretreated, overall response rates of 17, 30, and 31% and complete response rates of 0, 3, and 10%, were noted in patients treated with droloxifene at doses of 20 mg, 40 and 100 mg, respectively (60). Overall response rates vary from 15–47% in these Phase II trials and there does not appear to be a dose-response effect. However, in one study, 10 patients with advanced breast cancer, 40% of whom were pretreated, experienced response rates of 60 and 80%, following treatment with droloxifene at doses of 100 mg every 2 or 3 d, respectively (61).

In all studies, droloxifene was well-tolerated with gastrointestinal symptoms and hot flashes being the most commonly reported symptoms.

2.3. Idoxifene

Idoxifene (Fig. 1) was initially developed by the Cancer Research Campaign Laboratory in the UK and is currently being developed by SmithKline Beecham in the UK.

2.3.1. Preclinical Studies

Compared with tamoxifen, idoxifene binds to the ER with two times greater affinity, resulting in a small increase in its ability to inhibit the growth of ER-positive, MCF-7 breast-cancer cells, in vitro (66). Unlike tamoxifen, idoxifene is not metabolized to a 4-hydroxy derivative and therefore is a less potent antiestrogen (67). Idoxifene has less potent antiestrogenic activity than tamoxifen in immature rat uterine tests, but has less uterotropic activity than tamoxifen when administered alone (66).

Idoxifene inhibits the growth NMU-induced rat mammary carcinomas, at a dose range of 1–2 mg/kg (66). Higher doses than tamoxifen are required to inhibit tumor growth in this model, since idoxifene is not metabolically activated (66).

2.3.2. Toxicology

Idoxifene has not been evaluated as a rat liver carcinogen. However, tamoxifen's genotoxic effects on rat liver are likely due to its metabolites (68). As idoxifene is not metabolically activated, it is anticipated that it will not result in rat liver tumors.

2.3.3. Pharmacology

Preliminary studies in the laboratory demonstrate no metabolism of idoxifene over 48 h following administration (69). The most likely metabolite of idoxifene, 4-hydroxyidoxifene, has not been detected clinically. Idoxifene has an initial half-life of 15 h and a terminal half-life three times that of tamoxifen (70).

2.3.4. Clinical Studies

One clinical study involving 20 patients, with pretreated, advanced breast cancer treated with idoxifene has been reported (71). Idoxifene was administered at doses of 10, 20, 40, or 60 mg daily. The overall response rate was 14%, with no complete responses and a further 29% of patients experiencing stable disease (71). Toxicity was mild and not dose-related, with nausea, anorexia, and fatigue the most commonly reported symptoms.

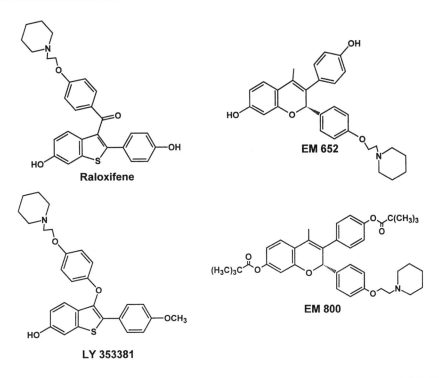

Fig. 2. Structures of raloxifene-like antiestrogens, LY 353,381, EM 800, and EM 652 (the active metabolite of EM 800), compared with raloxifene.

3. RALOXIFENE-LIKE ANTIESTROGENS

3.1. Raloxifene

Raloxifene (Fig. 2) is a selective estrogen-receptor modulator (SERM), which has recently been approved for the prevention of osteoporosis in post-menopausal women.

3.1.1. PRECLINICAL STUDIES

Raloxifene has been shown to have high affinity for the estrogen receptor and be a potent antiestrogen, as well as having little uterotrophic activity in the rodent uterus *(72)*. Raloxifene has been shown to preserve bone density in oophorectomized rats *(73–75)*. Raloxifene has antitumor activity against breast-cancer cells in vitro *(76)* and prevents rat mammary tumorigenesis *(77)*.

3.1.2. CLINICAL STUDIES

Raloxifene is not planned for use as a breast-cancer treatment. However, one small study demonstrated a 30% response rate in pretreated patients with advanced breast cancer *(78)*. In a large randomized trial where postmenopausal women were randomized to raloxifene or placebo, raloxifene significantly maintained bone density compared with placebo *(79)* and on the basis of this study, the drug is now approved for the prevention of osteoporosis in post-menopausal women. Additionally, this trial demonstrated that raloxifene, like tamoxifen, reduced circulating LDL cholesterol levels. Unlike tamoxifen, there was no significant difference in uterine thickness between the raloxifene-treated patients and the placebo group *(79)*.

Recent data suggest that raloxifene, like tamoxifen, may prevent breast cancer, through its antiestrogenic effects on the breast *(80,81)*. One of these studies actually noted a decrease in the rate of endometrial cancer in the raloxifene-treated patients compared with patients who received placebo *(81)*. On the basis of this data, the next large prevention study will randomize post-menopausal women at risk of breast cancer to tamoxifen or raloxifene.

3.2. LY 353,381

LY 353,381.HCL (Fig. 2) is a benzothiophene analog with selective estrogen receptor (ER) modulator activity similar to, but not identical with raloxifene, which is being developed for the treatment of breast cancer.

3.2.1. PRECLINICAL STUDIES

LY 353,381.HCL contains an ether linked basic side chain, which makes it a highly potent estrogen antagonist, and a methoxy group, which increases oral bioavailability *(82,83)*. In rats, LY 353,381.HCL prevents the ovariectomy-induced increase in body weight and serum cholesterol levels, in a dose-dependent manner, with efficacy similar to estrogen and raloxifene. *(84)*. In the rat uterus, LY 353,381.HCL has a marginal effect on uterine weight compared with ovariectomized controls *(84)*. This observation is similar to raloxifene, but opposite to that seen with estrogen. LY 353,381.HCL has little or no stimulatory effect on the rat endometrium, as demonstrated by no change in uterine epithelial-cell height *(84)*. LY 353,381.HCL prevents tibial bone loss and preserves the strength of the femoral neck in ovariectomized rats *(84)*. In uteri of immature rats treated with estrogen, LY 353,381.HCL antagonized the estrogen-induced elevation in uterine weight comparable to vehicle-dosed control levels *(84)*. Therefore, although similar to raloxifene, LY353,381 is more potent, has minimal uterine stimulation and preserves cortical bone, which may offer a therapeutic advantage over raloxifene in postmenopausal women.

3.2.2. CLINICAL STUDIES

To date, LY 353,381.HCL has been evaluated in one Phase I clinical trial *(85)*. In 32 patients with refractory metastatic breast cancer, there was one minor response and nine patients had stable disease *(85)*.

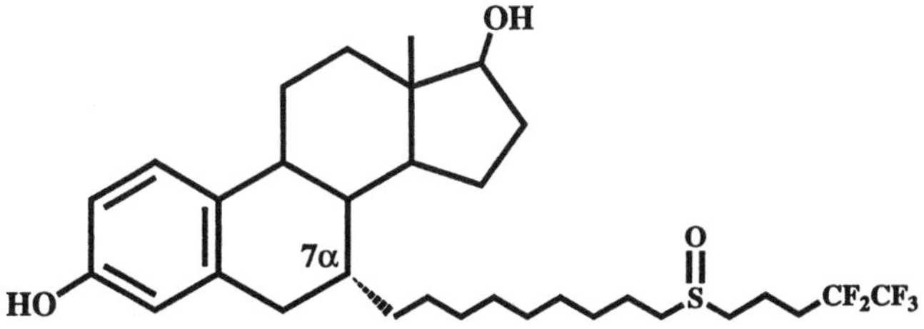

Fig. 3. Structure of the pure antiestrogen, ICI 182,780.

3.3. EM 800

EM 800 (or EM 652) (Fig. 2) is a SERM that is being developed as a treatment for breast cancer. Recent data suggest that EM 800 is a raloxifene-like agent rather that a pure antiestrogen.

3.3.1. PRECLINICAL STUDIES

EM 800, administered orally, acts as an antiestrogen on the breast, both inhibiting the growth of hormone-responsive breast cancer, in vitro *(86)* and in vivo *(87),* and preventing the growth of breast cancer in rats *(88).*

EM 800 appears act as a pure antiestrogen on the uterus. In both intact and ovariectomized mice, EM 800 administered for 24 wk did not result in estrogenic effects on the uterus or vagina *(89).* Additionally, in vitro studies using EM 652 (the active metabolite of EM 800) demonstrate that the drug is a potent antiestrogen in human endometrial cells, resulting in no increase in alkaline phosphatase activity even in the presence of estrogen *(86).* EM 800, like raloxifene, does not dramatically reduce bone density in rats *(82).*

3.3.2. CLINICAL STUDIES

EM 800 is currently being evaluated in a large randomized trial in patients with tamoxifen-refractory metastatic breast cancer who will receive EM 800 or anastrozole. No results are available from this trial.

3.4. Pure Antiestrogens

The pure antiestrogens were originally developed in the 1980s in the UK. One of the pure antiestrogens, ICI 182,780 (Faslodex) (Fig. 3), is currently being evaluated in two large, international, randomized trials. In the first trial patients with tamoxifen-refractory, metastatic breast cancer are randomized to anastrozole or Faslodex. In the second trial, patients with tamoxifen-naïve, metastatic breast cancer are randomized to tamoxifen or Faslodex.

3.4.1. PRECLINICAL STUDIES

ICI 182,780 competively blocks estrogen binding to the ER *(90)*, but has, additionally, been noted to cause a rapid loss of ER, in vitro *(91,92)*. ICI 182,780 inhibits the growth of ER-positive, MCF-7 breast-cancer cells *(90)*, more completely than tamoxifen *(93)*, and, like tamoxifen, does not inhibit the growth of ER-negative breast-cancer cells.

ICI 182,780 acts as a complete antiestrogen in the immature rat. ICI 182,780 has been demonstrated to inhibit the partial estrogen-like effects of tamoxifen on the rat uterus *(90)*. The pure antiestrogens inhibit the growth of tamoxifen-stimulated tumors in athymic mice for prolonged periods, although growth eventually occurs *(94,95)*. Additionally, in preliminary studies, ICI 182,780-resistant tumors have been developed *(95)*. ICI 182,780 inhibits the growth of tamoxifen-stimulated endometrial cancer in athymic mice *(17)*. In rats with established DMBA-induced breast cancers, the combination of a luteinizing hormone releasing hormone (LH-RH) analog and the pure antiestrogen, ICI 164,384, results in a more rapid decrease in tumor size and uterine weight than with the LH-RH analog alone *(96)*.

3.4.2. TOXICOLOGY

There are no proven reports of genotoxicity or carcinogenesis with ICI 182,780. ICI 182,780, as would be expected, results in a reduction of cancellous bone in rats *(97)*.

3.4.3. PHARMACOLOGY

ICI 182,780 must be given by subcutaneous or intramuscular injection due to poor oral bioavailabilty.

3.4.4. CLINICAL STUDIES

In a Phase II clinical study of postmenopausal women with advanced breast cancer who had failed tamoxifen, treated with ICI 182,780 each month by intramuscular injection, there was a 69% overall response rate *(98)*. The treatment was tolerated without major side-effects, the main toxicity being some pain and redness at the injection site. There is currently a large international study ongoing where postmenopausal women with advanced, tamoxifen-refractory breast cancer are randomized to ICI 182,780 or anastrozole. Preliminary results of this study should be available in the near future.

REFERENCES

1. Early Breast Cancer Trialists' Collaborative Group. Tamoxifen for early breast cancer: an overview of the randomized trials. *Lancet* 1998; 351:1451–1467.
2. Fisher B, Costantino JP, Wickerham DL, Redmond CK, Kavanah M, Cronin WM, et al. Tamoxifen for prevention of breast cancer: report of the National Surgical Adjuvant breast and Bowel Project P-1 Study. *J Natl Cancer Inst* 1998; 90:1371–1388.

3. Schafer JI, Liu H, Tonetti DA, Jordan VC. The interaction of raloxifene and the active metabolite of the antiestrogen EM-800 (SC 5705) with the human estrogen receptor (ER). *Cancer Res* 1999; 59:4308–4313.

4. Kangas L, Niemenen A.-L, Blanco G, Gronroos M, Kallio S, Karjalainen A, Perilla M, Soderwall M, Tiovola R. A new triphenylethylene compound Fc-1157a II antitumor effects. *Cancer Chemo Pharm* 1986; 17:109–113.

5. Warri AM, Huovinon RL, Laine AM, Mairtikainen PM, Harkonen PL. Apoptosis in toremifene growth inhibition of human breast cancer cells in vivo and in vitro. *J Natl Cancer Inst* 1993; 85:1412–1418.

6. Grenman RL, Laine KM, Klemi PJ, Grenman S, Hayashida DJ, Joensuu H. Effect of the antiestrogen toremifene on growth of human mammary carcinoma cell line MCF-7. *J Cancer Res Clin Oncol* 1991; 117:223–2268.

7. Robinson SP, Goldstein D, Witt PL, Borden EC, Jordan VC. Inhibition of hormone dependent and independent breast cancer growth in vivo and in vitro with the antiestrogen toremifene and recombinant human interferon α2. *Breast Cancer Res Treat* 1990; 15:95–101.

8. DiSalle E, Zaccheo T, Ornati G. Anioestrogenic and antitumor properties of the new tripphenylethylene derivative toremifene in the rat. *J Steroid Biochem* 1990; 36:203–206.

9. Huovinen R, Warri A, Collan Y. Mitotic activity, apoptosis and TRPM-2 messenger RNA expression in DMBA-induced rat mammary carcinoma treated with the antiestrogen toremifene. *Intl J Cancer* 1993; 55:685–691.

10. Huovinen R, Kellokumpu-Lehtinen PL, Collan Y. Evaluating the response to antiestrogen toremifene treatment in DMBA-induced rat mammary carcinoma *Intl J Exp Pathol* 1994; 75:257–263.

11. Huovinen RL, Alanen KA, Collan Y. Cell proliferation in dimethylbenz(A) anthracene-induced rat mammary carcinoma treated with antiestrogen toremifene. *Acta Oncol* 1995; 34:479–485.

12. Robinson SP, Mauel DA, Jordan VC. Antitumor actions of toremifene in the 7,12 dimethyl-benzanthracene (DMBA)-induced rat mammary tumor model. *Eur J Cancer* 1988; 24:1817–1821.

13. Robinson SP, Jordan VC. Antiestrogen action of toremifene on hormone-dependent, independent and heterogeneous breast tumor growth in the athymic mouse. *Cancer Res* 1989; 49:1758–1762.

14. Osborne CK, Jarman M, McCague R, Coronado EB, Hilsenbeck SG, Wakeling AE. The importance of tamoxifen metabolism in tamoxifen-stimulated breast tumor growth. *Cancer Chemo Pharmacol* 1994; 34:89–95.

15. Kangas L. Review of the pharmacological properties of toremifene. *J Steroid Biochem* 1990; 36:191–195.

16. Kangas L. Biochemical and pharmacological effects of toremifene metabolites. *Cancer Chemo Pharmacol* 1990; 27:8–12.

17. O'Regan RM, Cisneros A, England GM, MacGregor JI, Muenzner HD, Assikis V, et al. Growth characteristics of human endometrial cancer transplanted in athymic mice and treated with new antiestrogens, toremifene and ICI 182,780. *J Natl Cancer Inst* 1998; 90:1552–1558.

18. Hard GC, Iatropoulos MJ, Jordan K, Radi K, Kaltenberg OP, Imondi AR, Williams GM. Major differences in the hepatocarcinogenicity and DNA adduct forming ability between toremifene and tamoxifen in female Crl;CD (BR) rats. *Cancer Res* 1993; 53:4534–4541.

19. Hirsimaki P, Hirsimaki Y, Nieminen L, Payne BJ. Tamoxifen induces hepatocellular carcinoma in rat liver: A 1 year study with 2 antiestrogens. *Arch Toxicol* 1993; 67:49–59.

20. Dragan YP, Vaughan J, Jordan VC, Pitot HC. Comparison of tamoxifen and toremifene on liver and kidney tumor promotion in female rats. *Carcinogenesis* 1995; 16:2733–2741.

21. Antilla M, Valvaara R, Kivinen S, Maanpaa J. Pharmacokinetics of toremifene. *J Steroid Biochem* 1990; 36:249–252.

22. Jordan VC. Biochemical pharmacology of antiestrogen action. *Pharmacol Rev* 1984; 36:245–276.

23. Wiebe VJ, Benz C, Shemano I, Cadman TB, DeGregorio MW. Pharmacokinetics of toremifene and its metabolites in patients with advanced breast cancer. *Cancer Chemo Pharmacol* 1990; 25:247–251.

24. Webster LK, Crinis NA, Stokes KH, Bishop JF. High performance liquid chromatographic method for the determination of toremifene and its major human metabolites. *J Chromatogr B Biomed Appl* 1991; 565:482–487.

25. Berthou F, Dreano Y. High performance liquid chromatographic analysis of tamoxifen, toremifene and their major human metabolites. *J Chromatogr B Biomed Appl* 1993; 616:117–127.

26. Bishop J, Muray R, Webster L, Pitt P, Stokes K, Fennessy A, Olveri I, Leber G. Phase I clinical and pharmacokinetics study of high dose toremifene in postmenopausal patients with advanced breast cancer. *Cancer Chemo Pharmacol* 1992; 30:174–178.

27. Kohler PC, Hamm JF, Wiebe VJ, DeGregorio MW, Shemano I, Tormey DC. Phase I study of the tolerance and pharmacokinetics of toremifene in patients with cancer. *Breast Cancer Res Treat* 1991; 16:19–26.

28. Hamm JT, Tormey DC, Kohler PC, Haller D, Green M, Shemano I. Phase I study of toremifene in patients with advanced cancer. *J Clin Oncol* 1991; 9:2036–2041.

29. Tominga T, Abe O, Izuo M, Nomurga UT. A phase I study of toremifene. *Breast Cancer Res Treat* 1990; 16:27.

30. Valavaara R, Pyrhonen S, Heikkinen M, Rissanen P, Blanco G, Tholix E, et al. Toremifene, a new antiestrogenic treatment of advanced breast cancer Phase II study. *Eur J Cancer* 1988; 24:785–790.

31. Valavaara R, Pyrhonen S. Low-dose toremifene in the treatment of estrogen receptor-positive advanced breast cancer in postmenopausal women. *Curr Ther Res* 1989; 46:966–973.

32. Valavaara R. Phase II experience with toremifene in the treatment of ER-positive breast cancer of postmenopausal women. *Cancer Invest* 1990; 8:275–276.

33. Gunderson S. Toremifene, a new antiestrogenic compound in the treatment of advanced breast cancer. Phase II study. *Eur J Cancer* 1990; 24A:785–790.

34. Hietanen T, Baltina D, Johansson R, Numminen S, Hakala T, Helle L, Valavaara R. High dose toremifene (240mg daily) is effective as first line hormonal treatment in advanced breast cancer: an ongoing phase II multicenter Finnish-Latvian cooperative study. *Breast Cancer Res Treat* 1990; 16:37–40.

35. Modig H, Borgstrom M, Nilsson I, Westman G. Phase II clinical study of toremifene in patients with metastatic breast cancer. *J Steroid Biochem* 1990; 36:235–236.

36. Hayes DF, Van Zyl JA, Hacking A, Goedhals L, Bezwoda WR, Maillard JA, Jones SE, Vogel CL, Berus RF, Shemano I. Randomized comparison of tamoxifen and two separate doses of toremifene in postmenopausal patients with metastatic breast cancer. *J Clin Oncol* 1995; 113:2556–2566.

37. Konstantinova MM, Gershanovich ML. Results of comparative clinical evaluation of antiestrogens toremifene and tamoxifen in locally advanced and disseminated breast cancer [in Russian]. *Vopr Onkol* 1990; 36:1182–1186.

38. Nomura Y, Tominaga T, Abe O, Izuo M, Ogawa N. Clinical evaluation of NK 22 (toremifene citrate) in advanced or recurrent breast cancer: a comparative study by a double blind method with tamoxifen [in Japanese]. *Gan to Kagaku Ryoho* 1993; 20:247–258.

39. Stenbygaard LE, Herrstedt J, Thomsen JF, Svendsen KR, Engelholm SA, Dombernowsky P. Toremifene and tamoxifen in advanced breast cancer: a double-blind cross-over trial. *Breast Cancer Res Treat* 1993; 25:57–63.

40. Ebbs SR, Roberts J, Baum M. Response to toremifene (Fc-1157a) therapy in tamoxifen failed patients with breast cancer. Preliminary communication. *J Steroid Biochem* 1990; 36:239.

41. Hindy I, Juhos E, Szanto J, Szamel I. Effect of toremifene in breast cancer patients. Preliminary communication. *J Steroid Biochem* 1990; 36:225–226.

42. Jonsson PE, Malmberg M, Bergljung L, Ingvar C. Phase II study of high dose toremifene in advanced breast cancer progressing during tamoxifen treatment. *Anticancer Res* 1991; 11:873–876.

43. Asaishi K, Tominaga T, Abe O, Izuo M, Nomula Y. Efficacy and safety of high dose NK 622 (toremifene citrate) in tamoxifen failed patients with breast cancer [in Japanese]. *Gan to Kagaku Ryoho* 1993; 20:91–99.

44. Pyrrhonen S, Valavaara R, Vuorinen J, Hajba A. High dose toremifene in advanced breast cancer resistant to or relapsed during tamoxifen treatment. *Breast Cancer Res Treat* 1994; 29:223–228.

45. Vogel CL, Shemano I, Schoenfelder J, Gams RA, Green MR. Multicenter phase II efficacy trial of toremifene in tamoxifen refractory patients with advanced breast cancer. *J Clin Oncol* 1993; 11:345–350.

46. Perry JJ, Berry DA, Weiss RB, Hayes DM, Duggan DB, Henderson IC. High dose toremifene for estrogen and progesterone receptor negative metastatic breast cancer. A phase II trial of the Cancer and Leukemia Group B (CALGB). *Breast Cancer Res Treat* 1995; 36:35–40.

47. Saarto T, Blomquist C, Ehnholm C, Taskinen MR, Elomaa I. Antiatherogenic effects of adjuvant antiestrogens: A randomized trial comparing the effects of tamoxifen and toremifene on plasma lipid levels in postmenopausal women with node-positive breast cancer. *J Clin Oncol* 1996; 14:429–433.

48. Roos WK, Oeze L, Loser R, Eppenberger U. Antiestrogen action of 3-hydroxytamoxifen in the human breast cancer cell line MCF-7f. *J Natl Cancer Inst* 1993; 71:55–59.

49. Loser R, Seibel K, Eppenberger U. No loss of estrogenic and antiestrogenic activity after demethylation of droloxifene (3-OH tamoxifen). *Intl J Cancer* 1985; 36:701–701.

50. Loser R, Seibel K, Roos W, Eppenberger U. In vivo and in vitro antiestrogenic action of 3-hydroxytamoxifen, tamoxifen and 4-hydroxytamoxifen. *Eur J Cancer Clin Oncol* 1985; 21:900–985.

51. Eppenberger U, Wosikowski K, Kung W. Pharmacologic and biologic properties of droloxifene, a new antiestrogen. *Am J Clin Oncol* 1991; 14:s5–s14.

52. Kawamura I, Mizota T, Lacey E, Tanaka Y, Manda T, Shimomura K, Kohsaka M. Pharmacologic and biologic properties of droloxifene, a new antiestrogen. *Japn J Pharmacol* 1993; 63:27–34.

53. Hasman M, Rattel B, Loser R. Preclinical data for droloxifene. *Cancer Lett* 1994; 84:101–116.

54. Wosikowski K, Kung W, Hasmann M, Loser R, Eppenberger U. Inhibition of growth factor activated proliferation by antiestrogens and effects of early gene expression of MCF-7 cells. *Int J Cancer* 1993; 53:290–297.

55. Ke HZ, Simmons HA, Pirie CM, Crawford DT, Thompson DD. Droloxifene, a new estrogen antagonist/agonist, prevents bone loss in ovariectomized rats. *Endocrinology* 1995; 136:2435–2441.

56. Kawamura I, Mizota T, Kondo N, Shimomura L, Kohsaka M. Antitumor effects of droloxifene, a new antiestrogen drug against 7,12 dimethyl (a) anthracene-induced mammary tumor in rats. *Japn J Pharmacol* 1991; 57:215–224.

57. Winterfeld G, Hauff P, Grolich M, Arnold W, Fichtner I, Staab HJ. Investigations of droloxifene and other hormonal manipulations on N-nitrosomethlurea-induced rat mammary tumours. *J Cancer Res Clin Oncol* 1992; 119:91–96.

58. Grill HJ, Pollow K. Pharmacokinetics of droloxifene and its metabolites in breast cancer patients. *Am J Clin Oncol* 1991; 14:s21–s29.
59. Raushning W, Pritchard KI. Droloxifene, a new antiestrogen: its role in metastatic breast cancer. *Breast Cancer Res Treat* 1994; 31:83–94.
60. Bellmunt J, Sole L. European early phase II dose finding study of droloxifene in advanced breast cancer. *Am J Clin Oncol* 1991; 14:536–539.
61. Ahlemann LM, Staab HJ, Loser R, Seibel K, Huber HJ. Inhibition of growth of human cancer by intermittent exposure to the antiestrogen droloxifene. *Tumor Diagn Ther* 1988; 9:41–46.
62. Abe O, Enomote K, Fujiwara K, Izuo M, Iino Y, Tominaga T, et al. Phase I study of FK 435. *Japn J Cancer Clin* 1990; 36:903–913.
63. Abe O, Enomote K, Fugiwara K, Izumo M, Iino Y, Tominaga T, et al. Japanese early phase II study of droloxifene in the treatment of advanced bresat cancer. *Am J Clin Oncol* 1991; 14:540–541.
64. Haarstad H, Gundersen S, Wist E, Raabe N, Mella O, Kvinnsland S. Droloxifene: a new anti-estrogen phase II study in advanced breast cancer. *Acta Oncol* 1992; 31:425–428.
65. Buzdar AU, Kau S, Hortobagyi GN, Theriault RL, Booser D, Holmes FA, et al. Phase I trial of droloxifene in patients with metastatic breast cancer. *Cancer Chemother Pharmacol* 1994; 33:313–316.
66. Chander SK, McCague R, Lugmani Y, Newton C, Dowsett M, Jarman M, Coombes RC. Pyrrolidino-4-iodotamoxifen and 4-iodotamoxifen, new analogues of the antiestrogen tamoxifen for the treatment of breast cancer. *Cancer Res* 1991; 51:5851–5858.
67. McCague R, Parr IB, Haynes BP. Metabolism of the 4 iodo derivative of tamoxifen by isolated rat hepatocytes. Demonstration that the iodine atom reduces metabolic conversion and identification of four metabolites. *Biochem Pharmacol* 1990; 40:2277–2283.
68. White INH, deMatteis F, Davies A, Smith LL, Crofton-Sleigh C, Venitt S, Hewer A, Phillips DH. Genotoxic potential of tamoxifen and analogues in female Fischer 344/n rats, DBA/2 and C57BL/6 mice and human MCL-5 cells. *Carcinogenesis* 1992; 13:2197–2203.
69. Carnochan P, Trivedi M, Young H, Eccles S, Potter G, Haynes B, Ott R. Biodistribution and kinetics of pyrrolidino-4-iodotamoxifen and 4-iodotamoxifen, new analogues of the antiestrogen, tamoxifen, in the treatment of breast cancer. *J Nuclear Biol Med* 1994; 38:96–98.
70. Jordan VC, Gradishar WJ. Molecular mechanisms and future uses of antiestrogens. *Mole Aspects Med* 1997; 18:168–247.
71. Coombes RC, Haynes BP, Dowsett M, Quigley M, English J, Judson IR, Griggs LJ, Potter GA, McCague R, Jarman M. Idoxifene: report of a phase I study in patients with metastatic disease. *Cancer Res* 1995; 55:1070–1074.
72. Black LJ, Jones CD, Falcone JF. Antagonism of estrogen action with a new benzothiophene-derived antiestrogen. *Life Sci* 1983; 32:1031–1036.
73. Black LJ, Sato M, Rowley ER, Magee DE, Bekele A, Williams DC, et al. Raloxifene (LY 139481 HCL) prevents bone loss and reduces serum cholesterol without causing uterine hypertrophy in ovariectomized rats. *J Clin Invest* 1994; 93:63–69.
74. Jordan VC, Phelps E, Lindgren JU. Effects of antiestrogens on bone in castrated and intact female rats. *Breast Cancer Res Treat* 1987; 10:31–35.
75. Sato M, Kim J, Short LL, Szemenda CW, Bryant HU. Longitudinal and cross-setional analysis of raloxifene effects on tibiae from ovariectomized rats. *J Pharmacol Exp Ther* 1995; 272:1251–1259.
76. Scholl M, Huff KK, Lippman ME. Antiestrogenic effects of LY117018 in MCF-7 cells. *Endocrinology* 1983; 113:611–617.
77. Gottardis MM, Jordan VC. The antitumor action of keoxifene and tamoxifen in the N-nitrosomethylurea-induced rat mammary carcinoma model. *Cancer Res* 1987; 47:4020–4024.

78. Gradishar W, Glusman J, Lu Y, Vogel C, Cohen FJ, Sledge GW, Jr. Effects of high dose raloxifene in selected patients with advanced breast carcinoma. *Cancer* 2000; 88:2047–2053.

79. Delmas PD, Bjarnason NH, Mitlak BH, Ravoux AC, Shah AS, Huster WJ, et al. Effects of raloxifene on bone mineral density, serum cholesterol concentrations, and uterine endometrium in postmenopausal women. *N Engl J Med* 1997; 337:1641–1647.

80. Jordan VC, Glusman JE, Eckert S, Lippman M, Powles T, Costa A, et al. Incident primary breast cancers are reduced by raloxifene: integrated data from multicenter, double-blind, randomized trials in ~ 12,000 postmenopausal women. *Proc ASCO Abs* 1998; 466:122a.

81. Cummings SR, Eckert S, Krueger KA, Grady P, Poweles TJ, Cauley JA, et al. The effect of raloxifene on risk of breast cancer in postmenopausal women: results from the MORE randomized trial. Multiple Outcomes of Raloxifene Evaluation. *JAMA* 1999; 281:2189–2197.

82. Palkowitz AD, Glasebrook AL, Thrasher JK, Hauser KL, Short LL, Philips L, et al. Discovery and synthesis of [6-hydroxy-3-[4-(1-piperidinyl)-ethoxy-phenoxy]-2-(4-hydroxyphenyl)benzo[b]thiophene: a novel, highly potent selective estrogen receptor modulator (SERM). *J Med Chem* 1997; 40:1407–1416.

83. Bryant HU, Glasebrook AL, Knadler MP, Shetler PK, Short LL, Sato M, et al. LY 353,381.HCL: a highly potent, orally active selective estrogen receptor modulator. The Endocrine Society 79th Annual Meeting (Abstr.), 1997; 548:p3–446.

84. Sato M, Turner CH, Wang T, Dee Adrian M, Rowley E, Bryant HU. LY 353,381.HCL: A novel raloxifene analog with improved SERM potency and efficacy in vivo. *J Pharmacol Exp Ther* 1998; 287:1–7.

85. Munster PN, Buzdar A, Dhingra K, Enas N, Ni L, Major M, et al. Phase I study of a third-generation selective estrogen receptor modulator, LY353381.HCl, in metastatic breast cancer. *J Clin Oncol* 2001; 19,7:2002–2009.

86. Simard J, Labrie C, Belanger A, Gauthier S, Singh SM, Merand Y, Labrie F. Characterization of the effects of the novel non-steroidal antiestrogen EM-800 on basal and estrogen-induced proliferation of T-47D, ZR-75-1 and MCF-7 human breast cancer cells in vitro. *Intl J Cancer* 1997; 73:104–112.

87. Couillard S, Gutman M, Labrie C, Belanger A, Candas B, Labrie F. Comparison of the effects of the antiestrogens EM-800 and tamoxifen on the growth of human breast ZR-75-1 cancer xenografts in nude mice. *Cancer Res* 1998; 58:60–64.

88. Luo S, Stojanovic M, Labrie C, Labrie F. Inhibitory effect of the novel antiestrogen EM-800 and medroxyprogesterone acetate on estrone-stimulated growth of dimethylbenz[a]anthracene-induced mammary carcinoma in rats. *Intl J Cancer* 1997; 3:580–586.

89. Luo S, Sourla A, Labrie C, Gauthier S, Meraud Y, Belanger A, Labrie F. Effect of twenty-four-week treatment with the antiestrogen EM-800 on estrogen-sensitive parameters in intact and ovariectomized mice. *Endocrinology* 1998; 139:2645–2656.

90. Wakeling AE, Dukes M, Bowler J. A potent specific pure antiestrogen with clinical potential. *J Endocrinol* 1991; 99:455–464.

91. Dauvois S, Danielian PS, White R, Parker MG. Antiestrogen ICI 164,384 reduces cellular estrogen receptor by increasing its turnover. *Proc Natl Acad Sci USA* 1992; 89:4037–4041.

92. Gibson MK, Nemmers LA, Beckman WC, Davis VL, Curtis SW, Korach KS. The mechanism of ICI 164, 384 antiestrogenicity involves rapid loss of estrogen receptor in uterine tissue. *Endocrinology* 1991; 129:2000–2010.

93. Thompson EW, Katz D, Shima TB, Wakeling AE, Lipman ME, Dickson RB. ICI 164, 384, a pure antagonist of estrogen stimulated MCF-7 cell proliferation and invasiveness. *Cancer Res* 1989; 49:6929–6934.

94. Osborne CK, Coronado EB, Robinson JP. Human breast cancer in athymic nude mice: cytostatic effects of long-term antiestrogenic activity. *Eur J Cancer* 1987; 23:1189–1196.

95. Osborne CK, Coronado-Heinsohn EB, Hilsenbeck SG, McCue BL, Wakeling AE, McClelland RA, et al. Comparison of the effects of a pure steroidal aniestrogen with those of tamoxifen in a model of human cancer. *J Natl Cancer Inst* 1995; 87:746–750.
96. Nicholson RI, Walker KJ, Bouzukar N, Wills RJ, Gee JM, Rushmere NK, Davies P. Estrogen deprivation in breast cancer. Clinical, experimental and biological aspects. *Ann NY Acad Sci* 1990; 595:316–327.
97. Gallagher A, Chambers TJ, Tobias JH. The estrogen antagonist ICI 182,780 reduces cancellous bone volumes in female rats. *Endocrinology* 1993; 133:2787–2791.
98. Howell A, DeFriend D, Robertson J, Blamey R, Walton P (1995). Response to a specific antiestrogen (ICI 182780) in tamoxifen-resistant breast cancer. *Lancet* 1995; 345:29–30.

10 Breast-Cancer Prevention with Antiestrogens

Monica Morrow and V. Craig Jordan

CONTENTS

1. INTRODUCTION

In 1936 Lacassagne suggested that if breast cancer was caused by a special genetic susceptibility òf the breast to estrogen, then perhaps a therapeutic antagonist could be found to prevent the disease *(1)*. It is now 40 years since the first description of the target, the estrogen receptor (ER), by Elwood Jensen *(2)* and the report of the first nonsteroidal antiestrogen MER25 by Leonard Lerner *(3)*. Regrettably, MER25 was not useful clinically, but a related compound, tamoxifen, first reported by Harper and Walpole as an antifertility agent in animals *(4,5)*, subsequently has become the endocrine therapy of choice for all stages of breast cancer *(6,7)*. There are now more than 10 million woman-years of clinical experience with adjunct tamoxifen therapy, and there is unimpeachable evidence that the benefits

From: *Hormone Therapy in Breast and Prostate Cancer*
Edited by: V. C. Jordan and B. J. A. Furr © Humana Press Inc., Totowa, NJ

accrued in lives saved and the reduction of contralateral breast cancer far outweigh any risks *(8)*.

A focus on the toxicology and pharmacology of tamoxifen during the past decade has propelled the concept of antiestrogens to prevent breast cancer into clinical testing. Indeed, much of the impetus was catalyzed by the advocate community who demanded ideas be rapidly translated from the laboratory to the clinic. Tamoxifen is the first success in the effort to prevent breast cancer. The drug represents a triumph of translational research that, for the first time, provides options for women with risk factors for breast cancer.

However, not all women who develop breast cancer have recognized risk factors for the disease. Studies estimate that about half the women who present with a diagnosis of breast cancer would not have been preselected for special monitoring *(9)*. As a result of this observation, alternate breast cancer-prevention strategies have been devised to broaden the applicability of antiestrogens. Raloxifene, an antiestrogen paradoxically available for the prevention of osteoporosis *(10)*, is the first of a series of selective ER modulators that are planned to prevent osteoporosis and coronary heart disease in postmenopausal women but with the advantageous side effect of preventing breast and endometrial cancer *(11,12)*.

In this chapter we will first describe the biological rationale for the direct (tamoxifen) and indirect (raloxifene) strategies to prevent breast cancer in women. We will then consider the issue of a woman's risk to test an antiestrogen and finally discuss the results of current trials.

2. THE BIOLOGICAL BASIS FOR BREAST-CANCER PREVENTION WITH ANTIESTROGENS

Tamoxifen has been tested extensively in the laboratory and clinics for three decades. There are now estimated to be 10 million woman-years of experience in the use of tamoxifen for the treatment of breast cancer. However, the value of tamoxifen as a potential preventive requires special criteria and additional benefits over and above antitumor properties. The rationale for the use of tamoxifen as a preventive comes from proof that it prevents mammary cancer in the laboratory, evidence that it prevents contralateral breast cancer in adjuvant clinical trials, and a careful examination of clinical toxicology based on laboratory studies.

Tamoxifen prevents the development of mammary tumors in response to mammary carcinogens *(13–15)*. The antiestrogen is effective both at the time of carcinogen administration *(13)* and during the promotional phase of carcinogenesis *(14,15)*. Additionally, long-term tamoxifen treatment is superior to early ovariectomy in preventing the development of mammary tumors in high-risk strains of female mice *(16,17)*. This was Lacassagne's original experimental model *(1)* and is an important laboratory result because tamoxifen was originally classified as an estrogen in the mouse. One result could have been that tamoxifen increased mammary tumorigenesis in the mouse model, and would have introduced a note of caution for clinical testing. In fact, the results strongly supported clinical trials to test the worth of tamoxifen to prevent breast cancer in high-risk women.

The observation that tamoxifen reduced the incidence of contralateral breast cancer *(18)* acted as a catalyst, with the laboratory evidence *(13),* to go forward with a feasibility study to test the toxicology and compliance of patients in a small pilot study *(19,20).* The original observation *(18)* that tamoxifen prevents contralateral breast cancer has been confirmed in numerous individual trials *(8).* Indeed, these data provide the strongest proof that antiestrogens had the potential to be effective preventives in high-risk women. However, the safety of tamoxifen in well women was the most important issue a decade ago. If estrogen is essential to prevent osteoporosis and coronary heart disease, then perhaps the long-term use of an antiestrogen would predispose women to osteoporosis and coronary heart disease. However, a decade ago, a series of laboratory studies demonstrated the antiestrogens exhibited target-site specificity *(15,21–23).* They were estrogens in bone but were antiestrogens in breast. This laboratory demonstration of selective ER modulation translated to the clinic *(24)* and opened the door for the second strategic approach to prevent breast cancer in postmenopausal women with only age as a risk factor.

Tamoxifen is an antitumor agent with beneficial effects in maintaining bone density *(24–26)* and reducing circulating cholesterol *(27).* Indeed, there are suggestions from the literature that tamoxifen can reduce the incidence of cardiac conditions *(28–30).* A decade ago, based on laboratory evidence and emerging clinical studies, we suggested that drugs should be developed that prevent coronary heart disease or osteoporosis, but prevent breast and endometrial cancer as beneficial side effects *(6,22).* Additionally, an early concern about the carcinogenic potential of tamoxifen *(23,31)* suggested that this was not going to be the agent of choice for well women without risk factors for breast cancer. Tamoxifen produces only a modest increase in early-stage, low-grade endometrial cancer *(32),* and there is little evidence for complete carcinogenesis in human tumors *(33–36).* New agents that are completely antiestrogenic in the uterus would be ideal as agents in general medicine. This concept provided the scientific rationale for the subsequent development of raloxifene for the prevention of osteoporosis.

Despite the strong scientific rationale for the use of antiestrogens to prevent breast cancer, the demonstration of effectiveness is an enormous task. The key to success is the identification of high-risk women so that an evaluation of risks and benefits can be made in raloxifene clinical trials.

Although the cause of breast cancer is unknown, multiple factors that are associated with an increase in the risk of breast-cancer development have been identified. These can be grouped under the general headings of genetic and

Table 1
Probability of Developing and Dying
of Breast Cancer at Given Age Intervals

Age	Risk of developing breast cancer (%)	Risk of dying of breast cancer (%)
20–40	0.49	.09
35–55	2.53	.56
50–70	4.67	1.04
65–85	5.48	1.01
Birth–110	10.2	3.6
65–110	6.53	1.53

Adapted with permission from ref. *(37)*.

familial factors, hormonal factors, benign breast disease, and environmental factors. In addition, age is a major breast-cancer risk factor, with half a woman's lifetime risk of breast-cancer development occurring after age 65 *(37)* (Table 1).

3. BREAST-CANCER RISK FACTORS

Family history is probably the most well-recognized risk factor for breast cancer, and it is now known that two forms of risk are associated with a family history of the disease. A genetically inherited predisposition to breast cancer is believed to account for only 5–10% of breast-cancer cases *(38,39)*. Although infrequent, these mutations are significant since they are associated with a lifetime risk of breast-cancer development of 50–80% *(40,41)*. At present, two predisposition genes, BRCA1, located on chromosome 17q21 *(42)*, and BRCA2, located on chromosome 13q12-13 *(43)*, have been identified. Both genes are inherited in an autosomal dominant fashion and are characterized by an extremely high risk of breast-cancer development that begins at a young age. Both genes also confer an increased risk of ovarian cancer development, which in BRCA1 carriers is estimated to be 10% by age 60 *(44)*, and is lower in BRCA2 carriers. In addition, germ-line mutations of the tumor-suppressor gene p53, as seen in patients with the Li-Fraumeni syndrome, may account for about 1% of breast-cancer cases occurring in women age 40 and younger *(45,46)*.

Most women with a family history of breast cancer do not have the genetically transmitted form of the disease, and therefore their increase in risk is much less than that seen in women who have inherited a predisposition gene.

The cumulative probability that a 30-yr-old woman with a mother or sister with breast cancer will develop breast cancer by the age of 70 is reported to be between 7 and 18% *(47,48)*. While this risk increases as the number of relatives with breast cancer increases, the probability of cancer development if both a mother and sister have bilateral breast cancer has been reported to be only 25% *(46,48)*. The cumulative risk of breast-cancer development in women with a family history of breast cancer rarely exceeds 30%, making it critically important to distinguish those women with hereditary breast cancer from those with a family history of the disease. Factors that should increase the clinician's index of suspicion that a woman is at risk for genetically transmitted breast cancer include multiple relatives (maternal or paternal) with the disease, a family history of ovarian cancer in association with breast cancer, and a family history of bilateral and/or early onset of breast cancer. Although not all women with these factors will have genetically transmitted breast cancer, a referral for genetic counseling will allow the construction of a detailed pedigree to estimate both breast-cancer risk and the competing causes of death due to an increased risk of the development of other types of cancer.

Breast cancer is clearly related to endogenous hormones, and numerous studies have linked breast cancer risk to the age of menarche, menopause, and first pregnancy. Although the absolute age-specific incidence of breast cancer is higher in postmenopausal than premenopausal women *(49)*, the absolute rate of rise of the curve is greatest up to the time of menopause, then slows to one-sixth of that seen in the premenopausal period. Further support for the promotional role of estrogen in breast-cancer development comes from the observations that early menarche *(50)*, late menopause *(51)*, nulliparity, and late age at first birth *(52)*, all increase the risk of breast-cancer development. An increased number of ovulatory cycles is suggested to be the common mechanism of increased risk.

Other hormonal risk factors have been suggested, but are not as well-established. Abortion, whether spontaneous or induced, has been reported by some authors to increase risk *(53,54)*, while other studies have found no relationship between abortion and breast-cancer risk *(55,56)*. Studies of the effect of lactation on breast-cancer risk have also been inconclusive *(57,58)*, but recent studies have suggested that a long duration of lactation reduces breast-cancer risk in premenopausal women *(59)*. Physical activity in adolescence is reported to decrease risk, perhaps due to a higher rate of anovulatory cycles *(60,61)*, but an increased level of physical activity later in life has not been shown to reduce breast-cancer risk *(62)*. Postmenopausal obesity also has been shown to increase risk *(63)*, perhaps due to increased peripheral estrogen production, but this relationship between weight and risk is not observed in premenopausal women. In fact, some studies have reported an inverse relationship between weight and risk at a younger age *(64)*.

Table 2
Magnitude of Known Breast-Cancer Risk Factors

Relative Risk <2	Relative Risk 2–4	Relative Risk >4
Early menarche	Age >35 first birth	Gene mutations
Late menopause	1° relative with breast cancer	Lobular carcinoma *in situ*
Nulliparity	Radiation exposure	Ductal carcinoma *in situ*
Proliferative benign disease	Prior breast cancer	Atypical hyperplasia
Obesity		
Alcohol use		
Hormone replacement		

The effects of exogenous hormones in the form of oral contraceptives and hormone-replacement therapy on breast-cancer risk have been studied extensively, but few firm conclusions may be drawn. Overall, there is no convincing evidence of an increase in breast-cancer risk in women who have ever used oral contraceptives *(65)*. However, some studies have suggested that the long-term use of oral contraceptives in young women prior to first birth may increase breast-cancer risk *(66,67)*.

Two recent meta-analyses of the effect of estrogen-replacement therapy demonstrate small but statistically significant increases in risk for users *(68,69)*. However, Steinberg et al. *(68)* noted no increase in risk until after at least 5 yr of estrogen use, after which a proportional increase in risk for each year of estrogen use was observed, while Sillero-Arenas *(69)* did not observe a significant association between duration of hormone-replacement therapy and breast-cancer risk. In summary, although hormonal risk factors are clearly implicated in the pathogenesis of breast cancer, most of them are associated with a relative risk of breast-cancer development of three or less (Table 2), and the presence of a single hormonal risk factor is insufficient to classify a woman as high-risk.

The relationship of benign breast disease to breast carcinoma was a subject of confusion for many years. The use of a standard classification of benign breast diseases as nonproliferative, proliferative, or proliferative with atypia has resolved much of the controversy. The histologic diagnoses comprising these categories are shown in Table 3. Nonproliferative disease is associated with no increase in breast-cancer risk while proliferative disease increases risk by a factor of 1.5–2.0, and atypical hyperplasia by a factor of 4–5. Approximately 70% of palpable breast masses contain nonproliferative disease *(70)* and only 3.6% are atypical hyperplasia. The incidence of atypia is somewhat

Table 3
Classification of Benign Breast Disease

Nonproliferative no increase in risk	Proliferative RR 1.5–2.0	Proliferative with atypia RR 4.5–5.0
Cysts, micro or macro	Papilloma	Atypical ductal hyperplasia
Duct ectasia	Sclerosing adenosis	Atypical lobular hyperplasia
Fibroadenoma		
Moderate or sever hyperylasia		
Mastitis		
Fibrosis		
Metaplasia, squamous or apocrine		
Mild hyperplasia		

higher in biopsies performed for mammographic lesions, ranging from 7–10% *(71,72)*. However, the risk of breast-cancer development 15 yr after a diagnosis of atypical hyperplasia is only 8% in the absence of a family history of breast cancer. Proliferative breast disease is also noted more frequently in women with a significant family history of breast cancer than in controls, further supporting its role as a risk factor *(73)*.

Another benign breast lesion that is clearly associated with an increased risk of breast-cancer development is lobular carcinoma *in situ* (LCIS). In the past, LCIS was though to be a malignant lesion, albeit one with a favorable prognosis. However, the finding that LCIS is associated with a risk of breast-cancer development of approx 1% per year, the observation that the risk of carcinoma is equal in both breasts, and the finding that neither the extent of LCIS in the breast nor its presence at a margin of resection influence the risk of subsequent cancer have led LCIS to be regarded as a risk factor for breast-cancer development rather than the actual precursor of carcinoma *(74)*.

A number of environmental factors have also been linked to breast-cancer risk. Exposure to ionizing radiation, whether secondary to nuclear explosion or medical procedures, has been clearly demonstrated to increase breast-cancer risk *(75–77)*. The level of risk varies with the age of exposure, with a minimal increase in risk observed for exposure in women older than 40 yr. A large amount of attention has been directed towards the role of diet in the etiology of breast cancer. This link has been suggested by the large international variation in breast cancer-incidence rates, and the observation that national per capita fat consumption correlates with breast-cancer incidence and mortality. However, prospective studies of diet and breast-cancer risk have failed to identify a relationship between dietary fat intake and breast-cancer incidence for up to 10 yr of follow-up *(78)*. The lack of a relationship between dietary fat intake and cancer risk within the context of a Western diet is confirmed by a pooled analysis of seven cohort studies involving a total of 337,819 women that demonstrated no difference in risk for women with the lowest and highest quintile of fat intake *(79)*. However, all of these studies have addressed fat intake in adult life, and they do not exclude the possibility that fat intake during childhood and adolescence may influence subsequent breast-cancer risk.

Stronger evidence exists to support an association between alcohol and breast cancer. A meta-analysis of 12 case-control studies demonstrated a relative risk of 1.4 for each 24 g of alcohol consumed daily *(80)*. Defining a relationship between age of alcohol consumption and breast-cancer risk is more difficult, with conflicting data on the importance of drinking early in life *(81,82)*. A summary of the magnitude of increase in risk associated with the factors discussed is provided in Table 2.

4. INTERACTIONS AMONG RISK FACTORS

A major problem in the clinical identification of the "high-risk woman" is the lack of knowledge of the interactions among the various factors known to alter breast-cancer risk since the majority of studies have focused on defining individual risk factors. Most women have a combination of factors that both increase risk and are protective, complicating the assessment of an individual's level of risk. In addition, it is unclear whether the risk conferred by multiple risk factors is additive, multiplicative, or varies with the risk factor under study.

The interactions between a family history of breast cancer and other risk factors have been examined, often with conflicting results. Dupont and Page *(70)* observed that the combination of atypical hyperplasia and a family history of a first-degree relative with breast cancer increased the relative risk of breast cancer to 11 times that of an index population, compared to a relative risk of 4.4 for atypia alone. However, Rosen *(83)* found that the presence of a family history of breast carcinoma did not alter the level of risk after a diagnosis of LCIS, a lesion often considered part of a continuum with atypical hyperplasia. An analysis of data from the Nurses Health Study *(84)* found that in women with a mother or sister with breast cancer, known risk factors of age at menarche or menopause, parity, age at first birth, alcohol use, and the presence of benign breast disease did not further alter risk. In contrast, Anderson and Badzioch *(85)* and Brinton et al. *(86)* have reported that hormonal factors further modulate risk in women with a family history of breast cancer, although the effect varies with the factor under study.

Studies of the interaction between estrogen-replacement therapy and other known breast-cancer risk factors also have variable results, depending on the risk factor under study. In a meta-analysis of 16 published studies, Steinberg et al. *(68)* found that the effect of estrogen replacement did not differ among parous and nulliparous women and those with or without benign breast disease. However, an enhanced risk was observed in women with a family history of breast cancer. The analysis of the interaction among risk factors is further complicated by the fact that some factors may be important for the risk of premenopausal, but not postmenopausal, cancer, and vice versa, and these effects may not be constant over time.

A model to predict the risk of breast-cancer development in women at a given age over a defined time interval was developed by Gail et al. *(87)* using data from 4,496 matched pairs of cases and controls in the Breast Cancer Diagnosis and Demonstration Project. The model incorporates the risk factors of age at menarche, age at first live birth, number of first-degree relatives with breast cancer, and number of previous breast biopsies, and has been shown to predict risk accurately in two validation studies of women undergoing annual mammographic screening *(88,89)*. However, the model overpredicts breast cancer risk by 33% among women age 60 and younger who do not undergo annual screening. There are several other limitations of the model. Because only first-degree relatives are considered, it is not an appropriate model for women with extensive family histories of breast cancer, where risk may be underestimated. In women with risk due to LCIS, or atypical hyperplasia, the model underestimates risk, since the higher relative risk for breast biopsy is 2.0. Similarly, for the woman with nonproliferative disease, the model may overestimate risk. In spite of these limitations, the model is a clinically useful tool for identifying a woman's level of risk over a clinically relevant time period, after correction for competing causes of mortality.

5. IDENTIFICATION OF CANDIDATES FOR CHEMOPREVENTION

Women at increased risk for breast cancer would seem to be ideal candidates for chemoprevention initiatives. However, from the preceding discussion it is apparent that the problem of identification of the high-risk woman is far from solved. There is no consensus regarding what level of increase in risk is clinically relevant. The interactions among risk factors and their variability over time are poorly understood, and most of the data on risk comes from studies of white women, so little is known about the impact of ethnic diversity on risk. Finally, with the exception of women with mutations of breast cancer-predisposition genes, the majority of women with risk factors will not develop breast carcinoma. In addition, a recent study of the fraction of breast-cancer cases in the United States attributable to well-established risk factors identified only 47% of patients as having attributable risk factors *(90)*. A family history of breast cancer accounted for only 9.1% of cases, while relatively minor risk factors such as later age at first birth and nulliparity contributed 29.5% of cases. In a similar study, Seidman et al. *(91)* noted that only 21% of breast-cancer cases in women age 30–54 and 29% of cases in women age 55–84, occurred in women with one of 10 common breast-cancer risk factors. The majority of women in the studies described had minor risk factors that increase the relative risk of breast cancer only twofold, and most had only a single risk factor. This level of "increased risk" would not meet the entry criteria for the trials of breast-cancer prevention in high-risk women discussed below. This data suggests that even if women with a very small increase in breast-cancer risk were targeted for prevention initiatives, a large number of cases would continue to be missed.

6. RESULTS OF BREAST-CANCER PREVENTION TRIALS WITH ANTIESTROGENS

The results of four studies of the effect of antiestrogens on breast-cancer incidence have been published. Two of these were specifically targeted to women at increased risk for breast cancer development. The biggest study, the National Surgical Adjuvant Breast Project (NSABP) P1 study included 13,388 women aged 35 and older who were randomized to tamoxifen 20 mg daily or placebo *(92)*. Eligibility for the trial was based on the level of breast-cancer risk. Women aged 60 or older were eligible regardless of the presence of breast-cancer risk factors. For those age 35–59, the 5-yr risk of breast-cancer development, as calculated by the Gail model *(87),* had to be equal or greater than that of a 60-yr-old. The trial was reported at a mean follow-up of 3.6 yr. At that time, 175 cases of invasive carcinoma had occurred in the placebo group and 89 in the tamoxifen group, a 49% reduction in incidence. A statistically significant reduction in the rate of intraductal carcinoma from 69 to 35 cases, $p = 0.002$, was also noted. The major effect of tamoxifen was on the incidence of estrogen receptor (ER)-positive tumors. There were 130 ER-positive tumors in the control group and 41 in the tamoxifen group, with no differences noted in ER-negative tumors (31 and 38) or ER-unknown (14 and 10). The concern that patients on tamoxifen might develop unfavorable breast cancers was not supported by the stage data. Two-thirds of the cancers were 2 cm or less in size, and 60% were node-negative. The benefits of tamoxifen were seen across all age groups, with a relative risk of 0.65 for those aged 49 and younger, 0.52 for those 50–59, and 0.47 for women aged 60 and older. The effect of tamoxifen on women with mutations in breast cancer-predisposition genes has not been reported, although such an analysis is planned. The subset of women with LCIS has been analyzed, and tamoxifen reduced the risk of breast-cancer development by 57% in this group.

In addition to the reduction in breast-cancer incidence, a 19% reduction in the risk of hip, wrist, and spine fractures was noted in the tamoxifen arm of the trial. No difference in the risk of ischemic heart-disease endpoints was recorded. Toxicity in the tamoxifen arm was limited to women age 50 and older. A 2.5-fold increase in endometrial cancer (36 vs 15 cases) and an increased risk of venous thrombosis and pulmonary embolism (53 vs 28) were observed. Two additional deaths from pulmonary embolism occurred in the tamoxifen arm, although both patients had significant comorbidities.

The study reported by Powles and colleagues from the Royal Marsden hospital also randomized high-risk women to tamoxifen or placebo for 8 yr *(93)*. The sample size was 2,471, and eligibility criteria included one first-degree relative with breast cancer before age 50, a first-degree relative with bilateral breast cancer, or a first-degree relative of any age plus an additional first- or second-degree relative. Women with a prior benign breast biopsy and a first-degree relative of any age were also eligible. At a median follow-up of 70 mo, 34 breast cancers were noted in the tamoxifen group and 36 in the placebo group, 8 of which were ductal carcinoma *in situ* (DCIS), a relative risk of 1.06. In this study, 42% of participants received hormone-replacement therapy, but their outcome was no different than that observed for women not taking hormones. Data on other endpoints and toxicity was not reported.

The other two studies were not limited to high-risk women. Veronesi et al. *(94)* studied 5408 women aged 35–70 who had had a total hysterectomy for a non-neoplastic disease. Of the 5408 women randomized, 1422 withdrew from the study, leaving 3837 in the trial. When first reported, only 149 women (77 tamoxifen, 72 placebo) had completed 5 yr of treatment. Only 12.4% had a first-degree relative with breast cancer, compared to 55% in both the Marsden and NSABP trials. Only 41 cases of breast cancer occurred in the study population, 19 in the tamoxifen arm, and 22 in the placebo arm. Among women on treatment for at least 1 yr there were 19 breast-cancer cases in the placebo group and 11 in the tamoxifen group. Characteristics of breast-cancer cases including size, nodal status, histologic grade, and hormone-receptor status did not differ between groups. A significant increase in the incidence of venous thromboembolic problems was observed in the tamoxifen arm ($p = 0.005$), although the majority of these were superficial phlebitis.

The final study, reported by Jordan and colleagues *(95)*, analyzed breast-cancer cases in a population of 10,533 women in randomized trials of raloxifene. Patients were selected for study entry on the basis of risk factors for osteoporosis. Sixty-four percent of participants were over age 60, with a median age of 68.5 yr. The remaining 3767 had a median age of 54.6 yr. There was a two-to-one randomization to the raloxifene arm, with raloxifene given at doses of 60 mg or 120 mg daily. After a median follow-up of 33 mo, 58 breast cancers had occurred, with a relative risk of 0.46 for the raloxifene arm. When cases determined to have been present at study entry by review of mammograms and pathology were excluded, the relative risk of breast cancer decreased to 0.37 for

Table 4
Results of Breast-Cancer Chemoprevention Studies

Breast cancer/1000 woman-yr

Trial	High risk	# Subjects	Age	Placebo	Tamoxifen	RR (95% CI)
NSABP P1	Yes	13,388	≥35	6.5	3.6	0.55 (0.42–0.72)
Powles	Yes	2471	>30, ≤70	5.0	4.7	1.06 (0.7–1.7)
Veronesi	No	5408	≥35, ≤70	2.3	2.1	Not significant
Jordan	No	10,533	Post-menopausal	3.7	Raloxifene 1.7	0.46 (0.28, 0.75)

patients taking raloxifene. When only patients on raloxifene treatment for 18 mo or more were analyzed, the relative risk of breast cancer decreased to 0.32. A 70% reduction in the incidence of ER-positive tumors was observed in this study while the incidence of ER-negative tumors was unaffected. The data from the chemoprevention trials is summarized in Table 4 and shown graphically in Fig. 1. These data represent the rationale for testing raloxifene for the prevention of breast cancer in high-risk women.

7. STUDY OF TAMOXIFEN AND RALOXIFENE (STAR)

The STAR trial is a Phase III, double-blind trial that will assign eligible postmenopausal women to either daily tamoxifen (20 mg orally) or raloxifene (60 mg orally) therapy for 5 yr. Trial participants will also complete a minimum of two additional years of follow-up after therapy is stopped.

The STAR trial's primary aim is to determine whether long-term raloxifene therapy is effective in preventing the occurrence of invasive breast cancer in postmenopausal women who are identified as being at high risk for the disease. The comparison is to be made to the established drug, tamoxifen. Its secondary aim is to establish the net effect of raloxifene therapy, by a comparison of cardiovascular data, fracture data, and general toxicities with tamoxifen. It is clear that the activation or suppression of various target sites around a woman's body is similar for tamoxifen and raloxifene, but an evaluation of the overall comparative benefits of the agents will be an important new clinical data base for raloxifene in postmenopausal women.

Premenopausal women at risk for breast cancer are, currently, not eligible for the STAR trial. Although there is extensive information about the efficacy

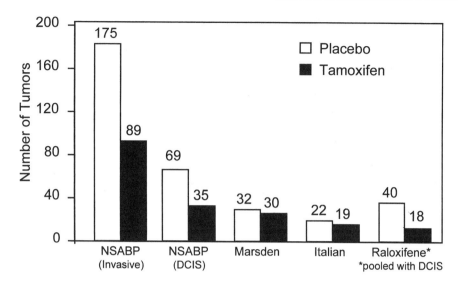

Fig. 1. Comparison of the evaluable events observed in the studies to reduce the incidence of breast cancer. The NSABP P-1 trial is the only prospective clinical trial designed to test the worth of an antiestrogen for preventing breast cancer in a large number (13,388) of high-risk women; the figure illustrates the effect of tamoxifen on both invasive and noninvasive (DCIS) breast cancer *(92)*. By contrast, the Royal Marsden Hospital study *(93)* is a pilot project originally designed to be a toxicity evaluation in 2,471 high-risk women, and the Italian Tamoxifen Prevention Study *(94)* reports 5-yr data on 5,408 normal-risk young women. The raloxifene data *(95)*, which can only be estimated from published abstracts, is a secondary end-point from 10,553 postmenopausal women in osteoporosis trials. The reported cases include both invasive and noninvasive (DCIS) breast cancers.

of tamoxifen in premenopausal breast-cancer patients *(8)* and women at risk for breast cancer *(92)*, clinical experience with raloxifene is confined to monitoring the action of the drug in postmenopausal women. Raloxifene is classified as an antiestrogen with less estrogen-like actions than tamoxifen *(96–98)*. However, tamoxifen has been shown to produce a small decrease in bone density in premenopausal women *(99)*, and there is concern that raloxifene might produce greater decreases in bone density. The National Cancer Institute is currently conducting a randomized study of raloxifene (60 mg daily and 300 mg daily) in high-risk premenopausal women to address the issue of raloxifene and bone density. Additionally, short-term raloxifene treatment (5 d or 28 d), causes elevations in circulating estradiol but does not prevent ovulation *(100)*, consistent with the known elevation of steroid hormones produced by tamoxifen in premenopausal breast-cancer patients *(101)*. The changes in endocrine function produced by raloxifene will also be assessed as a prelude to the recruitment of premenopausal high-risk women to the STAR trial.

The results from the STAR trial are anticipated by 2006. Clearly, it will be invaluable to establish the overall benefits of the drugs with regard to breast-cancer incidence, coronary heart disease, and osteoporosis. The comparisons of endometrial cancer will be most instructive because the standard of care, i.e., self-reporting, will be employed in the STAR trial rather than routine screening with annual biopsies.

8. CONCLUSIONS

During the past 60 years, Lacassagne's *(1)* suggestion that an antiestrogen could prevent breast cancer has become a reality. The success of tamoxifen and the promise of raloxifene have opened the door to the testing of a range of novel compounds and acted as a catalyst for the discovery of novel molecules to prevent multiple diseases associated with advancing age after the menopause.

REFERENCES

1. Lacassagne A. Hormonal pathogenesis of adenocarcinoma of the breast. *Am J Cancer* 1936; 243:217–225.
2. Jensen EV, Jacobson HI. Basic guides to the mechanism of estrogen action. *Recent Prog Horm Res* 1962; 18:387–414.
3. Lerner LJ, Holthaus JF, Thompson CR. A nonsteroidal estrogen antagonist 1-(p-2-diethy-laminoethoxyphenyl)-1-phenyl-2-p-methoxyphenylethanol. *Endocrinology* 1958; 63:295–318.
4. Harper MJK, Walpole AL. A new derivative of triphenylethylene: effect on implantation and mode of action in rats. *J Reprod Fertil* 1967; 13:101–119.
5. Harper MJK, Walpole AL. Mode of action of I.C.I. 46,474 in preventing implantation in rats. *J Endocrinol* 1967; 37:83–92.
6. Lerner LJ, Jordan VC. Development of antiestrogens and their use in breast cancer. Eighth Cain Memorial Award Lecture. *Cancer Res* 1990; 50:4177–4189.
7. Jordan VC. Current view of the use of tamoxifen for the treatment and prevention of breast cancer. Gaddum Memorial Lecture. *Br J Pharmacol* 1993; 110:507–517.
8. Early Breast Cancer Trialists Collaborative Group. Tamoxifen for early breast cancer: an overview of the randomized trials. *Lancet* 1998; 351:1451–1467.
9. Madigan MP, Ziegler RG, Benichou J, Byrne C, and Hoover RN. Proportion of breast cancer cases in the United States explained by well-established risk factors. *J Natl Cancer Inst* 1995; 87:1681–1685.
10. Delmas PD, Bjarnason NH, Mitlak BH, Ravoux A-C, Shah AS, Huster WJ, et al. Effects of raloxifene on bone mineral density, serum cholesterol concentrations and uterine endometrium in postmenopausal women. *N Engl J Med* 1997; 337:1641–1647.
11. Jordan VC, MacGregor JI, Tonetti DA. Tamoxifen: from breast cancer therapy to the design of a postmenopausal prevention maintenance therapy. *Osteoporos Int* 1997; 7:S52–57.
12. Jordan VC. Tamoxifen: the herald of a new era of preventive therapeutics. *J Natl Cancer Inst* 1997; 89:747–749.
13. Jordan VC. Effect of tamoxifen (I.C.I. 46,474) on initiation of growth of DMBA-induced rat mammary carcinoma. *Eur J Cancer* 1976; 12:419–424.

14. Jordan VC, Allen KE. Evaluation of the antitumor activity of the non-steroidal antioestrogen monohydroxytamoxifen in the DMBA-induced rat mammary carcinoma model. *Eur J Cancer* 1980; 16:231–251.

15. Gottardis MM, Jordan VC. Antitumor actions of keoxifene and tamoxifen in the N-nitrosomethylurea-induced rat mammary carcinoma model. *Cancer Res* 1987; 47:4020–4024.

16. Jordan VC, Lababidi MK, Mirecki DM. The anti-estrogenic and anti-tumor properties of prolonged tamoxifen therapy in C3H/OUJ mice. *Eur J Cancer* 1990; 26:718–721.

17. Jordan VC, Lababidi MK, Langan-Fahey S. Suppression of mouse mammary tumorigenesis by long-term tamoxifen therapy. *J Natl Cancer Inst* 1991; 83:492–496.

18. Cuzick J, Baum M. Tamoxifen and contralateral breast cancer. *Lancet* 1985; 2:282.

19. Powles TJ, Hardy JR, Ashley SE, Farrington GM, Cosgrove D, Davey JB, et al. A pilot trial to evaluate the acute toxicity and feasibility of tamoxifen for prevention of breast cancer. *Br J Cancer* 1989; 60:126–131.

20. Powles TJ, Tillyer CR, Jones AL, Ashley SE, Treleaven J, Davey JB, McKinna JA. Prevention of breast cancer with tamoxifen; an update of the Royal Marsden Pilot Program. *Eur J Cancer* 1990; 26:680–648.

21. Jordan VC, Robinson SP. Species specific pharmacology of antiestrogens: role of metabolism. *Fed Proc* 1987; 46:1870–1874.

22. Jordan VC, Phelps E, Lindgren JU. Effects of antiestrogens on bone in castrated and intact female rats. *Breast Cancer Res Treat* 1987; 10:31–35.

23. Gottardis MM, Robinson SP, Satyaswaroop PG, Jordan VC. Contrasting actions of tamoxifen on endometrial and breast tumor growth in the athymic mouse. *Cancer Res* 1988; 48:812–815.

24. Love RR, Mazess RB, Barden HS, Epstein S, Newcomb PA, Jordan VC, et al. Effects of tamoxifen on bone mineral density in postmenopausal women with breast cancer. *N Engl J Med* 1992; 326:852–6.

25. Ward RL, Morgan G, Dalley D, Kelly PJ. Tamoxifen reduces bone turnover and prevents lumbar spine and proximal femoral bone loss in early postmenopausal women. *Bone Miner* 1993; 22:87–94.

26. Kristensen B, Ejlertsen B, Dalgaard P, Larsen L, Holmegaard SN, Transbol I, Mouridsen HT. Tamoxifen and bone metabolism in postmenopausal low-risk breast cancer patients: a randomized study. *J Clin Oncol* 1994; 12:992–997.

27. Love RR, Wiebe DA, Newcomb PA, Cameron L, Leventhal H, Jordan VC, et al. Effects of tamoxifen on cardiovascular risk factors in postmenopausal women. *Ann Intern Med* 1991; 115:860–864.

28. McDonald CC, Stewart HJ. Fatal myocardial infarction in the Scottish tamoxifen trial. *Br Med J* 1991; 303:435–437.

29. Rutqvist LE, Matteson A. Cardiac and thromboembolic morbidity among postmenopausal women with early-stage breast cancer in a randomized trial of tamoxifen. The Stockholm Breast Cancer Study Group. *J Natl Cancer Inst* 1993; 85:1398–1406.

30. Costantino JP, Kuller LH, Ives DG, Fisher B, Dignam J. Coronary heart disease mortality and adjuvant tamoxifen therapy. *J Natl Cancer Inst* 1997; 89:776–782.

31. Williams GM, Iatropoulos MJ, Djordjevic MV, Kaltenberg OP. The triphenylethylene drug tamoxifen is a strong liver carcinogen in the rat. *Carcinogenesis* 1993; 14:315–317.

32. Assikis VJ, Neven P, Jordan VC, Vergote I. A realistic clinical perspective of tamoxifen and endometrial carcinogenesis. *Eur J Cancer* 1996; 32A;1464–1476.

33. Jordan VC. Tamoxifen and tumorigenicity: a predictable concern. *J Natl Cancer Inst* 1995; 87:623–626.

34. Martin EA, Rich KJ, White IN, Woods KL, Powles TJ, Smith LL. 32P-postlabelled DNA adducts in liver obtained from women treated with tamoxifen. *Carcinogenesis* 1995; 16:1651–1654.

35. Phillips DH, Carmichael PL, Hewer A, Cole KJ, Hardcastle IR, Poon GK, et al. Activation of tamoxifen and its metabolite alpha-hydroxytamoxifen to DNA-binding products: comparisons between human, rat and mouse hepatocytes. *Carcinogenesis* 1996; 17:89–94.

36. Dal Cin P, Timmerman D, Van den Berghe I, Wanschura S, Kazmierczak B, Vergote I, et al. Genomic changes in endometrial polyps associated with tamoxifen show no evidence for its action as an external carcinogen. *Cancer Res* 1998; 58:2278–2281.

37. Seidman H, Mushinski MH, Gelb SK, Silverberg E. Probabilities of eventually developing or dying of cancer: United States, 1985. *CA Cancer J Clin* 1985; 35:36–41.

38. Newman B, Austin MA, Lee M, King, MC. Inheritance of human breast cancer: evidence for autosomal dominant transmission in high risk families. *Proc Natl Acad Sci USA* 1988; 85:3044–3048.

39. Claus EB, Risch N, Thompson WD. Genetic analysis of breast cancer in the cancer and steroid hormone study. *Am J Hum Genet* 1991; 48:232–242.

40. Easton DF, Bishop DT, Ford D, Crockford GP, and the Breast Cancer Linkage Consortium. Genetic linkage analysis in familial breast and ovarian cancer: results from 214 families. *Am J Hum Genet* 1993; 52:678–701.

41. Struewing JP, Hartge P, Wacholder S, Baker SM, Berlin M, McAdams M, et al. The risk of cancer associated with specific mutations of BRCA1 and BRCA2 among Ashkenazi Jews. *N Engl J Med* 1997; 336:1401–1408.

42. Miki Y, Swenson J, Shattuck-Eidens D, Futreal PA, Harshman K, Tavtigian S, et al. A strong candidate for the breast and ovarian cancer susceptibility gene, BRCA 1. *Science* 1994; 266:66–71.

43. Wooster R, Neuhausen SL, Mangion J, Quirk Y, Ford D, Collins N, et al. Localization of a breast cancer susceptibility gene, BRCA 2, to chromosome 13q12–13. *Science* 1994; 265:2088–2090.

44. King MC, Rowell S, Love SM. Inherited breast and ovarian cancer. What are the risks? What are the choices? *JAMA* 1993; 269:1975–1980.

45. Malkin D, Li, FP, Strong LC, Fraumeni JF Jr., Nelson CE, Kim DH, et al. Germ line p53 mutations in a familial syndrome of breast cancer, sarcomas, and other neoplasms. *Science* 1990; 250:1233–1238.

46. Sidransky D, Tokino T, Helzlsouer K, Zehnbauer B, Rausch G, Shelton B, et al. Inherited p53 gene mutations in breast cancer. *Cancer Res* 1992; 52:2984–2986.

47. Ottman R, Pike MC, King MC, Henderson BE. Practical guide for estimating risk for familial breast cancer. *Lancet* 1983; 3:556–558.

48. Anderson DE, Badzioch MD. Risk of familial breast cancer. *Cancer* 1985; 56:383–387.

49. Ries LAG, Miller BA, Hankey BF, et al. (eds.) *SEER Cancer Statistics Review, 1973–1991*. NIH Pub. 94-2789. USDHHS National Cancer Institute, Bethesda, MD, 1994.

50. MacMahon B, Trichopoulos D, Brown J, Andersen AP, Aoki K, Cole P, et al. Age at menarche, probability of ovulation and breast cancer risk. *Intl J Cancer* 1982; 29:13–16.

51. Trichopoulos D, MacMahon B, Cole P. Menopause and breast cancer risk. *J Natl Cancer Inst* 1972; 48:605–613.

52. MacMahon B, Cole P, Lin TM, Lowe CR, Mirra AP, Ravnihar B, et al. Age at first birth and breast cancer risk. *Bull WHO* 1970; 43:209–221.

53. Daling JR, Malone KE, Voight LF, White E, Weiss, NS. Risk of breast cancer among young women: relationship to induced abortion. *J Natl Cancer Inst* 1994; 86:1584–1592.

54. Newcomb PA, Storer BE, Longnecker MP, Mittendorf R, Greenberg ER, Willett WC. Pregnancy termination in relation to risk of breast cancer. *JAMA* 1996; 275:283–287.

55. Harris BM, Eklund G, Meirik O, Rutqvist LE, Wiklund K. Risk of cancer of the breast after legal abortion during the first trimester: a Swedish register study. *BMJ* 1989; 299:1430–1432.

56. Melbye M, Wohlfahrt J, Olsen JH, Frisch M, Westergaard T, Helweg-Larsen K, Andersen PK. Induced abortion and the risk of breast cancer. *N Engl J Med* 1997; 336:81–85.
57. Layde PM, Webster LA, Baughman AL, Wingo PA, Rubin GL, Ory HW. The independent associations of parity, age at first full-term pregnancy, and duration of breastfeeding with the risk of breast cancer. *J Clin Epidemiol* 1989; 42:963–973.
58. Kvale G, Heuch I. Lactation and cancer risk: is there a relation specific to breast cancer? *J Epidemiol Community Health* 1988; 42:30–37.
59. Newcomb PA, Storer BE, Longnecker MP, Mittendorf R, Greenberg ER, Clapp RW, et al. Lactation and a reduced risk of premenopausal breast cancer. *N Engl J Med* 1994; 330:81–87.
60. Frisch RE, Gotz-Welbergen AV, McArthur JW, Albright T, Witschi J, Bullen B, et al. Delayed menarche and amenorrhea of college athletes in relation to age of onset of training. *JAMA* 1981; 246:1559–1563.
61. Bernstein L, Henderson BE, Hanisch R, Sullivan-Halley J, Ross RK. Physical exercise and reduced risk of breast cancer in young women. *J Natl Cancer Inst* 1994; 86:1403–1408.
62. Dorgan JF, Brown C, Barrett M, Splansky GL, Kreger BE, D'Agostino RB, et al. Physical activity and risk of breast cancer in the Framingham heart study. *Am J Epidemiol* 1994; 139:662–669.
63. de Waard F, Baanders-van Halewijn E. A prospective study in general practice on breast cancer risk in postmenopausal women. *Intl J Cancer* 1974; 14:153–160.
64. London SJ, Colditz GA, Stampfer MJ, Willett WC, Rosner B, Speizer FE. Prospective study of relative weight, height, and risk of breast cancer. *JAMA* 1989; 262:2853–2858.
65. Malone KE, Daling JR, Weiss NS. Oral contraceptives in relation to breast cancer. *Epidemiol Rev* 1993; 15:80–97.
66. Meirik O, Lund E, Adami HO, Bergstrom R, Christoffersen T, Bergsjo P. Oral contraceptive use and breast cancer in younger women. A joint national case control study in Sweden and Norway. *Lancet* 1986; 2:650–654.
67. UK National Case-Control Study Group. Oral contraceptive use and breast cancer risk in young women. *Lancet* 1989; 1:976–982.
68. Steinberg KK, Thacker SB, Smith SJ, Stroup DF, Zack MM, Flanders WD, Berkelman RL. A meta-analysis of the effect of estrogen replacement therapy on the risk of breast cancer. *JAMA* 1991; 265:1985–1990.
69. Sillero-Arenas M, Delgado-Rodriguez M, Rodigues-Canteras R, Bueno-Cavanillas A, Galvez-Vargas R. Menopausal hormone replacement therapy and breast cancer: a meta-analysis. *Obstet Gynecol* 1992; 79:286–294.
70. Dupont WD, Page D. Risk factors for breast cancer in women with proliferative breast disease. *N Engl J Med* 1985; 312:146–151.
71. Morrow M. Management of nonpalpable breast masses. *PPO Updates* 1990; 4:1–11.
72. Rubin E, Visscher DW, Alexander RW, Urist MM, Maddox WA. Proliferative disease and atypia in biopsies performed for nonpalpable lesions detected mammographically. *Cancer* 1988; 61:2077–2082.
73. Skolnick MH, Cannon-Albright LA, Goldgar DE, Ward JH, Marshall CJ, Schumann GB, et al. Inheritance of proliferative breast disease in breast cancer kindreds. *Science* 1990; 250:1715–1720.
74. Morrow M, Schnitt SJ. Lobular carcinoma in situ, in *Diseases of the Breast* (Harris JR, Lippman ME, Morrow M, Hellman S, eds). Lippincott-Raven, Philadelphia, PA, 1996; pp 369–374.
75. Land CE, McGregor DH. Breast cancer incidence among atomic bomb survivors: implications for radiobiologic risk at low doses. *J Natl Cancer Inst* 1979; 62:17–21.
76. Hildreth NG, Shore RE, Dvoretsky PM. The risk of breast cancer after irradiation of the thymus in infancy. *N Engl J Med* 1989; 321:1281–1284.

77. Miller AB, Howe GR, Sherman GJ, Lindsay JP, Yaffe MJ, Dinner PJ, et al. Mortality from breast cancer after irradiation during fluoroscopic examinations in patients being treated for tuberculosis. *N Engl J Med* 1989; 321:1285–1289.

78. Hunter DJ, Willett WC. Dietary factors, in *Diseases of the Breast* (Harris JR, Lippman ME, Morrow M, Hellman S, eds). Lippincott-Raven, Philadelphia, PA, 1996; pp 201–212.

79. Hunter DJ, Spiegelman D, Adami HO, Beeson L, van den Brandt PA, Folsom AR, et al. Cohort studies of fat intake and the risk of breast cancer: a pooled analysis. *N Engl J Med* 1996; 334:356–361.

80. Longnecker MP, Berlin JA, Orza MJ, Chalmers TC. A meta-analysis of alcohol consumption in relation to breast cancer risk. *JAMA* 1988; 260:652–656.

81. Young TB. A case-control study of breast cancer and alcohol consumption habits. *Cancer* 1989; 64:552–558.

82. Gapstur SM, Potter JD, Sellers TA, Folsom AR. Increased risk of breast cancer with alcohol consumption in postmenopausal women. *Am J Epidemiol* 1992; 136:1221–1231.

83. Rosen PP, Kosloff C, Lieberman PH, Adair F, Braun DW Jr. Lobular carcinoma in situ of the breast. Detailed analysis of 99 patients with average followup of 24 years. *Am J Surg Pathol* 1978; 2:225–251.

84. Colditz GA, Willett WC, Hunter DJ, Stampfer MJ, Manson JE, Hennekens CH, Rosner BA. Family history, age, and risk of breast cancer. Prospective data from the Nurses' Health Study. *JAMA* 1993; 270:338–343.

85. Anderson DE, Badzioch MD. Combined effect of family history and reproductive factors on breast cancer risk. *Cancer* 1989; 63:349–353.

86. Brinton LA, William RR, Hoover RN, Stegens NL, Feinleib M, Fraumeni JF Jr. Breast cancer risk factors among screening program participants. *J Natl Cancer Inst* 1979; 62:37–44.

87. Gail MH, Brinton LA, Byar DP, Coric DK, Green SB, Schairer C, Mulvihill JJ. Projecting individualized probabilities of developing breast cancer for white females who are being examined annually. *J Natl Cancer Inst* 1989; 81:1879–1886.

88. Bondy ML, Lustbader ED, Halabi S, Ross E, Vogel VG. Validation of a breast cancer risk assessment model in women with a positive family history. *J Natl Cancer Inst* 1994; 86:620–625.

89. Spiegelman D, Colditz GA, Hunter D, Hertzmark E. Validation of the Gail et al model for predicting individual breast cancer risk. *J Natl Cancer Inst* 1994; 86:600–607.

90. Madigan MP, Ziegler RG, Benichou J, Byrne C, Hoover RN. Proportion of breast cancer cases in the United States explained by well-established risk factors. *J Natl Cancer Inst* 1995; 87:1681–1685.

91. Seidman H, Stellman SD, Mushinski MH. A different perspective on breast cancer risk factors: some implications of the nonattributable risk. *CA Cancer J Clin* 1982; 32:301–312.

92. Fisher B, Costantino JP, Wickerham DL, Redmond CK, Kavanah M, Cronin WM, et al. Tamoxifen for prevention of breast cancer: report of the National Surgical Adjuvant Breast and Bowel Project P-1 Study. *J Natl Cancer Inst* 1998; 90:1371–1388.

93. Powles TJ, Eeles R, Ashley S, Easton D, Chang J, Dowsett M, Tidy A, Viggers J, Davey J. Interim analysis of the incidence of breast cancer in the Royal Marsden Hospital tamoxifen randomised chemoprevention trial. *Lancet* 1998; 352:98–101.

94. Veronesi U, Maisonneuve P, Costa A, Sacchini V, Maltoni C, Robertson C, et al. Prevention of breast cancer with tamoxifen: preliminary findings from the Italian randomised trial among hysterectomised women. *Lancet* 1998; 352:93–97.

95. Jordan VC, Glusman JE, Eckert S, et al. Incident primary breast cancers are reduced by raloxifene: integrated data from multicenter double blind, randomized trials in 12,000 postmenopausal women. *Proc Am Soc Clin Oncol* 1998; 17:122a.

96. Black LJ, Jones CD, Falcone JF. Antagonism of estrogen action with a new benzothiophene derived antiestrogen. *Life Sci* 1983; 32:1031–1036.
97. Black LJ, Goode RL. Uterine bioassay of tamoxifen, trioxifene and a new estrogen antagonist (LY117018) in rats and mice. *Life Sci* 1980; 26:1453–1458.
98. Jordan VC, Gosden B. Inhibition of the uterotropic activity of estrogens and antiestrogens by the short acting antiestrogen LY117018. *Endocrinology* 1983; 113:463–468.
99. Powles TJ, Hickish T, Kanis JA, Tidy VA, Ashley S. Effect of tamoxifen on bone mineral density measured by dual energy x-ray absorptiometry in healthy premenopausal and postmenopausal women. *J Clin Oncol* 1996; 14:78–84.
100. Baker VL, Draper M, Paul S, Allerheiligen S, Glant M, Shifren J, Jaffe RB. Reproductive endocrine and endometrial effects of raloxifene hydrochloride, a selective estrogen receptor modulator, in women with regular menstrual cycles. *J Clin Endocrinol Metab* 1998; 83:6–13.
101. Jordan VC, Fritz NF, Langan-Fahey S, Thompson M, Tormey DC. Alteration of endocrine parameters in premenopausal women with breast cancer during long term adjuvant therapy with tamoxifen as the single agent. *J Natl Cancer Inst* 1991; 83:1488–1491.

III   INHIBITION OF ESTROGEN SYNTHESIS

11 Aromatase Inhibitors

Paul E. Goss and Caroline C. Reid

1. INTRODUCTION

There are two biological subtypes of human breast carcinoma: those that are hormone-dependent and those that are hormone-independent. Estrogen is thought to be the primary mitogen for the hormone-dependent subtype, but the exact mechanism(s) by which it promotes and stimulates growth has not been fully established. In both the adjuvant and metastatic setting estrogen deprivation is beneficial in a proportion of patients. To this end, hypophysectomy and adrenalectomy have been performed in postmenopausal women while ovarian ablation (surgical or radiation-induced) remains a treatment in premenopausal women *(1)*. These irreversible procedures have significant morbidity and do not address estrogen biosynthesis occurring in extraglandular or peripheral tissues *(2,3)*.

Currently there are three medical approaches to estrogen deprivation of breast tumors. One is to block estrogen receptors (ER) with antagonists such as tamoxifen. A second is to inhibit gonadotrophins by continuous administration of gonadotrophin-releasing hormone (GnRH) or one of its analogues *(4)*. The third is to decrease circulating estrogens by inhibiting their biosynthesis. The

From: *Hormone Therapy in Breast and Prostate Cancer*
Edited by: V. C. Jordan and B. J. A. Furr © Humana Press Inc., Totowa, NJ

target of such inhibition is the aromatase enzyme, which catalyzes the final step in estrogen production in humans *(5,6)*.

In this chapter, estrogen synthesis with respect to therapeutic inhibition is examined in detail. Particular emphasis has been placed on the aromatase (estrogen synthetase) enzyme complex, which is responsible for the final step in the estrogen biosynthetic pathway. Firstly, the aromatase P450 gene, CYP19, and tissue-specific estrogen production regulated by alternate CYP19 promoter usage is described. The potential both for estrogen production within the breast to promote carcinogenesis, as well as for intratumoral estrogen synthesis to enhance breast-tumor growth, are then discussed. Subsequently, aromatase enzyme inhibitors, which have recently become available for the treatment, and possible prevention, of breast cancer in women, are introduced according to current classifications. Cell culture and in vivo models used for preclinical evaluation of aromatase inhibitors are described providing a background to their clinical development. Nonpharmacologic aromatase inhibitors are reviewed and targets of inhibition of the aromatase pathway other than enzyme inhibitors are proposed. The clinical experience and future potential of aromatase inhibitors are described in more detail in the next chapter.

2. AROMATASE AND ESTROGEN SYNTHESIS

2.1. The Aromatase Enzyme Complex

The initial step in estrogen biosynthesis is the cleavage of the cholesterol side chain to yield pregnenolone, a process catalyzed by the enzyme desmolase. A subsequent multi-step process culminates with the conversion of the androgens to estrogens by aromatase (estrogen synthetase) (Fig. 1). This enzymatic process is the rate-limiting step in estrogen biosynthesis and ultimately results in the conversion of C_{19} steroids, such as testosterone and androstenedione, into the C_{18} steroids, estradiol and estrone, respectively. Located in the endoplasmic reticulum, aromatase is an enzyme complex composed of two proteins: aromatase cytochrome P450 (aromatase P450) and reduced nicotinamide adenine dinucleotide diphosphate (NADPH)-cytochrome P450 reductase. Aromatase P450 binds androgen substrates and, in the presence of molecular oxygen and NADPH, catalyzes a series of slow steps to produce 2-beta-hydroxy-19-aldehydes, which then collapse rapidly and nonenzymatically to estrogens. NADPH-cytochrome P450 reductase, a ubiquitous flavoprotein component of the endoplasmic reticulum in most cells, transfers reducing equivalents from NADPH to aromatase P450. For every mole of C_{19} steroid metabolized, the aromatase reaction utilizes three moles of oxygen and three moles of NADPH *(7)*. The principal source of substrate presented to the aromatase enzyme complex in breast tissue is circulating androstenedione. As a result, the primary product of aromatization in the breast is estrone. Estrone may be converted locally to estra-

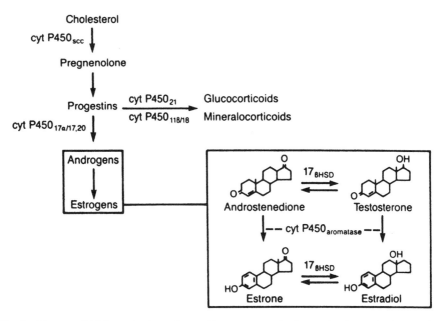

Fig. 1. The steroid biosynthetic pathway. Estrogen synthesis results from the irreversible conversion of androgens by the aromatase enzyme complex. Cyt, cytochrome; SCC, side-chain cleavage; HSD, hydroxysteroid dehydrogenase.

diol, the most biologically active estrogen, by 17β-hydroxysteroid dehydroge-nase *(8)*. Aromatization of androgens via the aromatase complex and aromatase P450 in particular, is a unique, rate-limiting reaction in steroidogenesis. It is therefore a logical target for the selective inhibition of estrogen synthesis cru-cial to the treatment of estrogen-dependent malignancy.

2.2. CYP19, the Aromatase Gene

Aromatase cytochrome P450 is the product of the CYP19 gene located on chromosome 15 *(9)*. CYP19 is a member of the cytochrome P450 gene super-family, which includes over 300 members in at least 36 families *(10)*. Since cloning of the complementary DNA (cDNA) a decade ago *(11,12)* the human CYP19 gene has been well-characterized *(13–21)*. The gene spans over 75 kb and consists of at least 16 exons (Fig. 2). The nine coding exons, exon II to exon X, are contained within a 35 kb region. Exon II contains 38 bp of the 5' untranslated sequence and 145 bp of the coding sequence including a putative membrane-spanning domain. Exon X contains a heme-binding region charac-teristic of the cytochrome P450 superfamily, the translational termination codon, 1336 bp of the 3' untranslated sequence and two polyadenylation sig-

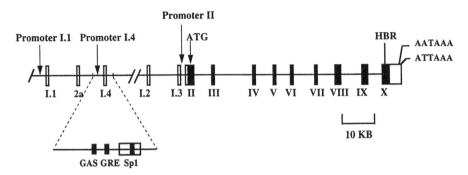

Fig. 2. The human CYP19 gene and promoter region. The closed bars represent translated sequences. Exon II encodes 38bp of the 5'untranslated sequence and 145bp of the amino-terminal protein-coding sequence. The septum in the open bar in exon II represents the 3'-acceptor splice junction for the untranslated exons. The sequence immediately to the left of the septum is that present in mature transcripts whose expression is driven by promoter II. The five untranslated exons I.1, 2a, I.2, I.3, and I.4 are indicated in their approximate locations. The location of exon I.5 and 1 f have not been determined at this time. Exon X encodes 1336bp of the 3' untranslated sequence and contains a heme-binding region (HBR) and two alternative polyadenylation signals (AATAAA, ATTAAA). The genomic region shown spans at least 75 kb. The distance indicated by the gap between I.4 and I.2 is unknown. Adapted with permission from ref *(25a)*.

nals. Alternate use of these polyadenylation signals produces two distinct mRNA species of 3.4 and 2.9 kb. Direct sequencing of polymerase chain reaction (PCR) products of exons III, VII, and X has shown that CYP19 contains common polymorphisms *(22)*

Tissue-specific expression of the CYP19 gene is determined, in part, by the use of distinct promoters in each tissue. Transcription initiation occurs via specific promoters upstream of each of the seven untranslated exons, I.1, 2a, I.4, I.2, I.3, I.5, and 1 f. Exons I.1, 2a, and I.2 are transcribed chiefly in the placenta. Exon 1.4 is transcribed in adipose tissue and fetal liver. Exon 1.3 is also transcribed in brain tissue. Exon I.5 is transcribed in fetal intestine and fetal liver *(23)* and exon 1 f is transcribed in brain tissue *(24)*. All transcripts, regardless of tissue type, are then spliced at a common 3'-splice junction upstream of the start of translation in exon II. Different tissues therefore contain mature transcripts which differ at their 5'-untranslated termini. The protein encoded by each of these transcripts is, however, always the same.

In the ovary, aromatase P450 expression is regulated by a proximal promoter, PII, located approx 140 bp upstream of the start of translation *(17,25)* (Fig. 2). Aromatase P450 expression from PII is controlled by follicle-stimulating hormone (FSH). When bound to its cell-surface receptor, FSH causes an increase in intracellular cAMP, which, in turn, stimulates aromatase P450 expression *(26)*.

cAMP-induced transcription results, in part, from binding of the steroid receptor Ad4BP/SF-1 to a single hexameric element upstream from the PII transcription start site. Further interactions possibly involving Ad4BP/SF-1 and other uncharacterized trans-activating factors have been suggested (27).

In adipose tissue, aromatase P450 expression is regulated by promoters I.4, II and I.3 (20,28). Exon I.4 contains a glucocorticoid response element (GRE) and an Sp 1 nuclear transcription-factor consensus sequence as well as a GAS (interferon-γ [IFN-γ] activation sequence) element (29) (see Fig. 2). Class I cytokines and glucocorticoids stimulate expression from promoter I.4 via a second-messenger pathway consisting of a Jak 1 kinase and a STAT 3 transcription factor that binds to the GAS element. Once glucocorticoid receptors are bound to the GRE and Sp1 is bound to its site, transcriptional activation from promoter I.4 is initiated (30). Though second-messenger pathways mediating aromatase P450 expression via promoters II and I.3 are not yet defined, the stimulatory action of cAMP and phorbol esters suggests that protein kinase A (PKA) and protein kinase C (PKC) pathways could be involved (31).

Adipose tissue is the main site of peripheral estrogen production by androgen aromatization. It consists of adipocytes and stromal-vascular cells. Aromatase P450 expression occurs primarily in the stromal component (32). Transcript expression patterns are constant with increasing age and at different body sites with exon I.4-specific transcripts occurring in greatest relative copy number (28). Age-related increases in conversion of androstenedione to estrone appear to be mostly due to observed progressive increases in adipose tissue aromatase P450 transcript levels (33). Interestingly, a different transcription expression pattern has been observed in breast adipose tissue from patients with breast cancer. In a significant number of breast-cancer patients, promoter II and I.3-specific transcripts appear in high copy number relative to I.4-specific transcripts (34,35). Cultured fibroblasts have been shown to produce exon I.4-specific transcripts when stimulated by Class 1 family cytokines in the presence of glucocorticoids. Alternatively, when aromatase expression is stimulated by dibutyrl cyclic AMP, PII and exon I.3-specific transcripts predominate (20,31).

Since it appears that expression levels of specific transcripts are influenced by the types of stimulatory factors present, the differences in transcript expression between malignant and nonmalignant tissue may reflect the factors secreted by malignant and nonmalignant cell types. It has also been suggested that increased expression of I.3-specific transcripts in malignant breast tissue may reflect induction of aromatase transcription in a subpopulation of the epithelial component of the tumor (36). It is also conceivable that if common polymorphisms, already identified within the CYP19 protein-coding region, also occur within the promoter region, then individual variations in tissue-specific promoter use and therefore individual differences in susceptibility to breast cancer, could occur.

Premenopausal   ### Postmenopausal

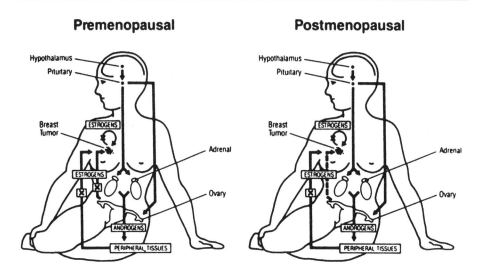

Fig. 3. Sources of estrogen in pre- and postmenopausal women.

2.3. Estrogen Production in Women

In premenopausal breast-cancer patients (Fig. 3), the ovaries, and in particular the granulosa cells of the ovarian follicle, are the most important source of estrogen production (37,38). Currently available aromatase inhibitors are unable to completely block ovarian estrogen production in premenopausal women (39–41). There is also concern that blocking ovarian estrogen production may cause a reflex increase in gonadotrophin levels and result in an ovarian hyper-stimulation syndrome. As a result, clinical use of aromatase inhibitors in the management of breast cancer is currently focused on their use as single agents in postmenopausal women. The role that they may have in combination with other hormonal agents in the treatment of premenopausal breast cancer has yet to be elucidated.

With the onset of menopause (Fig. 3), the ovaries secrete some testosterone and androstenedione but cease to produce significant estrogen and progesterone. Relative to premenopausal women, circulating plasma estrogen concentrations are drastically reduced in postmenopausal women. Production of estrogen essential to the growth of hormone-dependent breast tumors does continue however via aromatization of adrenal androgens in peripheral sites including muscle, liver and, most substantially, adipose tissue (42–45). Furthermore, adipose aromatase P450 activity increases both with age and with body weight (33,46,47). At peripheral sites, androstenedione, primarily produced in the adrenal glands, is converted into estrone. Conversion of testosterone into estradiol is a lesser contributor to peripheral estrogen production

(48). The extraglandular sites of estrogen production in postmenopausal women are more amenable to inhibition by aromatase inhibitors than the ovaries of younger women.

2.4. Estrogen Production in Normal and Malignant Breast Tissue

In contrast to the low plasma estrogen levels that occur in post-menopausal women with and without breast cancer *(49)*, high estrogen concentrations are present in both normal and malignant breast tissue. Furthermore, intratumoral estrogen concentrations are higher than those in normal breast tissue *(8,50–52)*. Aromatase activity is detectable in biochemical assays of normal breast tissue and 40–70% of breast tumors *(53–57)*. Immunocytochemical, radiometric, and *in situ* hybridization studies examining the location of aromatase P450 in normal and malignant breast tissue have detected the enzyme complex and mRNA transcripts in both stromal *(57–60)* and epithelial cells *(57,60,61)*.

Though there has been considerable controversy *(62)* regarding the clinical relevance of intratumoral estrogen production, a growing body of evidence from both in vitro and in vivo studies suggests that intratumoral aromatase synthesizes sufficient estrogen to stimulate estrogen-dependent tumor growth *(63–66)*. Furthermore, studies designed to determine whether intratumoral aromatase-derived estrogen plays a functional role in stimulating tumor-cell proliferation have shown a positive relationship between markers of intratumoral-cell proliferation such as DNA polymerase α and proliferating-cell nuclear antigen (PCNA), and aromatase P450 activity *(60,67)*. This relationship has also been shown to be abrogated by aromatase inhibitors in in vitro studies of tumor samples from patients before and after treatment with aromatase inhibitors *(68)*. Not surprisingly, studies suggest that those patients with breast carcinomas that express aromatase activity respond best to treatment with aromatase inhibitors *(69,70)*.

As illustrated in Fig. 4, studies have shown that areas of increased aromatase activity *(70)* and mRNA levels *(71)* in normal breast tissue occur most often in the same quadrant in which breast tumors have been detected. Augmented aromatase activity detected in tissue surrounding a breast tumor, as well as within the tumor itself, may be caused by stimulatory factors released from the tumor. Alternatively, inherently higher aromatase activity in breast tissue may be the primary event initiating tumorigenesis. Evidence exists that supports both of these hypotheses.

In the first instance, breast tumors often produce a desmoplastic reaction, which involves recruitment and stimulation of fibroblasts and smooth-muscle cells resulting in interspersing of stromal and tumor cells *(72)*. Proliferating stromal cells involved in the desmoplastic reaction express significant aromatase activity *(58)*. In vitro studies of stromal cells have shown that aro-

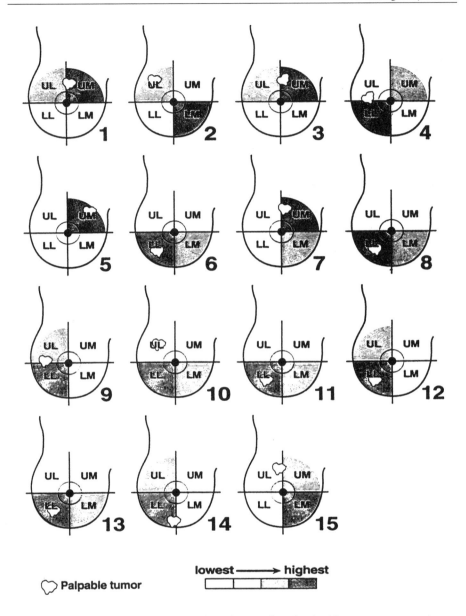

Fig. 4. Aromatase P450 transcript levels and tumor location in 15 mastectomy specimens. In 10 out of 15 cases, the highest aromatase P450 transcripts levels (as determined by reverse transcriptase-PCR) were found in breast quadrants bearing a tumor. In five cases where tumor occupied two adjacent quadrants, the index quadrant was chosen to be the one bearing the largest bulk of the tumor. Adapted with permission from ref. *(71)*.

matase activity can be regulated by a variety of factors including members of the class I cytokine family (e.g., interleukin-1 [IL-1], IL-6, or tumor necrosis factor-α [TNF-α], reviewed ref. 73) and prostaglandin E_2 (31). These factors are produced by malignant breast cells as well as macrophages and lymphocytes, which can represent up to 50% of breast-tumor volume (74). Indeed cytosol prepared from breast tumors or activated macrophages and lymphocytes, but not normal breast tissue, has been shown to stimulate aromatase activity significantly (75,76). It is conceivable then that stromal-cell-derived estrogen functions in a positive feedback mechanism by acting through the estrogen receptor (ER) on tumor cells to stimulate growth factor and cytokine production and secretion (77). These stimulatory factors may then promote further tumor growth in an autocrine and paracrine fashion while stimulating further neighboring and intratumoral stromal-cell proliferation and aromatase P450 expression (78,79). Finally, estrogen produced by ER-positive breast-tumor epithelial cells may stimulate growth via an autocrine action (72).

On the other hand, a number of studies suggest that increased aromatase P450 activity in normal breast tissue precedes, and may promote, tumorigenesis. Aromatase P450 mRNA transcript analysis has shown a similar magnitude of variability in aromatase P450 activity between quadrants from mastectomy specimens that do not contain malignancy compared to those that do, suggesting that variable aromatase activity is a feature of normal breast tissue (71). Furthermore, one study has shown that the highest levels of aromatase P450 transcripts occur in the lateral regions of normal breasts where cancer most commonly arises (80). Recent studies of transgenic mice that overexpress the aromatase P450 gene under the control of mouse mammary tumor virus enhancer/promoter have shown that increased aromatase expression leads to a range of histological abnormalities in mammary tissue indicative of preneoplastic changes (81). This suggests that enhanced expression of aromatase P450 could predispose mammary tissue to preneoplastic changes, which may, in turn, increase the risk of developing breast cancer.

These mechanisms of breast aromatase involvement in estrogen-dependent tumor growth are not necessarily exclusive. Enhanced aromatase expression in breast tissue may be related to tumor promotion in a number of ways: by occurring in normal tissue thereby providing a favorable environment for carcinogenesis, by occurring as a result of factors produced by breast tumors, and by occurring as a result of factors produced by tumor-induced infiltrating macrophages and lymphocytes. In light of the current focus on development and clinical use of aromatase P450 inhibitors as described below and in the next chapter, elucidation of the role aromatase P450 in both normal and malignant breast tissue is essential.

Table 1
Aromatase Inhibitor Classification

Type of aromatase inhibition	Drug or natural product	Structure	Generation
Competitive	Aminoglutethimide	Nonsteroidal	First
	Rogletimide (pyridoglutethimide)	Nonsteroidal	Second
	Fadrozole (CGS 16949)	Imidazole	Second
	Letrozole (CGS 20267)	Triazole	Third
	Vorozole	Triazole	Third
	Anastrozole (Arimidex®)	Triazole	Third
	Lignans	Diphenolic Phytoestrogens	Natural compound
	Flavonoids	Diphenolic Phytoestrogens	Natural compound
	Sesquiterpene lactones	Phytoestrogen	Natural compound
Suicide	Testololactone	Steroidal	First
	Formestane (4-hydroxyandrostenedione)	Steroidal	Second
Exemestane	Steroidal	Third	

3. AROMATASE ENZYME INHIBITORS

3.1. Classification

There are two main types of aromatase enzyme inhibitors: the competitive type and the mechanism-based or suicide inhibitors (Table 1). Competitive inhibitors compete with the substrate (i.e., androstenedione) for reversible noncovalent binding to the active site of aromatase P450. Inhibitors in this class may be either steroidal or nonsteroidal. Suicide inhibitors also compete for the active site of aromatase P450, but are converted to reactive, alkylating species by the enzyme. These then form covalent bonds at or near the active site, thus irreversibly inactivating the enzyme (82). All suicide inhibitors described to date are steroids.

Steroidal inhibitors, which usually have an androgen structure, associate with the substrate-binding site of aromatase. Nonsteroidal inhibitors, which include aminoglutethimide, its analogues, several imidazoles, and a number of triazoles, interact with the cytochrome P450 moiety of the system. Although steroidal inhibitors are capable of inhibiting the aromatase enzyme specifically, they have the potential to induce unwanted agonist or antagonist effects, especially on estrogen, glucocorticoid, androgen, or progesterone receptors. Furthermore, suicide-type steroidal inhibitors may show long-lasting effects in vivo, since the affected enzyme should remain inactivated even after free inhibitor is no longer present

(83). Interestingly, the steroidal suicide-type inhibitors formestane and exemestane do not appear to have significant effects on plasma levels of cortisol, aldosterone, 17-hydroxyprogesterone, DHEAS, LH, and FSH *(84–86)*.

Unlike steroidal aromatase inhibitors, nonsteroidal inhibitors are more likely to exhibit lack of specificity, as they have the potential to block several cytochrome P-450-mediated steroid hydroxylations. Their potential advantage is that they are less likely to exhibit agonist or antagonist properties observed with steroids and are more likely to be orally absorbed. Aminoglutethimide, a first generation nonsteroidal aromatase inhibitor, not only inhibits aromatase but also inhibits cholesterol side-chain cleavage in the adrenal glands. The resulting suppression of cortisol synthesis creates the need for administration of replacement corticosteroid. Rogletimide, a second-generation nonsteroidal aromatase inhibitor, is a less potent analog of aminoglutethimide, which does not inhibit cholesterol side-chain cleavage *(87,88)*. Another second-generation nonsteroidal drug, fadrozole, does not appear to affect levels of aldosterone and cortisol when used in low dosages *(89,90)*. Letrozole, anastrozole, and vorozole are all third-generation nonsteroidal aromatase inhibitors. These triazole derivatives have no discernible effects on adrenal function at dosages that effectively inhibit aromatase *(91,93)*.

3.2. Models for Preclinical Evaluation of Aromatase Inhibitors

3.2.1. IN VITRO

Microsomal preparations from rat ovaries (stimulated with pregnant mare serum gonadotrophin) or from human placenta provide a useful source of aromatase *(94–96)*. Triitiated androgens are added to these preparations in the presence of an NADPH-generating system and estrogen synthesis is measured indirectly by the amount of tritiated water released. Incubation of this test system in the presence of a prospective inhibitor allows the potency of the inhibitor to be determined. Subsequently washing the microsomal preparations with dextran-coated charcoal, reincubating them with androgen precursor, and measuring residual enzyme inhibition also allows for classification of the inhibitor as reversible or irreversible. Data from studies in the rat ovarian granulosa model which demonstrate dose dependent inhibition of aromatase by vorozole and aminoglutethimide is shown in Fig. 5.

Cell lines have also been explored as a mechanism for characterizing aromatase inhibitors. Human MCF-7 breast-cancer cells in particular can convert physiological concentrations of androgens to estrogens via the aromatase enzyme. Autocrine stimulation of DNA synthesis occurs in this cell line when estrogen binds to ER. As a result, aromatase-enzyme inhibition can be observed in this system either directly, by the tritiated water method described previously, or indirectly, by its biological influence on DNA synthesis. Furthermore, measurement of aromatase activity following pre-incubation of MCF-7 cells with an aromatase inhibitor can allow for differentiation between competitive and suicide inhibitors.

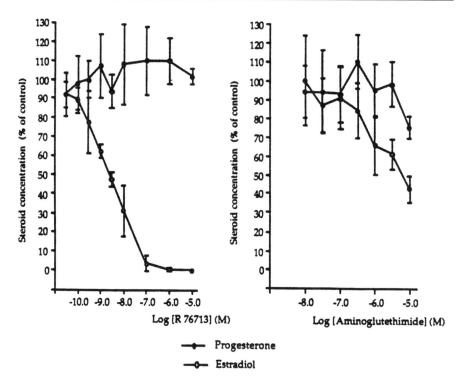

Fig. 5. Effect of increasing concentrations of vorozole and aminoglutethimide on estradiol and progesterone synthesis in rat granulosa cells. Rat ovarian granulosa cells were cultured and steroid synthesis was stimulated with an FSH preparation. The effects of increasing concentrations of vorozole and aminoglutethimide were tested and compared in this system. At the end of incubation, estradiol and progesterone were measured by radio-immunoassay. Estradiol synthesis was inhibited with an IC_{50} value of 3.0 ± 0.2 nM for vorozole and 3900 ± 2800 nM (mean $\pm$ SD) for aminoglutethimide. Adapted with permission from ref *(96a)*.

As shown in Fig. 6, pre-incubation with the competitive class of inhibitors can cause an augmentation of subsequent androgen stimulation of aromatase activity and DNA synthesis whereas suicide inhibitors cause a decrease *(97)*.

Though the inherent, low-level aromatase activity expressed by MCF-7 breast carcinoma-cell line has proved extremely useful for the identification of aromatase inhibitors, it does not mimic the enhanced intratumoral aromatization, which is believed to play a significant role in the growth of human breast carcinomas. Stable transfection of MCF-7 cells with the human aromatase P450 gene produces clonal lines that can express aromatase P450 at 1,000 times the endogenous level in wild-type MCF-7 cells *(64)*. Androstenedione-supported growth of these cells is dependent on aromatase P450 and is blocked in the presence of aro-

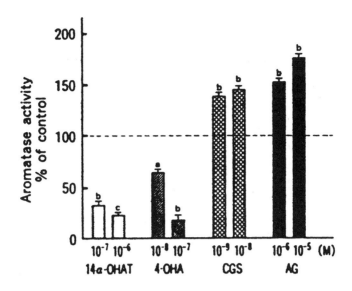

Fig. 6. Aromatase activity of MCF-7 cells after exposure to aromatase inhibitors. The cells were preincubated for 24 h with aromatase inhibitors. Activity was compared to controls incubated with androgen alone. 14α-OHAT (14α-hydroxy-4-androstene-3,6,17-trione) and 4-OHA (4-hydroxyandrostenedione or formestane) are suicide inhibitors. AG (aminoglutethimide) and CGS (fadrozole) are competitive inhibitors. [a]$p < 0.05$; [b]$p < 0.01$; [c]$p < 0.001$ vs androgen alone. Adapted with permission from ref. *(97)*.

matase inhibitors. Not only is this in vitro model of augmented aromatase activity useful for screening of aromatase inhibitors, growth of these cells in vivo, as described below, provides a model of intratumoral aromatase activity.

3.2.2. In Vivo

Though in vitro models provide the means to examine the biochemical pharmacology of aromatase inhibitors, they do not provide information regarding the more complex aspects of a living system such as drug bioavailability, drug metabolites, intratumoral effects, or interactions with other hormones. In vivo models of hormone-dependent tumor growth are therefore essential to preclinical drug evaluation.

Induction of mammary tumors in cycling female rats with dimethylbenz(a)anthracene (DMBA) or dimethylnitrosourea (NMU) provides a model of premenopausal breast cancer. These carcinogens induce mammary tumors, approx 80–90% of which are ovarian hormone-dependent *(96)*, within 6–8 wk of administration *(98,99)*. The ability of aromatase inhibitors to inhibit ovarian estrogen secretion, to cause mammary tumor regression, or to halt tumor growth can be assessed in these animals. Figure 7 provides an example of the distinct

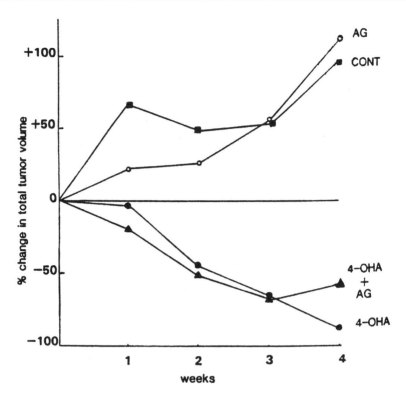

Fig. 7. Effect of 4-hydroxyandrostenedione (formestane) and aminoglutethimide on DMBA-induced, hormone-dependent mammary tumors in the rat. Percentage change in tumor volume in rats treated with 4-hydroxyandrostenedione, aminoglutethimide or 4-hydroxyandrostenedione plus aminoglutethimide vs controls. ■, 8 animals injected with vehicle; ●, 10 animals injected with 4-hydroxyandrostenedione (50 mg/kg/d); ○, 8 animals injected with aminoglutethimide (50 mg/kg/d); ▲, 6 animals injected with 4-hydroxyandrostenedione and aminoglutethimide (50 mg/kg/d each). Adapted with permission from ref. *(100).*

effects of 4-hydroxyandrostenedione (formestane) and aminoglutethimide on tumor growth in this model. Tumor volume in animals treated with 4-hydroxyandrostenedione (formestane), a suicide inhibitor, is decreased markedly within 2 wk, whereas tumor volume in animals treated with only aminoglutethimide, a competitive inhibitor, increases over the study period. Tumor regrowth in the presence of aminoglutethimide has been attributed to increased gonadotrophin levels, occurring as a result of feedback regulatory mechanisms triggered by the initial estradiol suppression, which stimulate aromatase synthesis by the ovaries. On the other hand, 4-hydroxyandrostenedione appears to suppress the hypothalamus-pituitary axis as well as estrogen synthesis, thereby enabling sustained tumor regression in this premenopausal model *(100).*

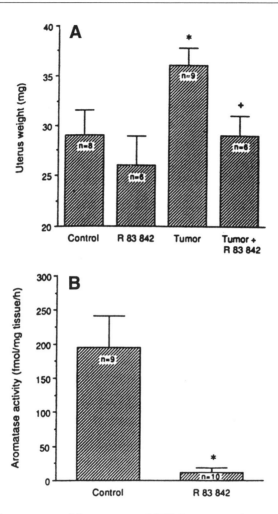

Fig. 8. Effect of the presence of the presence of JEG-3 tumors and treatment with vorozole on the uterus weight (**A**) and aromatase activity (**B**) in ovariectomized mice. Vorozole was administered orally once a day for 5 d. Uterus weight and aromatase activity was measured 1 h from the last drug administration. Results are expressed as a mean ± SEM. * $p < 0.005$ vs control; +$p < 0.005$ vs tumor. Adapted with permission from ref. (*102*).

Models of postmenopausal breast cancer in which estrogen is produced by nonovarian aromatization of androgens have been developed in ovariectomized athymic mice carrying hormone-dependent human tumors. For example, the JEG-3 human choriocarcinoma-cell line exhibits aromatase activity and is tumorigenic in nude mice (*101*). As illustrated in Fig. 8, aromatization of circulating androgens to estrogens by JEG-3 xenografts can be assessed in

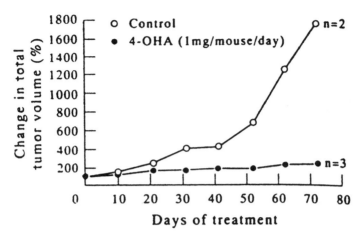

Fig. 9. The effect of formestane on tumor growth in athymic mice co-inoculated with MCF-7 cells and Matrigel. 2.1×10^6 MCF-7 cells in Matrigel suspension were injected subcutaneously into each flank of the mice. Subcutaneous injections of 1 mg formestane/mouse/d were begun 45 d after inoculation. Adapted with permission from ref. *(103)*.

ovariectomized nude mice by uterine weight as well as by direct measurement of enzyme activity in tumor explants *(101,102)*.

Though the JEG-3 tumor grown in nude mice provides a good model to study the action of aromatase inhibitors on local tumor estrogen production, models composed of human breast tumors better simulate the clinical application of aromatase inhibitors. Athymic mice coinoculated with MCF-7 cells and Matrigel, a basement membrane preparation that enhances tumorigenicity, provides an in vivo model of hormone-dependent human breast-cancer suitable for screening aromatase inhibitors *(103)*. Treatment of these mice with either the aromatase inhibitor formestane (shown in Fig. 9) or the antiestrogen tamoxifen results in significant suppression of tumor growth.

As previously discussed, estrogen is synthesized in the postmenopausal women in peripheral, extraglandular sites. Furthermore, intratumoral aromatase activity may play a significant role in hormone-dependent breast-tumor growth. Two comparable models have been developed from the MCF-7 mouse model using ovariectomized athymic mice to simulate hormone-dependent breast-tumor growth in postmenopausal women. In one model ovariectomized athymic mice are co-inoculated with human aromatase gene-transfected MCF-7 cells and Matrigel *(66)*. In the other, established aromatase gene-transfected MCF-7 tumors are transplanted to the animals *(104)*. When supplemented with androstenedione, the growth rate of the aromatase gene-transfected MCF-7 tumors in these models is greater than or equal to growth in intact mice. These models demonstrate the ability of aromatase to provide an endogenous source of estrogen to stimulate tumor growth and may be useful in assessing both the biological significance of intratumoral aromatase as well as the effect of aromatase inhibitors on intratumoral aromatase. They have been used to study the effect of a number of aromatase inhibitors, either alone or in combination with the anti-estrogen tamoxifen, on tumor growth, intratumoral aromatase activity, hormone-receptor expression, and uterine weight *(104,105)*. Tumor growth data from experiments with formestane, tamoxifen, and letrozole in this model are shown in Fig. 10.

The effect of aromatase inhibitors on peripheral aromatization in vivo can be studied in male rhesus or cynomolgus monkeys, in whom most of the circulating estrogen is extragonadal in origin *(106)*. Following a continuous infusion of [7^3H]androstenedione and [4^{14}C]estrone, both the rate and extent of conversion of androstenedione to estrone and estradiol in plasma can be measured. In this model, vorozole has been shown to cause a dose-dependent inhibition of in vivo peripheral aromatization with 50% inhibition observed at an intravenous dose of 130 ng/kg *(107)*.

Recently, transgenic mice that overexpress the aromatase gene under the control of mouse mammary tumor virus enhancer/promoter have been developed *(81)*. This model provides the opportunity to study the effects of locally produced estrogen on mammary epithelial cells. Histological abnormalities indicative of preneoplastic changes occur in the mammary epithelial cells of these mice suggesting that overexpression of the aromatase gene may lead to an increased risk of developing neoplasia and increased susceptibility to environmental carcinogens. Studies of the aromatase gene and other oncogenes such as *myc, ras,* and *int-2* *(108–110),* which have been shown to act in combination with hormonal stimulation to produce breast cancer, may be possible using a bitransgenic version of this model. The ability of aromatase inhibitors to block development of morphological abnormalities in this model and any future bitransgenic versions will be useful in assessing their use in the prevention of breast cancer.

3.2.3. IN VOLUNTEERS

The same double-label continuous infusion technique with [7^3H]androstenedione and [4^{14}C]estrone employed in animal models has been used to measure inhibition of peripheral aromatase activity in male and postmenopausal female volunteers. In Fig. 11, vorozole administered 4 h prior to isotope infusion is shown to inhibit peripheral aromatization in healthy female volunteers *(111)*.

4. CLINICAL APPLICATIONS OF AROMATASE INHIBITORS

4.1. Treatment of Newly Diagnosed (Adjuvant) and Advanced Breast Cancer

Antagonizing the effects of estrogen is a major strategy in the treatment and, more recently, in the prevention of breast cancer. The anti-estrogen tamoxifen has been shown to cause significant remission of cancer and delay in time to pro-

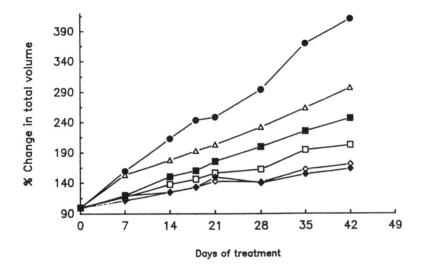

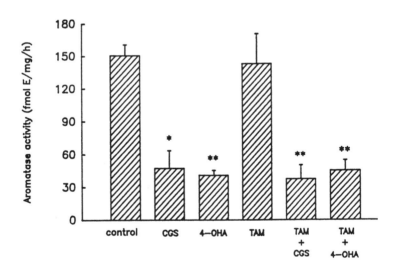

Fig. 10. (A) Growth curve of aromatase gene-transfected MCF-7 tumors in ovariectomized athymic mice receiving combined or single agent treatment with aromatase inhibitor and/or antiestrogen. Aromatase-transfected MCF-7 cells suspended in Matrigel were inoculated into the mice 1 d prior to initiation of daily 0.1 mg androstenedione supplementation. Treatment was with formestane (□; 0.5 mg/d), letrozole (◇; 0.25 mg/d), tamoxifen (Δ; 3 µg/d), formestane + tamoxifen (■; 0.5 mg/d + 3 µg/d), letrozole + tamoxifen (◆; 0.25 mg/d + 3µg/d), or, as a control, vehicle alone (●; 0.1 mL/d) and continued for 6 wk. There were four mice in each group. **(B)** Effect of combined or single agent treatment with aromatase inhibitor and/or antiestrogen on aromatase activity in aromatase gene-transfected MCF-7 tumors. Tumors were removed from animals described in (A). TAM, tamoxifen; CGS, CGS 16949 (letrozole); * $p < 0.05$; ** $p < 0.001$ vs control. Adapted with permission from ref. *(105).*

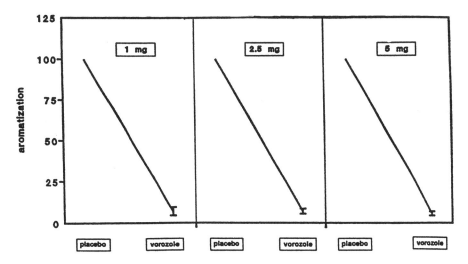

Fig. 11. Effect of different doses of vorozole on in vivo peripheral aromatization in normal postmenopausal women. Twelve healthy postmenopausal women were treated with a single dose of either 1, 2.5, or 5 mg of vorozole. Four h after dosing [^{14}C]-androstenedione and [^{3}H]-estrone were infused and the percentage of conversion of androstenedione to estrone was assessed. Each woman acted as her own control by performing the same experiment with placebo. Percentage conversion obtained with placebo was normalized as 100%. After administration of active compound, conversion decreased by an average of 94%. Adapted with permission from ref. *(111)*.

gression of ER-positive advanced breast cancer in both pre- and postmenopausal women. Likewise, tamoxifen has been shown to increase both disease-free and overall survival of women when given after primary treatment for breast cancer.

The efficacy of aromatase inhibitors in the treatment of patients who progress after tamoxifen has been established *(112–114)*. At present they are being tested in the adjuvant setting. Their interaction with tamoxifen and other pure anti-estrogens, when administered either in combination or sequentially, as well as the order in which to give them, remains to be determined. Current clinical applications of aromatase inhibitors in breast cancer will be discussed in more detail in the next chapter.

4.2. Prevention

Since the antiestrogen tamoxifen has been shown to lower the incidence of contralateral breast cancer in women with breast cancer *(115–118)*, multiple large international trials have been launched to determine its use in the prevention of breast cancer in healthy women. As discussed previously in this chapter, increased basal aromatase activity and estrogen levels in normal breast tissue may predispose to breast cancer. This and the apparent protective effect of tamoxifen, suggest that aromatase inhibitors, which abrogate the effects of estrogen by blocking its synthesis, may be useful in the prevention of breast tumorigenesis. Prior to consideration of prolonged aromatase inhibitor use in healthy individuals however, the long-term effects of estrogen deprivation on bone density and blood cholesterol levels must be investigated.

5. NATURAL PRODUCT AROMATASE ENZYME INHIBITORS

A number of natural products are known to exert hormonal effects including the suppression of aromatase activity. Plant-derived flavonoids *(119–123)*, lignans *(119,123)*, sesquiterpene lactones *(124)*, and tobacco alkaloids *(125)* have all been shown to inhibit aromatase-enzyme function significantly. Of these phytoestrogens, flavonoids and lignans, which are diphenolic compounds found in a variety of fruits, vegetables, legumes, and whole grains, have been studied most extensively with respect to dietary prevention of estrogen-dependent cancers.

A normal human diet is estimated to contain an average of 1 g flavonoids/d *(126)*. The main flavonoids in humans are equol and its precursor daidzein, and genistein. Lignans are formed from structural modification of plant precursors contained in fiber-rich foods by intestinal bacteria *(127)* and are excreted in urine in levels proportional to dietary fiber consumption *(128)*. Epidemiological studies have found low urinary lignan excretion in breast-cancer patients *(128)*. The primary mammalian lignans are enterolactone and enterodiol, which are derived from precursors matairesinol and secoisolari-ciresinol respectively.

Lignans and flavonoids have been shown to inhibit estrogen synthesis in human placental microsomes *(119–121)* and preadipocytes *(122,123)* by competitive aromatase inhibition *(123)* (Table 1). In preadipocytes, enterolactone and its precursors had K_i values between 10 and 30 times that of aminoglutethimide and were indicated to bind aromatase less than 1% as tightly as androstenedione. K_i values for various flavonoids ranged from 0–54 times the K_i of aminoglutethimide. Their affinities for aromatase were less than 3% than that of androstenedione *(123)*. Since these natural compounds have such a low affinity for aromatase it is likely that very high circulating concentrations would be required to compete with androstenedione and testosterone. The low circulating levels of any one of these compounds recorded in humans to date appear insufficient for significant aromatase inhibition *(129)* It is possible, however, that the long-term, total effect of these compounds together may be of physiological relevance *(123)*. In addition, flavonoids and lignans have been shown to compete with estradiol for binding to the ER as well as the nuclear type II estrogen-binding sites *(130,131,132)*. Lignans in particular have also been shown to stimulate sex hormone-binding globulin production *(132)* and to inhibit estrogen-induced RNA synthesis *(133)* and proliferation of breast cancer-cell lines *(134,135)*. The effect of weak aromatase inhibition by these phytoestrogens must be considered in the context of these additional antiestrogenic properties. Clearly, further research is required to characterize fully the ability of these natural compounds, when consumed on a regular and prolonged basis, to aid in both the treatment and prevention of breast cancer.

6. OTHER POTENTIAL TARGETS FOR AROMATASE INHIBITION

In this and the following chapter consideration is given to the agents that inhibit estrogen synthesis by interfering directly with aromatase P450 catalysis. However, the complex and unique regulatory mechanisms that govern aromatase P450 gene transcription and mRNA stability may also be considered as potential targets of inhibition. The second-messenger pathways that control transcription initiation from tissue-specific promoters consist of a variety of cofactors and costimulators that have not yet been fully characterized. As discussed previously, transcription from aromatase P450 promoters II and I.3 appears to be increased in breast adipose tissue in patients with breast cancer *(34,35)*. PKA and/or PKC pathways are thought to be involved in transcription from these promoters. In addition, interactions involving the steroid receptor Ad4BP/SF-1 and other uncharacterized trans-activating factors are believed to play a role in transcription from the PII promoter *(27)*. Inhibition of transcription from PII and I.3 promoters may be possible by removing or modifying factors such as Ad4BP/SF-1 or by impairing phosphorylation reactions. The potential to interfere with breast tissue-specific aromatase exclusively may achieve a local anti-tumor effect while avoiding unwanted inhibition of ovarian or peripheral aromatization. Specific inhibition of aromatization in breast tumors may also be possible by injecting PII and I.3 promoter-specific inhibitors or monoclonal antibodies (MABs). Local delivery of aromatase inhibitory agents may be necessary if it is determined that the current aromatase inhibitors are not potent enough to block intratumoral estrogen synthesis.

Finally, in vitro experiments showing increased aromatase activity with no change in aromatase P450 mRNA levels suggest that regulation of aromatase activity may occur by alterations in mRNA stability, rates of translation, post-translational processing, or aromatase P450 protein half-life *(72)*. Development of alternative mechanisms of inhibiting aromatase activity will be possible once the pathways controlling transcription from promoters PII and I.3 and post-transcriptional regulation are elucidated.

7. SUMMARY

Antagonizing the effect of estrogen is a major strategy in the treatment and prevention of breast cancer. Inhibition of estrogen synthesis is one important way of achieving this. Currently the aromatase P450 protein is the target of aromatase inhibition however other steps in this pathway may provide additional options for blockage of estrogen synthesis.

A number of useful in vitro and in vivo tests have been developed to screen enzyme inhibitors. At least four new third-generation orally available inhibitors have been shown to have effect in advanced breast-cancer patients and are now being investigated as adjuvant therapies.

The role of normal breast and tumor aromatase remains controversial. Whether enhanced aromatase activity in the breast is a feature of cancer progression or initiation is yet to be clarified. Furthermore, genetic and environmental influences on estrogen production and regulation have not been determined.

Natural products which inhibit aromatase have been identified. Dietary intake of these may play a role in cancer prevention and treatment. The next chapter focuses on the clinical development of aromatase inhibitors.

REFERENCES

1. Dowsett M. Inhibitors of steroidogenic enzymes for the treatment of breast cancer. *J Steroid Biochem Mol Biol* 1991; 39:805–809.
2. Ratzkowski E, Adler B, Hochman A. Survival time and treatment results of patients with disseminated breast cancer especially after adrenalectomy and hypophysectomy. *Oncology* 1973; 28:385–397.
3. Miller WR. Aromatase inhibitors in the treatment of advanced breast cancer. *Cancer Treat Rev* 1989; 16:83–93.
4. Conn PM, Crowley WF. Gonadotropin-releasing hormone and its analogues. *N Engl J Med* 1991; 324:93–103.
5. Thompson EA, Siiteri PK. The involvement of human placental microsomal cytochrome P-450 in aromatization. *J Biol Chem* 1974; 249:5373–5378.
6. Thompson EA, Siiteri PK. Utilization of oxygen and reduced nicotinamide adenine dinucleotide phosphate by human placental microsomes during aromatization of androstenedione. *J Biol Chem* 1974; 249:5364–5372.
7. Brueggemeier RW. Biochemical and molecular aspects of aromatase. *J Enzym Inhib* 990; 4:101–111.
8. Bonney RC, Reed MJ, Davidson K, Beranek PA, James VHT. The relationship between 17b hydroxysteroid dehydrogenase activity and oestrogen concentrations in human breast tumors and in normal breast tissue. *Clin Endocrinol* 1983; 19:727–739.
9. Chen S, Besman MJ, Sparkes RS, Zollman S, Klisak I, Mohandas T, Hall PF, Shively JE. Human aromatase: cDNA cloning. Southern blot analysis, and assignment of the gene to chromosome 15. *DNA* 1988; 7:27–38.
10. Nelson DR, Kamataki T, Waxman DJ, Guengerich FP, Estabrook RW, Feyereisen R, et al. The P450 superfamily: update on new sequence, gene mapping, accession numbers, early trivial names of enzymes, and nomenclature. *DNA Cell Biol* 1993; 12:1–51.
11. Corbin CJ, Graham-Lorence S, McPhaul M, Mason JI, Mendelson CR, Simpson ER. Isolation of a full length cDNA insert encoding human aromatase system cytochrome P-450 and its expression in non-steroidogenic cells. *Proc Natl Acad Sci USA* 1988; 85:8948–8952.
12. Harada N. Cloning of a comparative cDNA encoding human aromatase: immunochemical identification and sequence analysis. *Biochem Biophys Res Commun* 1988; 156:725–732.

13. Means GD, Mahendroo MS, Corbin CJ, Mathis JM, Powell FE, Mendelson CR, Simpson ER. Structural analysis of the gene encoding human aromatase cytochrome P450, the enzyme responsible for estrogen biosynthesis. *J Biol Chem* 1989; 264:19385–19391.

14. Harada N, Yamada K, Saito K, Kibe N, Dohmae S, Takagi Y. Structural characterization of the human estrogen syntetase (aromatase) gene. *Biochem Biophys Res Commun* 1990; 166:365–372.

15. Toda K, Terashima M, Kawamoto T, Sumimoto H, Yokoyama Y, Kuribayashi I, et al. Structural and functional characterization of human aromatase P450 gene. *Eur J Biochem* 1990; 193:559–565.

16. Mahendroo MS, Means GD, Mendelson CR, Simpson ER. Tissue-specific expression of human P450arom: the promoter responsible for expression in adipose is different from that utilized in placenta. *J Biol Chem* 1991; 266:11276–11281.

17. Means GD, Kilgore MW, Mahendroo MS, Mendelson CR, Simpson ER. Tissue-specific promoters regulate aromatase cytochrome P450 gene expression in human ovary and fetal tissues. *Mol Endocrinol* 1991; 5:2005–2013.

18. Kilgore MW, Means GD, Mendelson CR, Simpson ER. Alternative promotion of aromatase cytochrome P450 expression in the human placenta. *Mol Cell Endocrinol* 1992; 83:R6–R16.

19. Toda K, Shizuta Y. Molecular cloning of cDNA showing alternative splicing of the 5′-untranslated sequence of mRNA for human aromatase P450. *Eur J Biochem* 1993; 213: 383–389.

20. Mahendroo MS, Mendelson CR, Simpson ER. Tissue-specific and hormonally-controlled alternative promoters regulate aromatase cytochrome P450 gene expression in human adipose tissue. *J Biol Chem* 1993; 268:19463–19470.

21. Harada N, Utsumi T, Takagi Y. Tissue-specific expression of the human aromatase cytochrome P450 gene by alternative use of multiple exon 1 and promoters, and switching of tissue-specific exon 1 in carcinogenesis. *Proc Natl Acad Sci USA* 1993; 90:11321–11316.

22. Sourdaine P, Parker MG, Telford J, Miller WR. Analysis of the aromatase cytochrome P450 gene in human breast cancers. *J Molec Endocrinol* 1994; 13:331–337.

23. Toda K, Simpson ER, Mendelson CR, Shizuta Y, Kilgore MW. Expression of the gene encoding aromatase cytochrome P450 (CYP19) in fetal tissues. *Mol Endocrinol* 1994; 8:210–217.

24. Honda SI, Harada N, Takagi Y. Novel exon 1 of the aromatase gene specific for aromatase transcripts in human brain. *Biochem Biophys Res Commun* 1994; 198:1153–1160.

25. Jenkins C, Michael D, Mahendroo M, Simpson ER. Exon-specific Northern analysis and rapid amplification of cDNA ends (RACE) reveal that the proximal promoter II (PII) is responsible for aromatase cytochrome P450 (CYP19) expression in human ovary. *Mol Cell Endocrinol* 1993; 97:R1–R6.

25a. Simpson ER, Bulun SE, Nichols JE, Zhao Y. Estrogen biosynthesis in adipose tissue: regulation by paracrine and autocrine mechanisms. *J Endocrinol* 1996; 150:S51–S57.

26. Carr BR. in *Williams Textbook of Endocrinology* (Wilson JD, Foster DW, eds). WB, Saunders, Philadelphia, 1992, pp 733–798.

27. Michael MD, Kilgore MW, Morohashi K, Simpson ER. Ad4BP/SF-1 regulates cyclic AMP-induced transcription from the proximal promoter (PII) of the human aromatase P450 (CYP19) gene in the ovary. *J Biol Chem* 1995; 270:13561–13566.

28. Agarwal VR, Ashanullah CI, Simpson ER, Bulun SE. Alternatively spliced transcripts of the aromatase cytochrome P450 (CYP19) gene in adipose tissue of women. *J Clin Endocrinol Metab* 1997; 82:70–74.

29. Zhao Y, Mendelson CR, Simpson ER. Characterization of the sequences of the human CYP19 (aromatase) gene that mediate regulation by glucocorticoids in adipose stromal cells and fetal hepatocytes. *Mol Endocrinol* 1995; 9:340–349.

30. Zhao Y, Nichols JE, Bulun SE, Mendelson CR, Simpson ER. Aromatase P450 gene expression in human adipose tissue. Role of the Jak/STAT pathway in regulation of the adipose-specific promoter. *J Biol Chem* 1995; 270:16449–16457.

31. Zhao Y, Agarwal VR, Mendelson CR, Simpson ER. Estrogen biosynthesis proximal to a breast tumor is stimulated by PGE_2 via cyclic AMP, leading to activation of promoter II of the CYP19 (aromatase) gene. *Endocrinology* 1996; 137:5739–5742.

32. Price TM, O'Brien SN. Determination of estrogen receptor messenger ribonucleic acid and cytochrome P450 aromatase mRNA levels in adipocytes and adipose stromal cells by competitive polymerase chain reaction amplification. *J Endocrinol Metab* 1993; 77:1041–1045.

33. Bulun SE, Simpson ER. Competitive RT-PCR analysis indicates levels of aromatase cytochrome P450 transcripts in adipose tissue of buttocks, thighs and abdomen of women increase with advancing age. *J Clin Endocrinol Metab* 1994; 78:428–432.

34. Agarwal VR, Bulun SE, Leitch M, Rohrich R, Simpson ER. Use of alternative promoters to express the aromatase cytochrome P450 (CYP19) gene in breast adipose tissue of cancer-free and breast cancer patients. *J Clin Endocrinol Metab* 1996; 81:3843–3849.

35. Harada N, Honda S. Molecular analysis of aberrant expression of aromatase in breast cancer tissues. *Breast Cancer Res Treat* 49:515–521.

36. Utsumi T, Harada N, Maruta M, Takagi Y. Presence of alternatively spliced transcripts of aromatase gene in human breast cancer. *J Clin Endocrinol Metab* 1996; 81:2344–2349.

37. McNatty KP, Baird DT, Boltan A, Chambers P, Corker CS, McLean H. Concentration of oestrogens and androgens in human ovarian follicular fluid throughout the menstrual cycle. *J Endocrinol* 1976; 71:77–85.

38. Sasano H, Okamoto M, Mason JI, Simpson ER, Mendelson CR, Sasano N, Silverberg SC. Immunolocalization of aromatase. 17 alpha-hydroxylase and side-chain cleavage cytochromes P450 in human ovary. *J Reprod Fertil* 1989; 85:163:169.

39. Santen RJ. Clinical use of aromatase inhibitors in human breast carcinoma. *J Steroid Biochem Mol Biol* 1991; 40:247–253.

40. Harris AL, Dowsett M, Jeffcoate SL, McKinna JA, Morgan M, Smith IE. Endocrine and therapeutic effects of aminoglutethimide in premenopausal patients with breast cancer. *J Clin Endocrinol Metab* 1982; 55:718–720.

41. Wander HE, Blossey HCH Nagel GA. Aminoglutethimide in the treatment of premenopausal patients with breast cancer. *Eur J Cancer Clin Oncol* 1986; 22:1371–1374.

42. MacDonald PC, Rombaut RP, Siiteri PK. Plasma precursors of estrogen. I. Extent of conversion of plasma delta^4-androstenedione to estrone in normal males and nonpregnant normal, castrate and adrenalectomized females. *J Clin Endocrinol Metab* 1967; 27:1103–1111.

43. Longcope C. Metabolic clearance and blood production rates of estrogens in postmenopausal women. *Am J Obstet Gynecol* 1971; 111:778–781.

44. Grodin JM, Siiteri PK, MacDonald PC. Source of estrogen production in postmenopausal women. *J Clin Endocrinol Metab* 1973; 36:207–214.

45. Judd HL, Judd GE, Lucas WE, Yen SS. Endocrine function of the postmenopausal ovary: concentration of androgens and estrogens in ovarian and peripheral vein blood. *J Clin Endocrinol Metab* 1974; 39:1020–1024.

46. Santen RJ. Potential clinical use of new aromatase inhibitors. *Steroids* 1987; 50:575–593.

47. Edman CD, MacDonald PC. Effect of obesity on conversion of plasma androstenedione to estrone in ovulatory and anovulatory young women. *Am J Obstet Gynecol* 1978; 130:456–461.

48. Lonning PE, Dowsett M, Powles TJ. Postmenopausal estrogen synthesis and metabolism: alterations caused by aromatase inhibitors used for the treatment of breast cancer. *J Steroid Biochem* 1990; 35:355–366.

49. Reed MJ, Beranek PA, Cheng RW, Ghilchik MW, James VHT. The distribution of oestradiol in plasma from postmenopausal women with or without breast cancer: relationship with metabolic clearance rates of oestradiol. *Intl J Cancer* 1985; 35:457–460.

50. Van Landeghem AAJ, Poortman J, Nabuurs M, Thijssen JHH. Endogenous concentrations and subcellular distribution of androgens in normal and malignant breast tissue. *Cancer Res* 1985; 45:2907–2912.

51. Vermeulen A, Deslypere JP, Paridaens R, Leclercq G, Roy F, Heuson JC. Aromatase, 17b hydroxysteroid dehydrogenase and intratissular sex hormone concentrations in cancerous and normal glandular breast tissue in postmenopausal women. *Eur J Cancer Clin Oncol* 1986; 22:515–525.

52. Recchione C, Venturelli E, Manzari A, Cavalleri A, Martinetti A, Secreto G. Testosterone, dihydrotestosterone and oestradiol levels in postmenopausal breast cancer tissue. *J Steroid Biochem Mol Biol* 1995; 52:541–546.

53. Miller WR, Forrest APM. Oestradiol synthesis from C19 steroids by human breast cancers. *Br J Cancer* 1976; 33:116–118.

54. Lipton A, Santen RJ, Santen SJ, Harvey HA, Peil PD, White-Hershey D, et al. Aromatase activity in primary and metastatic human breast cancer. *Cancer* 1987; 59:779–783.

55. Li K, Adams JB. Aromatization of testosterone and oestrogen receptor levels in human breast cancer. *J Steroid Biochem Mol Biol* 1981; 14:269–272.

56. Silva MC, Rowlands MG, Dowsett M, Guterson B, McKinna JA, Fryatt I, Coombes RC. Intra-tumoral aromatase as a prognostic factor in human breast carcinoma. *Cancer Res* 1989; 49:2588–2591.

57. Santen RJ, Martel J, Hoagland M, Naftolin F, Roa L, Harada N, et al. Demonstration of aromatase activity and its regulation in breast tumor and benign breast fibroblasts. *Breast Cancer Res Treat.* 49:593–599.

58. Sasano H, Nagura H, Harada N, Goukon Y, Kimura M. Immunolocalization of aromatase and other steroidogenic enzymes in human breast disorders. *Human Pathol* 1994; 25:530–535.

59. Santen RJ, Martel J, Hoaland F, Naftolin F, Roa L, Harada N, et al. Stromal spindle cells contain aromatase in human breast tumors. *J Clin Endocrinol Metab* 1994; 79:627–632.

60. Brodie A, Long B, Lu Q. Aromatase expression in the human breast. *Breast Cancer Res Treat.* 49:585–591.

61. Esteban JM, Warsi Z, Haniu M, Hall P, Shivley JE, Chen S. Detection of intratumoral aromatase in breast carcinomas. *Am J Pathol* 1992; 140:337–343.

62. Bradlow HL. A reassessment over the role of breast tumor aromatase. *Cancer Res* 1982; 42:S3382–S3386.

63. Reed MJ, Owen AM, Lai LC, Coldham NG, Ghilchik MW, Shaikh NA, James VHT. *In situ* oestrone synthesis in normal breast and breast tumor tissues: effect of treatment with 4-hydroxyandrostenedione. *Int J Cancer* 1989; 44:233–237.

64. Macaulay VM, Nicholls JE, Gledhill J, Rowlands MG, MacLennan K, Dowsett M, Ashworth A. Biological effects of stable overexpression of aromatase in hormone-ddependent breast cancer cells. *Br J Cancer* 1994; 69:77–83.

65. Santner SJ, Chen S, Zhou D, Korsunsky Z, Martel J, Santen RJ. Effect of androstenedione on growth of untransfected and aromatase-transfected MCF-7 cells in culture. *J Steroid Biochem Mol Biol* 1993; 44:611–616.

66. Yue W, Zhou D, Chen S, Brodie A. A new nude mouse model for postmenopausal breast cancer using MCF-7 cells transfected with the human aromatase gene. *Cancer Res* 1994; 54:5092–5095.

67. James VHT, Reed MJ, Adams EF, Ghilchik MW, Lai LC, Coldham NG, et al. Oestrogen uptake and metabolism in vivo. *Proc Royal Soc Edinburgh* 1989; 95B:185–193.

68. Reed MJ, Lai LC, Owen AM, Singh A, Coldham NG, Purohit A, et al. Effect of treatment with 4-hydroxyandrostenedione on the peripheral conversion of androstenedione to estrone and in vivo tumor aromatase activity in postmenopausal women with breast cancer. *Cancer Res* 1990; 50:193–196.

69. Bezwoda WR, Manson R, Dansey R. Correlation of breast tumor aromatase activity and response to aromatase inhibition with aminoglutethimide. *Oncology* 1987; 44:345–349.

70. Miller WR, O'Neill J. The importance of local synthesis of oestrogen within the breast. *Steroids* 1987; 50:537–548.

71. Bulun SE, Simpson ER. Regulation of aromatase expression in human tissues. *Breast Cancer Res Treat* 1994; 30:19–29.

72. Santner SJ, Pauley RJ, Tait L, Kaseta J, Santen RJ. Aromatase activity and expression in breast cancer and benign breast tissue stromal cells. *J Endocrinol Metab* 1997; 82:200–208.

73. Reed MJ, Purohit A. Breast cancer and the role of cytokines in regulating estrogen synthesis: an emerging hypothesis. *Breast Cancer Res Treat.* In press.

74. Kelly PMA, Davison RS, Bliss E, McGee J'OD. Macrophages in human breast disease: a quantitative immunohistochemical study. *Br J Cancer* 1988; 57:174–177.

75. Reed MJ, Topping L, Coldham NG, Purohit A, Ghilchik MW, James VHT. Control of aromatase activity in breast cancer cells: the role of cytokines and growth factors. *J Steroid Biochem Mol Biol* 1993; 44:589–596.

76. Purohit A, Ghilchik MW, Duncan L, Wang DY, Singh A, Walker MM, Reed MJ. Aromatase activity and interleukin-6 production by normal and malignant breast tissue. *J Clin Endocrinol Metab* 1994; 80:3052–3058.

77. Dickson RB, Lippman ME. Estrogenic regulation of growth and polypeptide growth factor secretion in human breast carcinoma. *Endocrine Rev* 1987; 8:29–43.

78. Bulun SE, Simpson ER. Regulation of the CYP19 (P450arom) gene expression in breast adipose tissue and breast cancer. *Trends Endocrinol Metab* 1994; 5:113–120.

79. Simpson ER, Bulun SE, Nichols JE, Zhao Y. Estrogen biosynthesis in adipose tissue: regulation by paracrine and autocrine mechanisms. *J Endocrinol* 1994; 150:S51–S57.

80. Bulun SE, Sharda G, Rink J, Sharma S, Simpson ER. Distribution of aromatase P450 transcripts and adipose fibroblasts in the human breast. *J Clin Endocrinol Metab* 1996; 81:1273–1277.

81. Tekmal RR, Ramachandra N, Gubba S, Durgam VR, Mantione J, Toda K, Shizuta Y, Dillehay DL. Overexpression of *int-5/aromatase* in mammary glands of transgenic mice results in the induction of hyperplasia and nuclear abnormalities. *Cancer Res* 1996; 56:3180–3185.

82. Santen RJ. Clinical use of aromatase inhibitors: current data and therapeutic perspectives. *J Enzym Inhib* 1990; 4:79–99.

83. O'Neal Johnson J, Metcalf BW. Aromatase: a target enzyme in breast cancer, in *Novel Approaches to Cancer Chemotherapy* (Sunkara PS, ed). Academic, New York, 1984, pp 307–328.

84. Coombes RC, Goss PE, Dowsett M, Gazet J-C, Brodie A. 4-hydroxyandrostenedione in treatment of postmenopausal patients with advanced breast cancer. *Lancet* 1984; ii:1237–1239.

85. Pickles T, Perry L, Murray P, Plowman P. 4-hydroxyandrostenedione: further clinical and extended endocrine observations. *Br J Cancer* 1990; 62:309–313.

86. Di Salle E, Ornati G, Giudici D, Lassus M, Evans TRJ, Coombes RC. Exemestane (FCE 24304), a new steroidal aromatase inhibitor. *J Steroid Biochem Mol Biol* 1992; 43:137–143.

87. Foster AB, Jarman M, Leung C-S, Rowlands MG, Taylor GN, Plevey RG, Sampson P. Analogues of aminoglutethimide: Selective inhibition of aromatase. *J Med Chem* 1985; 28:200–204.

88. Leung C-S, Rowlands MG, Jarman M, Foster AB, Griggs LJ, Wilman DE. Analogues of 3-ethyl-3-(4-pyridyl)piperidine-2,6-dione as selective inhibitors of aromatase: derivatives with variable 1-alkyl and 3-alkyl substituents. *J Med Chem* 1987; 30:1550–1554.

89. Demers LM, Melby JC, Wilson TE, Lipton A, Harvey HA, Santen RJ. The effects of CGS 16949A, an aromatase inhibitor on adrenal mineralocorticoid biosynthesis. *J Clin Endocrinol Metab* 1990; 70:1162–1166.

90. Santen RJ, Demers LM, Lynch J, Harvey H, Lipton A, Mulagha M, et al. Specificity of low dose fadrozole hydrochloride (CGS 16949A) as an aromatase inhibitor. *J Clin Endocrinol Metab* 1991; 73:99–106.

91. Wouters W, Snoeck E, De Coster R. Vorozole, a specific non-steroidal aromatase inhibitor. *Breast Cancer Res Treat* 1994; 30:89–94.

92. Iveson TJ, Smith IE, Ahern J, Smithers DA, Trunet PF, Dowsett M. Phase I study of the oral non-steroidal aromatase inhibitor CGS 20267 in postmenopausal patients with advanced breast cancer. *Cancer Res* 1993; 53:266–270.

93. Dowsett M, Yates RA, Lindsay A, et al. Endocrine effects of arimidex, a potent aromatase inhibitor, in men and postmenopausal women. *Breast Cancer Res Treat* 1993; 27:152, (abstr 87).

94. Ryan KJ. Biological aromatization of steroids. *J Biol Chem* 1959; 234:268–272.

95. Brodie AMH, Schwarzel WC, Brodie HJ. Studies on the mechanism of estrogen biosynthesis in the rat ovary-I. *J Steroid Biochem* 1976; 7:787–793.

96. Brodie AMH, Wing LY, Goss P, Dowsett M, Coombes RC. Aromatase inhibitors and their potential clinical significance. *J Steroid Biochem* 1986; 25:859–865.

96a. Vorozole Investigators Brochure 1989, 1st ed., p. 6.

97. Kitawaki J, Kim T, Kanno H, Noguchi T, Yamamoto T, Okada H. Growth suppression of MCF-7 human breast cancer cells by aromatase inhibitors: a new system for aromatase inhibitor screening. *J Steroid Biochem Mol Biol* 1993; 44:667–670.

98. Geyer RP, Bryant JE, Bliesch VR, Peirce EM, Stare FJ. Effect of dose and hormones on tumor production in rats given 9,10-dimethyl-1,2-benzanthracene intravenously. *Cancer Res* 1953; 13:503–506.

99. Guillino PM, Pettigrew HM, Grantham FH. Nitrosomethylurea as mammary gland carcinogen in rats. *J Natl Cancer Inst* 1975; 54:401–409.

100. Wing LY, Garrett WM, Brodie AMH. Effects of aromatase inhibitors, aminoglutethimide, and 4-hydroxyandrostenedione on cyclic rats and rats with 7,12-dimethylbenz(a)anthracene-induced mammary tumors. *Cancer Res* 1985; 45:2425–2428.

101. Krekels MDWG, Wouters W, DeCoster R, Van Ginckel R, Leonaers A, Janssen PAJ. Aromatase in the human choriocarcinoma JEG-3: inhibition by R76 713 in cultured cells and in tumors grown in nude mice. *J Steroid Biochem Mol Biol* 1991; 38:415–422.

102. Krekels MDWG, Wouters W, Van Ginckel R, Janssen B, Callens M, DeCoster R. Aromatase inhibition by R 83 842, the dextroisomer of R 76 713, in JEG-3 choriocarcinoma grown in ovariectomized nude mice. *J Steroid Biochem Mol Biol* 1992; 41:761–764.

103. Yue W, Brodie A. MCF-7 human breast cell carcinomas in nude mice as a model for evaluating aromatase inhibitors. *J Steroid Biochem Mol Biol* 1993; 44:671–673.

104. Lee K, Macauley VM, Nicholls JE, Detre S, Ashworth A, Dowsett M. An in vivo model of intratumoral aromatase using aromatase-transfected MCF7 human breast cancer cells. *Intl J Cancer* 1995; 62:297–302.

105. Yue W, Wang J, Savinov A, Brodie A. Effect of aromatase inhibitors on growth of mammary tumors in a nude mouse model. *Cancer Res* 1995; 55:3073–3077.

106. Brodie AM, Romanoff LP, Williams KIH. Metabolism of the aromatase inhibitor 4-hydroxy-4-androstenedione by male rhesus monkeys. *J Steroid Biochem* 1981; 14:693–696.

107. Tuman RW, Morris DM, Wallace NM, Bowden CR. Inhibition of peripheral aromatization in the male cynomolgus monkey by a novel nonsteroidal aromatase inhibitor (R76713). *J Endocrinol Metab* 1991; 72:755–760.

108. Leder A, Pattengale PK, Kuo A, Stewart TA, Leader P. Consequences of widespread deregulation of the c-myc gene in transgenic mice: multiple neoplasms and normal development. *Cell* 1986; 45:485–495.

109. Andres A-C, Schonenberger C-A, Groner B, Hennighausen L, LeMeur M, Gerlinger P. Ha-*ras* oncogene expression directed by a milk protein gene promoter: tissue specificity, hormonal regulation, and tumor induction in transgenic mice. *Proc Natl Acad Sci USA* 1987; 84:1299–1303.

110. Muller WM, Lee FS, Dickson C, Peters G, Pattengale P, Leader P. The *int-2* gene product acts as an epithelial growth factor in transgenic mice. *EMBO J* 1990; 9:907–913.

111. van der Wall E, Donker TH, de Frankrijker E, Nortier HW, Thijssen JH, Blankenstein MA. Inhibition of the in vivo conversion of androstenedione to estrone by the aromatase inhibitor vorozole in healthy postmenopausal women. *Cancer Res* 1993; 53:4563–4566.

112. Buzdar A, Jonat W, Howell A, Jones SE, Blomqvist C, Vogel CL, et al. Anastrozole (ARIMIDEX), a potent and selective aromatase inhibitor, versus megestrol acetate (MEGACE) in postmenopausal women with advanced breast cancer: results of overview analysis of two phase III trials. *J Clin Oncol* 1996; 14:2000–2011.

113. Goss PE, Wine E, Tannock I, Schwartz IH, Kremer AB. Vorozole vs. Megace® in post-menopausal women with metastatic breast carcinoma who had relapsed following tamoxifen. *Proc Amer Soc Clin Oncol* 1997; 16:155a (abstract 542).

114. Marty M, Gershanovich M, Campos B, Romieu G, Lurie H, Bonaventura T, et al. Letrozole, a new potent, selective inhibitor (AI) superior to aminoglutethimide (AG) in postmenopausal women with advanced breast cancer (ABC) previously treated with antiestrogens. *Proc Amer Soc Clin Oncol* 1997; 16:156a (abstr 544).

115. Fisher B, Costantino J, Redmond C, Poisson R, Bowman D, Couture J, et al. A randomized clinical trial evaluating tamoxifen in the treatment of patients with node-negative breast cancer who have estrogen-receptor-positive tumors. *N Engl J Med* 1989; 320:479–484.

116. Breast Cancer Trials Committee, Scottish Cancer Trials Office. Adjuvant tamoxifen in the management of operable breast cancer: the Scottish trial. *Lancet* 1987; 2:171–175.

117. Fornander T, Rutqvist LE, Cedermark B, Glas U, Mattson A, Silfverward C, et al. Adjuvant tamoxifen in early breast cancer: occurrence of new primary cancers. *Lancet* 1989; 1:117–120.

118. Abram WP, Baum M, Berstock DA. Cyclophosphamide and tamoxifen as adjuvant therapies in the management of breast cancer. Preliminary analysis by the CRC Adjuvant Breast Trial Working Party. *Br J Cancer* 1988; 57:604–607.

119. Adlercreutz H, Bannwart C, Wähälä K, Mäkelä T, Brunow G, Hase T, et al. Inhibition of human aromatase by mammalian lignans and isoflavonoid phytoestrogens. *J Steroid Biochem Mol Biol* 1993; 44:147–153.

120. Ibrahim A-R, Abul-Hajj YL. Aromatase inhibition by flavonoids. *J Steroid Biochem Mol Biol* 1990; 37:257–260.

121. Kellis JT, Nesnow S, Vickery LE. Inhibition of aromatase cytochrome P450 (estrogen synthetase) by derivitaves of α-napthoflavone. *Biochem Pharmac* 1986; 35:2887–2891.

122. Campbell DR, Kurzer MS. Flavonoid inhibition of aromatase activity in human preadipocytes. *J Steroid Biochem Mol Biol* 1993; 46:381–388.

123. Wang C, Mäkelä T, Hase T, Adlercreutz H, Kurzer MS. Lignans and flvonoids inhibit aromatase enzyme in human preadipocytes. *J Steroid Biochem Mol Biol* 1994; 50:205–212.

124. Blanco JG, Gil RR, Alvarez CI, Patrito LC, Genti-Raimondi S, Flury A. A novel activity for a group of sesquiterpene lactones: inhibition of aromatase. *FEBS Lett* 1997; 409: 396–400.

125. Barbieri RL, Gochberg J, Ryan KJ. Nicotine, cotine, and anabasine inhibit aromatase in human trophoblasts in vitro. *J Clin Invest* 1986; 77:1727–1733.

126. Singleton VL. Naturally occurring food toxicants: phenolic substances of plant origin common in foods. *Adv Food Res* 1981; 27:149–242.

127. Borriello SP, Setchell KDR, Axelson M, Lawson AM. Production and metabolism of lignans by human fecal flora. *J Appl Bact* 1985; 58:37–43.

128. Adlercreutz H, Fotsis T, Heikkinen R, Dwyer JT, Woods M, Goldin BR, Gorbach SL. Excretion of the lignans enterolactone and enterodiol and of equol in omnivorous and vegetarian postmenopausal women and in women with breast cancer. *Lancet* 1982; 2: 1295–1299.

129. Adlercreutz H, Fotsis T, Lampe J, Wähälä K, Mäkelä T, Brunow G, Hase T. Quantitative determination of lignans and isoflavonoids in plasma of omnivorous and vegetarian women by isotope dilution gas chromatography-mass spectrometry. *Scand J Clin Lab Invest* 1993; 53 suppl. 215:5–18.

130. Martin PM, Horwiz KB, Ryan DS, McGuire WL. Phytoestrogen interaction with estrogen receptors in human breast cancer cells. *Endocrinology* 1978; 103:1860–1867.

131. Ranelletti FO, Ricci R, Larocca LM, Maggiano N, Caoelli A, Scambia G. Growth-inhibitory effect of quercetin and presence of type-II estrogen binding sites in human colon-cancer lines and primary colorectal tumors. *Intl J Cancer* 1992; 50:486–492.

132. Adlercreutz H, Mousavi Y, Clark J, Höckerstedt K, Hämäläinen E, Wähälä K, Mäkelä T, Hase T. Dietary phytoestrogens and cancer: in vitro and in vivo studies. *J Steroid Biochem Mol Biol* 1992; 41:331–337.

133. Waters AP, Knowler JT. Effect of lignan (HPMF) on RNA synthesis in the rat uterus. *Reprod Fertil* 1982; 66:379–381.

134. Hirano T, Fukuoka K, Oka K, Naito T, Hosaka K, Mitsuhashi H, Matsumoto Y. Antiproliferative activity of mammalian lignan derivatives against the human breast carcinoma cell line ZR-75-1. *Cancer Invest* 1990; 8:595–602.

135. Mousavi Y, Adlercreutz H. Enterolactone and estradiol inhibit each other's proliferative effects in breast cancer cells in culture. *J Steroid Biochem Mol Biol* 1992; 41:615–619.

12 Clinical Utility of Aromatase Inhibitors

K. Shenton, Mitchell Dowsett, and Michael Dukes

1. INTRODUCTION

Over the last 30 years, aromatase inhibitors have progressed from the status of experimental agents to that of established second-line treatment of advanced breast cancer, and their use in the adjuvant setting is currently being tested in large multicenter trials. The contrast between the chance discovery of the prototype inhibitor, aminoglutethimide, and the intensive development of the new third-generation compounds could not be more striking. Aminoglutethimide was developed in the 1950s as a derivative of the anticonvulsant glutethimide *(1);* having been found to have a superior therapeutic index to its parent compound, it was marketed in the USA for the treatment of epilepsy in1960. How-

From: *Hormone Therapy in Breast and Prostate Cancer*
Edited by: V. C. Jordan and B. J. A. Furr © Humana Press Inc., Totowa, NJ

ever, between 1963 and 1965, several cases of severe endocrine disturbance in children treated with the drug were reported, leading the Food and Drug Administration (FDA) to withdraw its licence in 1966. Its continued use as an "investigational agent" was fortunately allowed and intensive research demonstrated its inhibitory actions on steroid synthesis. This led in 1969 to the first use of aminoglutethimide in the treatment of postmenopausal advanced breast cancer *(2)*. Further studies ensued with responses thought to occur as a result of "medical adrenalectomy" *(3)*, but in 1978 the key action of aminoglutethimide in the suppression of estrogen synthesis via inhibition of the aromatase enzyme was recognized *(4)*.

The cytochrome P-450 enzyme aromatase is responsible for the conversion of androgens to estrogens. It is present in the ovaries but is also found in peripheral tissues such as fat, skin, and muscle and, following the menopause, significant amounts of estrogen continue to be produced from adrenal and ovarian androgens by aromatase in these peripheral tissues. In addition, it has been shown that approx two-thirds of breast tumors are themselves able to produce estrogens by virtue of the presence of aromatase *(5–7)*. Concentrations of estrogens in tumors from postmenopausal women have been found to be 10 times higher than those in the plasma *(8,9)*; locally produced estrogen may have a role in maintaining this gradient.

Approximately two-thirds of breast cancers in postmenopausal women are considered to depend on estrogens for their growth *(10)*. The therapeutic efficacy of blocking estrogenic activity is well-demonstrated by the clinical benefits of the estrogen "antagonist" tamoxifen, both in advanced breast cancer and in the adjuvant setting *(11,12)*. Thus the rationale for the treatment of postmenopausal breast cancer with aromatase inhibitors is clear: the inhibition of aromatase would be expected to produce clinical benefits by suppressing the production of estrogen peripherally and also potentially within the tumor itself. The case for their use in premenopausal breast cancer is not so straightforward, as their action may be potentially reversed by endocrine feedback causing increased gonadotrophin stimulation of the functional ovary. However, their use in association with other agents such as gonadotrophin hormone-releasing hormone agonists remains a possibility; this will be discussed later.

Studies with aminoglutethimide served to demonstrate that aromatase inhibition was potentially as effective as other endocrine treatments such as tamoxifen *(13)* and progestins *(14)* in advanced breast cancer, but aminoglutethimide's lack of specificity for aromatase, which necessitates concomitant administration of replacement glucocorticoid, side effects, and poor pharmacokinetics made it an unattractive drug and motivated the development of more potent and selective aromatase inhibitors. The potential to avoid certain of the side effects associated with tamoxifen, notably its partial agonist action on the uterus, and the weight gain and cardiovascular complications of the progestins further enhances the attractiveness of aromatase inhibition as a therapeutic approach.

In recent years a number of new aromatase inhibitors have been developed with improved potency, selectivity, and pharmacokinetics in comparison with aminoglutethimide. They have been studied extensively and are being used increasingly in the treatment of breast cancer. In this chapter we will describe the knowledge to date of their use in the treatment of advanced breast cancer and in the primary medical and adjuvant settings; possible resistance mechanisms, patient selection, non-breast cancer usage, and future prospects will also be discussed.

2. ADVANCED BREAST CANCER

2.1. Aminoglutethimide

The standard daily dose of aminoglutethimide (AG) of 1000 mg/d plus hydrocortisone in postmenopausal women with advanced breast cancer results in 90–95% inhibition of aromatase (4,15) and response rates similar to those seen with other endocrine therapies (13,14). Response rates vary depending on inclusion criteria such as previous endocrine treatment, estrogen receptor (ER) status and site of metastasis, but overall about one-third of patients experience either complete or partial response with a further 15% benefiting from disease stabilization (16). This latter category is of clinical importance since stable disease gives equivalent palliation and survival to that from objective response (17). Median duration of response is 12–15 mo, with soft-tissue and lymph-node metastases tending to respond better than those in visceral sites. AG has been reported to produce a high level of response in bone (18,19), and in particular a high incidence of relief of bone pain (20). A direct effect on prostaglandin metabolism rather than aromatase inhibition may contribute to the latter effect (21), but it should be noted that the large randomized trials of AG vs other endocrine therapy that are needed to confirm these observations have not been conducted.

AG is effective second-line therapy in patients who have previously responded to tamoxifen, adrenalectomy, or hypophysectomy and then relapsed (22). Studies of sequential use of tamoxifen and AG have demonstrated similar first-line responses to both agents, but when tamoxifen is used after AG, response rates may be lower than those seen with AG after tamoxifen (13,23). Combination of the two drugs is not more effective than either given alone (24–27). This may be due to the induction of tamoxifen metabolism by AG (28). With the possible exception of patients with bone pain, it has, therefore, been preferred management to give tamoxifen before AG. An additional reason for this sequence of treatment is the greater incidence of side effects with AG. These occur in approx 35% of patients and require discontinuation of treatment in 5% (22). The most important of these side effects include lethargy, vertigo, ataxia, depression, insomnia, nystagmus, rash, pruritus, and, rarely, blood dyscrasias. Clinical experience suggests, however, that side effects tend to improve with time and are on the whole tolerated in this group of patients.

The optimum dose of AG, and the role of glucocorticoid replacement in its mechanism of action and its possible contribution to antitumor efficacy have been the subject of detailed study, but much of the available data is from non-randomized studies, and, in those studies that are randomized, patient numbers are probably too small to show differences of 5–10%. These studies do not suggest any major role for glucocorticoids in the mechanism of action of AG, but glucocorticoid is still given because of the reduction in cortisol reserve by AG and to obviate reflex adrenal stimulation. While dose-response relationships in efficacy have not been definitively demonstrated, it is now generally accepted that reducing the dose of AG to 500 mg/d reduces side-effects while maintaining antitumor efficacy *(29)*.

2.2. Steroidal Aromatase Inhibitors

The steroidal group of inhibitors are all analogues of androstenedione or testosterone, the primary substrates of aromatase, and are mainly mechanism-based irreversible inhibitors. The group includes 4-hydroxyandrostenedione (formestane), which is clinically available in most European countries, and newer agents such as exemestane, currently completing Phase III trials.

Because of extensive first-pass hepatic glucuronidation, the bioavailibilty of orally administered formestane is low *(30,31)*, so in clinical use it is given parenterally to achieve optimal estrogen suppression. Formestane has low systemic toxicity *(32,33);* the most common side effects are local with pain and induration at injection sites and, more rarely, sterile abscesses, which have required discontinuation of therapy in 4.5% of patients in some studies *(33)*. Comparative pharmacology *(30,31)* and minimization of local side effects have made fortnightly administration of 250 mg intramuscularly the dosage regime of choice. At this dosage, aromatase is inhibited in patients by about 85% *(34)*. Formestane is highly specific for aromatase with no other significant endocrine effects when given parenterally.

In postmenopausal patients with advanced breast cancer, formestane produced tumor responses in 23–39% of patients and stabilized disease in a further 14–29% *(30,31,35–38)*. As with AG, those patients who have previously responded to endocrine therapy are more likely to benefit and the response is better in soft-tissue lesions than bony metastases or visceral disease *(34)*. Responses have also been observed in patients relapsing on AG *(35)*, suggesting that aromatase inhibition with different types of inhibitor may produce a second response. A recent comparison of formestane and tamoxifen as first-line treatment in advanced disease showed similar response rates for both drugs *(40),* but a longer duration of response with tamoxifen.

Exemestane is a potent, orally active, selective aromatase inhibitor. It achieved around 98% suppression of aromatase at a dose of 25 mg/d *(41)*. It is generally well-tolerated, but androgenic side effects have been reported in 4% of patients treated with the standard dose of 25 mg/d, increasing to 10% at 200 mg/d. Other side effects such as hot flushes, sweating, and nausea are seen in 11, 4, and 3% of patients treated with exemestane at 25 mg/d and 23, 14, and 19% treated with 200 mg/d, respectively. Two large multicenter trials comprising a total of 265 postmenopausal patients failing on tamoxifen therapy have shown an objective response rate of 22%, with 47% of patients benefiting if stable disease is included. Studies of exemestane as third-line treatment in patients failing on megestrol acetate or AG have shown response rates of 13 and 24%, respectively. Respective stable disease rates were 14 and 24%. Further studies of exemestane as third-line treatment are in progress along with dose escalation studies and a Phase III trial comparing exemestane at 25 mg/d with megestrol acetate *(42)*.

2.3. Nonsteroidal Aromatase Inhibitors

2.3.1. FADROZOLE

The nonsteroidal imidazole-derivative fadrozole has been reported to produce comparable estrogen suppression to the standard regime of AG 1000 mg hydrocortisone/d when given at a dose of 2 mg/d *(43)*. However, using the more sensitive measure of inhibition of whole-body aromatization, at 2 mg/d fadrozole had lower pharmacological activity than full-dose AG *(43)*. A double-blind randomized dose-finding multicenter study showed objective responses in 16% of women given fadrozole as second-line treatment *(44,45)*. No difference was demonstrated between doses of 1, 2 or 4 mg/d. In Phase II trials, response rates of 14 and 17% for second-line *(46,47)* and 50% as first-line treatment have been reported *(48)*. A Phase III trial comprising 683 patients randomized to receive either fadrozole or megestrol acetate showed no difference in overall response, response duration, time to progression, or survival with similar tolerability, except that weight gain, fluid retention, and dyspnoea were more common with megestrol acetate and nausea and vomiting more frequent with fadrozole *(49)*. A Phase III study with 212 patients comparing fadrozole to tamoxifen reported similar response rates of 20 and 27%, respectively. Time to treatment failure was longer in patients randomized to tamoxifen but the difference did not reach statistical significance, while fadrozole had a significantly lower percentage of clinically relevant toxic effects *(50)*. However, fadrozole is not completely selective for the aromatase enzyme and some suppressive effects on the synthesis of cortisol and aldosterone have been observed at doses as low as 1 mg bd *(51,52)*. This, in association with the slightly disappointing response rates and the development of the new potent and specific triazole inhibitors, means fadrozole is unlikely to come into widespread clinical use. It is licensed for use in Japan, but its development else-where has been curtailed.

2.3.2. TRIAZOLES

With the development of the third-generation triazole family of aromatase inhibitors, including anastrozole, letrozole, and vorozole, the aim of achieving highly potent and specific aromatase inhibition has been fulfilled. At the doses chosen for clinical use, they can each suppress plasma estradiol and estrone levels to below the limit of detection of highly sensitive assays *(53–55),* with anastrozole at 1 mg/d and letrozole at 2.5 mg/d inhibiting whole-body aro-matase activity by 96.7 and >98.9%, respectively *(56,57).*

Data on the clinical utility of these agents is available from recent reports of six large randomized trials each comparing one of these aromatase inhibitors with one of the established second-line endocrine agents, megestrol acetate, or AG. Only the studies of anastrozole vs megestrol acetate *(58)* and letrozole vs megestrol acetate *(59)* are published in peer-reviewed journals; the others have been presented in abstract form *(60–62).*

All three drugs are well absorbed orally and can be given on a once-daily basis. The Phase III trials confirm the conclusions of earlier studies that they are well-tolerated, with minor gastrointestinal disturbances such as anorexia and nausea being the most frequent adverse events, other than those related to estrogen deprivation. All three drugs caused less weight gain than megestrol acetate, which is a particular advantage in this group of women for whom unwanted changes in body image can result in significant psychological mor-bidity. There were also fewer thromboembolic or cardiovascular serious adverse events with the aromatase inhibitors than with megestrol acetate, and the trials of letrozole and vorozole vs AG demonstrated substantially improved tolerability with the new compounds.

The identical design of the two trials of anastrozole (1 mg/d vs 10 mg/d vs megestrol acetate 160 mg/d) allowed the data from the total of 764 patients to be combined. There were no significant differences in response, time to progression, or time to treatment failure between the treatment arms in the initial reports, but analysis at a median follow-up time of 31 mo revealed a statistically significant survival advantage for anastrozole 1 mg/d over megestrol acetate *(63,64).*

The studies of letrozole vs megestrol acetate 160 mg/d (551 patients) and aminoglutethimide 250 mg bd plus glucocorticoid replacement (555 patients) have shown the 2.5 mg/d dose of letrozole to be superior in response, time to progression, and time to treatment failure. A significant survival advantage for letrozole (2.5 mg/d) over AG was demonstrated, but not in respect of mege-strol acetate. In both studies the lower dose of letrozole (0.5 mg/d) was found not to be as effective as the higher dose but to have comparable efficacy to both megestrol acetate and AG.

Vorozole (2.5 mg/d) demonstrated trends towards improved efficacy over megestrol acetate (452 patients) and significantly better response rates with prolonged time to treatment failure in comparison with AG (556 patients). No significant survival differences have as yet been found. Vorozole was withdrawn from further development in late 1997.

2.4. Combination Treatments

In the 1980s several studies were conducted of aromatase inhibitors (chiefly AG) combined with other endocrine agents such as tamoxifen, a progestin, or danazol. In a few of these studies, marginally improved response rates were achieved but there was no improvement in survival. There is a general consensus that this type of combination in postmenopausal women with advanced breast cancer has been largely unhelpful *(65)*. The lack of improved efficacy may in some cases be explained by adverse drug interactions *(28)*, known to be possible with AG, a powerful inducer of hepatic P450 activity. If such effects are not induced by the newer aromatase inhibitors, it is possible that improved response rates from combining them with other endocrine treatments may yet be seen. Already, though, an adverse interaction between letrozole and tamoxifen has been demonstrated *(29)*, with plasma levels of letrozole being reduced by about 40% on the addition of tamoxifen. It is clear, therefore, that potential interactions need to be investigated carefully before larger studies are carried out. However, addition of anastrozole to breast-cancer patients already receiving tamoxifen had no affect on plasma concentrations of tamoxifen *(65a)*.

Combinations that have proved useful are those where a second agent has been added to a first to which the patient has responded but then acquired resistance. Examples include the addition of AG to 4-OHA, with two of seven postmenopausal women deriving a further response *(66)*, and the addition of 4-OHA to premenopausal patients relapsing on goserelin, a gonadotrophin-releasing hormone agonist, with response in four of six patients *(66)*. It is possible that these additional responses may be due to the tumors having acquired hypersensitivity to estrogen as has been demonstrated in vitro with breast-cancer cells grown under conditions of long-term estrogen deprivation *(67)*. Whether greater long-term disease control will be obtained by stepwise estrogen deprivation or by immediate complete deprivation using such combinations is a question that remains to be answered.

Another combination that may be worthy of further investigation is that of one of the new triazole inhibitors with a glucocorticoid. At first sight this may appear a retrograde step since one of the reasons for the development of new inhibitors was the desire to avoid the glucocorticoid replacement required with AG. However, there are two reasons why this combination may be useful. Firstly, the adrenal so-called androgen, $\Delta 5$-androstene-3β, 17β-diol, also has estrogenic activity in laboratory models *(68)* and the addition of glucocorticoid therapy would be expected to reduce production of this steroid by 80%. Secondly, since about 80 and 70%, respectively, of plasma levels of androstenedione and testosterone result from adrenal synthesis in postmenopausal women, glucocorticoid therapy would also bring about a substantial reduction in levels of these steroids and thereby reduce the available substrate for any residual aromatase. The improved clinical outcome reported to occur with the addition of prednisolone to tamoxifen treatment *(69)* may in part be dependent on the adrenal suppressive effects of prednisolone.

2.5. Summary

The development of the third-generation aromatase inhibitors offers the opportunity for improvements in both quality of life and survival in postmenopausal women with advanced breast cancer. They are the agents of choice for second-line therapy following relapse on tamoxifen.

3. PRIMARY MEDICAL/NEOADJUVANT TREATMENT

It has been suggested that in elderly patients who present with primary breast cancer, it may be preferable to avoid surgery and its associated risks and to treat with endocrine therapy alone. This has generally entailed the use of tamoxifen, but other agents, including aromatase inhibitors, could potentially be equally useful. However, while there is no evidence that survival is compromised by this approach, the rate of local recurrence is significantly higher in those treated nonsurgically *(70,71),* and on the whole it is generally reserved for those patients for whom surgery is not possible on medical grounds. If, however, it were possible to identify reliably those patients who would respond, primary endocrine therapy could be used with greater confidence.

A modification of this approach that is of interest currently is the use of neoadjuvant therapy: medical treatment for a limited period, usually about 3 mo, prior to surgery. The rationale for this is twofold. Firstly it may be possible to reduce the need for mastectomy in patients with large tumors and also to render inoperable tumors operable. Secondly, as indicated by a series of animal studies *(72),* improved survival may be possible with this approach. Most neoadjuvant studies to date have used chemotherapy, but the animal studies suggest that endocrine therapy in this context would have equivalent efficacy. Clinical studies of this type with aromatase inhibitors are limited, but the results are increasingly encouraging, particularly with the triazole inhibitors, as described below.

3.1. Aminoglutethimide

In a study of 81 patients with operable breast cancer of 4 cm or greater diameter treated with neoadjuvant therapy, 61 received endocrine therapy, 10 of these with AG (500 mg daily) plus hydrocortisone, for 12 wk prior to surgery *(73)*. Twenty-four patients treated with initial endocrine therapy (39%) showed significant tumor regression, with a median time to reach half volume of 44 d. One tumor showed a complete clinical response. All those patients who responded had ER-rich tumors ($\geq$ 20 fmol mg^{-1} cytosol protein). The proportion of patients achieving regression did not vary greatly according to the type of endocrine therapy received.

3.2. Steroidals

As part of a neoadjuvant study, 34 ER-positive postmenopausal patients were treated with 4-OHA (250 mg two-weekly) for 3 mo prior to surgery *(74)*. Twelve patients (35%) achieved a clinical response, which was complete in five patients. Thirteen patients showed no change and nine progressed on treatment. The authors concluded that in appropriate patients neoadjuvant endocrine therapy was useful to downgrade the tumor, increasing the opportunity for more conservative surgery.

3.3. Triazoles

To date there are no studies published in peer-review journals of neoadjuvant studies using the new triazole inhibitors, but a study with very encouraging results using letrozole has been presented in abstract form *(75,76)*. Twenty-four postmenopausal patients with ER-positive tumors >3cm were treated with a 3-mo course of letrozole at either 2.5 mg or 10 mg daily. Overall, based on ultrasound measurements of tumor volume, response rate was 92%. With the 2.5 mg dose there were two complete responses (CR) and 10 partial responses (PR). There was one complete histological response. With the 10 mg dose there were 2 CR, 8 PR, and 2 patients with static disease. Median reductions of tumor volume were 87% with 2.5 mg and 74% with 10 mg. After 3 mo of treatment with letrozole, 15 patients who would have required mastectomy at outset, had they been deemed operable, were all operable and none required mastectomy. Similar studies are underway with anastrozole and comparing vorozole with tamoxifen.

Much information concerning mechanism of drug action can be gained in these studies from sequential tumor biopsies and measurement of various biological markers. They also provide an opportunity to study effects of aromatase inhibitors on bone without the confounding effect of metastatic bone disease.

4. ADJUVANT TREATMENT

The evidence that tamoxifen provides a survival benefit in the adjuvant setting is clear *(11)* but equally so is the reality that many women still die from metastatic breast cancer despite receiving this treatment. Thus the need for alternative therapies is obvious and aromatase inhibitors would seem suitable candidates. One advantage that aromatase inhibitors may possess in this context is that, since they do not interact with the ER, it is unlikely that the disease could become stimulated by these drugs (cf. tamoxifen *[77]*). An early double-blind study that randomized 322 postmenopausal patients with primary breast cancer and ipsilateral node involvement to receive AG plus hydrocortisone or placebo for 2 yr failed to show any survival advantage of treatment over placebo *(78)*. The more powerful aromatase inhibition and much improved tolerability of the new orally active aromatase inhibitors make them an attractive option for re-evaluating this concept. A number of trials are underway or in the late stages of protocol development. These include a direct comparison of anastrozole against tamoxifen alone or a combination of the two (ATAC) and the use of sequential tamoxifen followed by an aromatase inhibitor or vice versa, the rationale for this being taken from the usefulness of the sequential approach in the advanced setting.

However, there are several concerns that remain to be addressed. First, it will be important to exclude any disadvantageous pharmacokinetic or pharmacological interactions between the drugs, such as those between AG or letrozole and tamoxifen as discussed earlier. Second, the effects of long-term estrogen deprivation on postmenopausal patients are presently unknown. In particular, the risk of accelerated osteoporotic changes and deleterious effects on plasma lipids with consequent increased cardiovascular disease cannot be ruled out at present. These issues are of particular importance in view of the protective effects of tamoxifen on both the skeleton and the cardiovascular system. However, should these concerns be confirmed with the aromatase inhibitors alone it is possible that combination with tamoxifen or one of the more recently developed selective estrogen-response modulators (SERMs) might abrogate them.

5. PREMENOPAUSAL BREAST CANCER

The majority of data available on the use of aromatase inhibitors has been obtained from studies in postmenopausal patients. Their use in premenopausal patients is theoretically complicated by negative feedback resulting in increased gonadotrophin stimulation of the ovaries and failure to suppress oestrogen levels completely. Early studies with AG in premenopausal patients demonstrated that, even at the full dose of 1000 mg/d, plasma estradiol levels were not suppressed reproducibly into the postmenopausal range *(79–80)*. Nevertheless, disturbance of menstrual activity and increases in gonadotrophin levels provided evidence of some inhibition of estrogen synthesis. More recently it has been reported that one of the triazole inhibitors (vorozole) markedly suppressed estrogen levels in premenopausal women over a 24-h period after administration of a single dose of 20 mg *(82)*, and another, letrozole, markedly suppressed follicular-phase estrogen levels in macaque monkeys *(83)*, suggesting that it may be possible to use these agents alone as estrogen suppressants in premenopausal women. However, the latter study also demonstrated that letrozole treatment during the follicular phase resulted in the development of multiple mature ovarian follicles, which would probably be unacceptable in patients.

It is possible that major suppression of plasma estrogen levels may not be necessary in order to achieve tumor regression in premenopausal women. In one of the studies described earlier, a response rate of 28% (5 out of 18 patients) was obtained in premenopausal women with advanced breast cancer treated with AG *(81)*. A plausible explanation of this is that response in these patients was dependent on suppression of local aromatase activity within, or adjacent to, the breast cancers themselves and not entirely on suppression of circulating estrogen levels *(84)*.

6. PATIENT SELECTION

As with other endocrine therapy, the best available predictor of response to aromatase inhibitors is the presence of ER within the tumor. Thus the majority of responses occurs in patients whose tumors are ER-positive, with very few in ER-negative tumors *(22,85)*. However, only about 50% of tumors that are ER-positive respond; it would, therefore, be desirable to find other markers with improved predictive value. An obvious target for study is the aromatase activity within the breast carcinoma itself. Some early studies have found that the response of breast tumors to aromatase inhibitors is greater when the tumors possess detectable aromatase activity. The aromatase activity in tumors from 23 postmenopausal women with advanced breast cancer whose tumors were known to be ER-positive was measured prior to treatment with AG and hydrocortisone *(84)*. Eleven of 18 patients with aromatase-positive tumors showed response to treatment, while none of five whose tumors possessed no aromatase activity responded ($p = 0.047$). A similar pattern of response was found in a group of 25 patients with primary breast cancer treated with either AG or 4-OHA *(86)*, achieving statistical significance when the results for both drugs were combined. Positive correlation of aromatase levels with response to treatment with AG has also been demonstrated by a second group *(87)*. These studies all involved biochemical measurement of aromatase activity which to date has been the accepted gold standard method. Unfortunately, these assays require approx half a gram of fresh or frozen tissue, which is often not available, and are time-consuming to perform and therefore difficult to apply to large numbers of patients. Recently, however, several groups have been working on the development of reliable immunohistochemical techniques for assaying aromatase present in paraffin blocks of tumors, including specimens as small as needle-core biopsies *(88–90)*. The validation of one of these antibodies for application to response prediction would be of great importance in the future application of aromatase inhibitors, particularly in the adjuvant context.

7. MECHANISMS OF RESISTANCE TO AROMATASE INHIBITORS

While a considerable number of patients benefit from treatment with aromatase inhibitors, many, particularly unselected patients in the advanced setting, do not. Furthermore, when response is achieved it is not usually permanent and disease almost invariably returns in a resistant form. Aromatase inhibitors are not unique in this, a similar pattern being observed with all forms of endocrine therapy and thus many of the mechanisms of resistance are probably common to estrogen deprivation in general. It is possible, however, that in certain patients resistance is specific to the use of aromatase inhibition and even to the type of inhibitor used.

7.1. General Mechanisms

Many breast cancers, particularly those that have no or only low concentrations of ER, are not dependent on estrogens for their growth and are unlikely to respond to aromatase inhibitors or other hormonal therapies aimed at mitigating estrogen stimulation. It follows that acquired resistance, after initially successful treatment with aromatase inhibitors, may result from the selection and outgrowth of estrogen-independent clones of cells that had been present from the start of treatment. While intratumoural heterogeneity of hormone-receptor status and sensitivity has been documented *(91,92)*, this theory of clonal selection has not been backed up by clinical data. If successful treatment with aromatase inhibitors were to be associated with destruction of ER-positive cells with the consequent emergence of receptor-negative clones, ER content of tumors should fall progressively during therapy. However, sequential studies on tumors from patients treated with either AG or 4-OHA have shown that in the majority of cases ER levels following response are similar to those before treatment *(93)*.

It is also clear that the mechanism or mechanisms through which tumors become resistant to tamoxifen do not result in resistance to aromatase inhibitors in a high proportion of cases. Indeed, prior response to tamoxifen is a good indicator of likely response to an aromatase inhibitor following relapse on or after tamoxifen *(24,54)*. Although considerable work has been conducted on tamoxifen resistance and numerous mechanisms suggested, much less work has been performed with aromatase inhibitors.

Work with cytotoxic chemotherapeutic agents has suggested that some tumors may possess or acquire resistance by mechanisms such as the presence of efflux pumps or metabolic activity, which reduce effective drug levels within tumor cells *(55)*. While it may be possible that a similar phenomenon is associated with resistance to aromatase inhibitors, no evidence of this has so far been presented. Furthermore, in contrast to other hormonal and chemotherapeutic agents whose antitumor action is directed at tumor cells, aromatase inhibitors achieve their reduction of systemic estrogen levels, and probably also of the greater part of the tumor estrogen levels, through effects on normal estrogen-synthesizing tissues. Unlike tumor cells, these normal tissues are genetically stable and not under survival pressures and are, therefore, less prone to the development of efflux and related resistance mechanisms.

As with many drugs, variations in response among patients or over time can result from differing or changing metabolic processing. Although acetylated derivatives are major metabolites of AG *(94)*, tumor response to this drug has been shown not to be related to patients' capacity to acetylate *(95)* but to induction of hepatic enzymes *(85)*, which accounts for its increased clearance and reduced plasma half-life during acute administration *(96)*. As data on plasma levels of AG at the time of relapse have not been published, the possibility that resistance may be associated with reduced drug levels cannot be excluded, but if this were the case, plasma estrogen levels would be expected to rise before or at the time of relapse. The data on this issue have been conflicting, with one study failing to detect a rise *(97)* while a larger study demonstrated a modest but significant rise in plasma estrone levels prior to relapse *(98)*. "Hormone escape" could therefore have contributed to relapse in some patients taking AG. If this is the case, further suppression of estrogen levels would be expected to elicit further responses. In this context it should be noted that second- or third-line therapies such as higher doses of AG *(99)* more potent aromatase inhibitors *(108)*, and hypophysectomy *(101)* have produced considerable response rates in patients relapsing on AG.

7.2. Specific Mechanisms

Intratumoral aromatase has been found to be a predictor of response to aromatase inhibitors *(84,86,87)*. Paradoxically, in patients treated with AG, levels of aromatase activity within the tumor have been shown to rise on treatment by as much as 25-fold *(84)*. This is consistent with the ability of AG to induce cytochrome p450 hydroxylases *(85)*, but it is also possible that the effect may relate to stabilisation of the enzyme following binding of the drug reducing its degradation. These elevated levels of enzyme activity could potentially reduce the efficacy of AG.

A further question is whether, in spite of circulating estrogens being reduced to very low, and, by the new inhibitors, often undetectable levels, there may still be sufficient residual estrogen to stimulate tumor growth. It has recently been demonstrated that the growth of long-term estrogen-deprived human breast-cancer cells in vitro can be stimulated by concentrations of estradiol as low as 10^{-14} to 10^{-15} M *(67)*. If similar sensitization of estrogen-deprived tumor cells occurs in vivo, hormone-dependent tumor growth may resume even with the near-complete aromatase inhibition provided by the latest drugs.

Mutations in the gene encoding aromatase leading to alterations in the structure of the enzyme represent another potential mechanism of resistance to aromatase inhibitors. Structure-function studies of site-specific mutations *(102)*, have revealed one such mutation that decreases the sensitivity of the enzyme to 4-OHA without changing its sensitivity to AG or the intrinsic activity of the enzyme itself. It is known that a subset of breast tumors appears to be relatively insensitive to the effects of 4-OHA while maintaining sensitivity to other inhibitors *(103)*, and it may be that these tumors contain mutations in the aromatase gene similar to those induced artificially. However other molecular evidence from human tumors does not support this as being clinically important *(104)*.

Finally, although specific aromatase inhibitors effectively reduce the availability of estradiol, estrone, estriol, and estrone sulphate, they do not affect other sources of estrogenic activity such as Δ5 androgens, which are produced in large quantities by the adrenals and are capable of producing estrogenic effects *(105)* including stimulating hormone-dependent breast-cancer growth *(106)*, and exogenous dietary estrogens. Any tumors capable of exploiting these alternative sources of estrogen stimulation would probably be resistant to treatment with aromatase inhibitors.

8. NONBREAST-CANCER USAGE

8.1. Prostatic Carcinoma

Initial endocrine therapy for patients with prostate cancer is castration, either surgical or medical, which removes approx 90% of plasma testosterone *(107)* and achieves clinical response in about 70–80% of patients *(108)*. Further hormonal treatment has generally been aimed at suppressing residual androgen stimulation provided by adrenal androgens. Early approaches used bilateral adrenalectomy or hypophysectomy *(109,110)*. Based on its inhibitory effects on adrenal steroidogenesis, AG has been used in prostate cancer in an attempt to achieve a medical adrenalectomy in castrated patients *(111,112)* and several studies have shown both subjective and objective responses to AG plus hydrocortisone *(113)*. However, AG does not suppress plasma androgen levels in castrated males and even in combination with hydrocortisone suppression is relatively minor *(114–116)*. Subjective responses to AG based on pain reduction may be due to inhibition of prostaglandin synthesis *(21)*.

The possibility that aromatase occurs in prostatic carcinomas and that estrogens produced within the prostate may be of biological importance in stimulating prostate cancer-cell growth has been raised *(117,118)*. This would provide a further explanation for the effectiveness of AG. Evidence for this mode of action is provided by studies of the more specific aromatase inhibitor 4-OHA in castrated patients with advanced prostatic cancer: subjective responses were reported in 12/19 *(119)* but data on objective response is currently not available.

8.2. Benign Prostatic Hyperplasia

Many observations in humans and animals have implicated estrogens as a principal underlying causative factor in the development of benign prostatic hyperplasia (BPH). These included the relative increase in the ratio of concentrations of estrogens and androgens in blood and prostate tissues with age in men *(120–122)*, synergism between estrogens and androgens in stimulating stromal growth and BPH in dogs and monkeys *(123,124)*, and stimulation by estrogens of periurethral hyperplasia in monkeys *(125)* and humans *(126)*. As well as effects on prostate growth, estrogens also increase the contractility of the neck of the bladder *(127)* and might further contribute to the symptomology of BPH by directly increasing resistance to bladder emptying. The capacity of aromatase inhibitors to block the development of BPH in animal models *(123–125,128)*, and to produce promising reductions in prostate volume and symptoms in two open clinical trials *(129,130)* provided further support for estrogen being an aetiological factor and aromatase inhibitors a potential remedy.

However, this early promise for aromatase inhibition has not been confirmed by two large, randomized, controlled trials that failed to demonstrate any therapeutic benefit of the steroidal aromatase inhibitor atamestane over placebo *(131,132)*. One possible explanation may lie in the degree of estrogen suppression achieved with the doses of atamastane used in these trials. Reductions in estrone and estradiol were of the order of 50–70% and 30–40%, respectively, and did not show a strong dose relationship over the range of doses (100–400 mg) used. It is still possible therefore that more complete estrogen suppression with one of the more potent triazole inhibitors may provide significant benefit.

However, a further possible explanation for the absence of benefit in the atamastane trials was the 30–60% increase in circulating testosterone and dihydrotestosterone, an inevitable consequence of the disturbance to gonadotrophin feedback, which, in males, is at least part regulated by hypothalamic aromatization of testosterone to estradiol. This increase in potential androgenic stimulation may be sufficient to reverse any benefits of reduced estrogenic stimulation, and if this is the more important explanation for the poor performance of atamastane, then even more potent aromatase inhibitors are unlikely to deliver greater efficacy as monotherapy. Combined treatment using an aromatase inhibitor and an antiandrogen or 5α-reductase inhibitor ought, theoretically, to provide maximal control of prostate growth, but will only be acceptable therapy provided any further increase in gonadotrophin secretion does not cause adverse testicular stimulation and that libido is not extinguished.

8.3. Endometrial Carcinoma

This common female cancer often contains hormone receptors *(133)*, and it is widely accepted that estrogen is one of the contributing factors to its development and growth. *In situ* estrogen synthesis has also been reported to be higher in endometrial-cancer tissue as compared with normal endometrium *(134)*. Thus, aromatase inhibitors might theoretically be of use in its management. In a study of nine patients given AG who had relapsed while receiving progestogens, an objective response was observed in two and stable disease in a further three *(135)*. To our knowledge, there are no data available on similar studies with other inhibitors, but such research may prove of interest in future.

8.4. Endometriosis

Aromatase activity has been detected in both uterine and ectopic endometrial tissue of women with endometriosis *(136)* and it has been postulated that locally synthesized estrogen may affect the growth of such deposits. A study in rats treated with the nonsteroidal aromatase inhibitor fadrozole has shown dose-dependent decrease in the size of cystic endometrial transplants *(137)* and anastrozole has recently been reported to be "extraordinarily successful" in treating severe postmenopausal endometriosis in a 57-yr-old woman *(138)*. Although aromatase inhibitors appear an attractive option for treating endometriosis, and other benign gynecological conditions, their use in premenopausal women is complicated by the disturbance to ovarian-pituitary feedback, increased gonadal stimulation, and risk of ovarian-cyst formation, as discussed earlier in the context of premenopausal breast cancer.

8.5. Malignant Melanoma

Aromatase activity has been described in malignant melanoma *(139)* and therefore a number of small studies have looked into the use of aromatase inhibitors in its management. In one study, two of nine patients with metastatic malignant melanoma treated with AG had disease stabilization, but no objective tumor shrinkage was seen *(140)*. A more recent study failed to demonstrate any response in 15 heavily pretreated patients treated with AG, and the authors concluded that AG was very unlikely to be useful in melanoma patients *(141)*.

8.6. Excessive Peripheral Aromatisation

This endocrinopathy, first described in the 1970s *(142)*, is characterized by gynecomastia of prepubertal onset, contrasexual precocity, and hypogonadism in boys; in girls it may give rise to isosexual precocity. Familial forms have subsequently been reported *(143)*. In one 17-yr-old boy with gynecomastia of prepubertal onset, extremely high circulating estrone, and estradiol levels were shown to be due to a conversion rate of androstenedione to estrone in the periphery of 55%, 50 times that of normal young men *(144)*. Treatment with anastrozole has been reported to be promising in such conditions *(145)*.

8.7. Ovulation Induction

Antiestrogens, particularly clomiphene citrate, are used to induce ovulation in women with hypogonadotrophic hypogonadism. There are no data relating to the use of aromatase inhibitors in this context, but their investigation would seem worthwhile. Antiestrogens have a long tissue half-life, theoretically having a negative impact on the integrity of the luteal phase of the cycle. The use of an aromatase inhibitor with a short half-life could potentially avoid this possible complication.

9. PROSPECTS FOR PREVENTION OF BREAST CANCER

An area of particular interest for possible future application of aromatase inhibitors is in breast-cancer prevention. There are several pieces of evidence that suggest that abating estrogen stimulation may have a specific role in preventing the emergence of this disease.

Epidemiological data has provided clear evidence that, in premenopausal women, estrogen deprivation in the form of ovarian ablation leads to a markedly reduced incidence of breast cancer *(146)*. More recent epidemiological data also support the proposed association between increased plasma estrogen levels and higher postmenopausal breast-cancer risk: a recent overview has been published of six prospective studies in which estradiol levels were measured in plasma samples collected several years prior to the development of breast cancer *(147)*. Estradiol levels were significantly higher in the women who have subsequently developed breast cancer. As the aromatase enzyme is responsible for the production of all steroidal estrogens, it seems likely that it may play a key role in the relationship between high estrogen levels and breast cancer.

In premenopausal patients with primary breast cancer, oophorectomy results in a much-reduced incidence of second primary breast cancers *(148)*, and in postmenopausal patients tamoxifen significantly reduces the incidence of contralateral breast tumors *(11,149)*. Tamoxifen's efficacy and comparative safety in the treatment of breast cancer prompted investigation of the possibility that it may be an effective prophylactic for breast cancer in women at high risk of developing the disease *(150)*. Large controlled trials in Europe and North America were begun in 1989 and 1992, respectively, and, shortly after the North American trial reached its target of 13,000 participants in late 1997, an interim review demonstrated a 49% reduction in the occurrence of breast cancer after an average duration of treatment of 4 yr in the tamoxifen arm of the study *(72)*. This is the most compelling evidence to date that pharmacological abatement of estrogen stimulation can at least delay the occurrence of breast cancer.

Aromatase inhibitors have not yet been explored as preventative agents against breast cancer in humans. They do, however, reduce the incidence of spontaneous tumors in rats *(151)*, and other recent observations suggest that targeting aromatase directly might be advantageous. One of the most compelling pieces of evidence that increased aromatase activity may lead to breast cancer was the discovery that the site of integration of the mouse mammary tumor virus is the aromatase gene *(152)*. The aromatase gene is identical to the gene called int-5 and the deregulation of aromatase caused by the integration of the virus evidently promotes the development of mammary cancer in mice. More recently, additional support for an association between mutations in the aromatase gene and increased breast-cancer risk has been provided by the demonstration that a polymorphism within the aromatase gene in humans is associated with increased breast cancer risk *(153)*. Several studies are underway to confirm this important observation.

Thus, there are several pieces of evidence that suggest that aromatase activity may be associated with breast-cancer risk and that aromatase inhibitors should be investigated as preventative agents. In comparison with tamoxifen and the newer SERMs, aromatase inhibitors clearly cannot offer the former's selective, partial estrogen-agonist actions, which are beneficial for maintaining bone mineral and favorable plasma lipid profiles. On the other hand, it is possible that partial estrogen agonist activity may limit efficacy in relation to breast-cancer prevention. With their capacity to extinguish more than 95% of endogenous estrogen synthesis, the latest aromatase inhibitors may prove effective in a higher proportion of women and/or for longer. However, such extreme estrogen depletion will probably exacerbate menopausal bone and lipid changes, and measures to control them, such as calcitonin or bisphosphonates for bones and "statins" for lipids, may have to be considered. The possibility of using a SERM in combination with an aromatase inhibitor might also be considered and the tamoxifen plus anastrozole arm of the current ATAC adjuvant trial may provide some indication of the potential of such combinations.

10. SUMMARY

Aromatase inhibition has moved forward from the use of nonspecific drugs to the development of rationally designed, highly potent and specific, well-tolerated agents with a clearly defined clinical role as second-line agents in postmenopausal advanced breast cancer. This role is likely to expand into other areas of breast-cancer management in the near future and the increased use of these agents, particularly in the context of clinical trials, may yield important information about the role of aromatase in the development and growth of human breast cancer. It is difficult to see a need for even more potent inhibitors until the full potential of the present generation has been fully assessed. Similarly, it is difficult to predict which of the new generation of inhibitors will prove the most useful; at present they are relatively similar in terms of potency, selectivity, tolerability, and clinical efficacy. Direct comparisons in large blinded randomized clinical trials will be required to reveal any significant differences between them. Breast-cancer prevention is an exciting possibility for future investigation.

REFERENCES

1. Hughes S, Burley D. ASantnarminoglutethimide: a 'side-effect' turned to therapeutic advantage. *Postgrad Med J* 1970; 46:409–416.
2. Hall T, Barlow J. Treatment of metastatic breast cancer with aminoglutethimide. *Clin Res* 1969; 17:402.
3. Lipton A, Santen R. Medical adrenalectomy using aminoglutethimide and dexamethasone in advanced breast cancer. *Cancer* 1974; 33:503–512.
4. Santen R, Santner S, Davis, B, Veldhuis, J, Samojlik, E, Ruby, E. Aminoglutethimide inhibits extraglandular estrogen production in postmenopausal women with breast carcinoma. *J Clin Endocrinol Metab* 1978; 47:1257–1265.
5. Miller WR, Forrest AP. Oestradiol synthesis from C19 steroids by human breast cancer. *Br J Cancer* 1974; 33:16–18.
6. Silva M, Rowlands M, Dowsett M, Gasterson B, McKinna JA Fryatt I, et al. Intratumoral aromatase as a prognostic factor in human breast carcinoma. *Cancer Res* 1989; 49:2588–2591.
7. Lipton A, Santer RJ, Santner S, Harvey HA, Sanders SI, Matthews YL. Prognostic value of breast cancer aromatase. *Cancer* 1992; 70:1951–1955.
8. Thorsen T, Tangen N, Stoa KF. Concentrations of endogenous estradiol as related to estradiol receptor sites in breast tumour cytosol. *Eur J Cancer Clin Oncol* 1982; 18:333–337.
9. van Landeghem AA, Poortman J, Nabuun M, Thijssen JH. Endogenous concentration and subcellular distribution of estrogens in normal and malignant breast tissue. *Cancer Res* 1985; 45:2900–2906.
10. James V, Reed M. Steroid hormones and human cancer. *Prog Cancer Res Ther* 1980; 14:471–487.
11. Early Breast Cancer Trialists' Collaborative Group (EBCTCG). Systemic treatment of early breast cancer by hormonal, cytotoxic and immune therapy. *Lancet*1992; 339:1–15, 71–85.
12. Jaiyesimi I, Buzdar A, Decker DA, Hortobaggi GN. Use of tamoxifen for breast cancer: twenty-eight years later. *J Clin Oncol* 1995; 13:513–529.
13. Gale K, Anderson J, Tonneg DC, Mansow EG, Davis TE, Horton J, et al. An Eastern Cooperative Oncology Group Phase III trial comparing aminoglutethimide to tamoxifen. *Cancer* 1994; 73:354–361.
14. Garcia-Giralt E, Ayme Y, Carton M, Daban A, Delozier T, Fargeot P, et al. Second and third line hormonotherapy in advanced post-menopausal breast cancer: a multicenter randomized trial comparing medroxyprogesterone acetate with aminoglutethimide in patients who have become resistant to tamoxifen. *Breast Cancer Res Treatment* 1993; 24:139–145.
15. MacNeill F, Jones A, Jacobs S, Lonning PE, Powles TJ, Dowsett M. The influence of Aminoglutethimide and its analogue Rogletimide on peripheral aromatisation in breast cancer. *Br J Cancer* 1992; 66:692–697.
16. Miller W. Aromatase inhibitors. *Endoc-Rel Cancer* 1996; 3:65–79.

17. Howell A, Mackintosh J, Jones M, Redford J, Wagstaff J, Sellwood RA. The definition of the "no change" category in patients treated with endocrine therapy and chemotherapy for advanced carcinoma of the breast. *Eur J Cancer Clin Oncol* 1988; 24:1567–1572.

18. Santen R, Worgul T, Samojlik E, Interrante A, Boucher AE, Lipton A, et al. A randomised trial comparing surgical adrenalectomy with aminoglutethimide plus hydrocortione in women with advanced breast cancer. *N Engl J Med* 1981; 305:545–551.

19. Lipton A, Harvey HA, Santer RJ, Boucher A, White D, Bernatt A. A randomised trial of aminoglutethimide versus tamoxifen in metastatic breast cancer. *Cancer* 1982; 50:2265–2268.

20. Harris AL, Dowsett M, Jeffcoate SL, McKenna JA, Morgan M, Smith IE. Endocrine and therapeutic effects of aminoglutethimide in premenopausal patients with breast cancer. *J Clin Endocrinol Metab* 1982; 55:718–720.

21. Harris AL, Dowsett M, Smith JE, Powles TJ. Suppression of plasma 6-keto-prostaglandin F1-alfa and 13, 14-dihydro-15-ketoprostaglandin F2-alfa by aminoglutethimide in advanced breast cancer. *Br J Cancer* 1983; 48:595–598.

22. Harris A. Aminoglutethimide: a new endocrine therapy in breast cancer. *Exp Cell Biol* 1985; 53:1–8.

23. Smith I, Harris A, Morgan M, Ford HT, Gazet JC, Harmer CL, et al. Tamoxifen versus aminoglutethimide in the treatment of advanced breast cancer. A controlled randomised cross-over trial. *BMJ* 1981; 283:1432–1434.

24. Smith I, Harris A, Morgan M, Gazet JC, McKinna JA. Tamoxifen versus amino-glutethimide versus combined tamoxifen and amiaoglutethimide in the treatment of advanced breast cancer. *Cancer Res* 1982; 42:3430S–3433S.

25. Milsted R, Habeshaw T, Kaye S, Sangster G, Macbeth F, Cambell-Ferguson J, et al. A randomized trial of tamoxifen versus tamoxifen with aminoglutethimide in postmenopausal women with advanced breast cancer. *Cancer Chemother Pharmacol* 1985; 14:272–273.

26. Ingle J, Green S, Ahmann DL, Long HJ, Edmonson JH, Rubin J, et al. Randomized trial of tamoxifen alone or combined with aminoglutethimide and hydrocortisone in women with metastatic breast cancer. *J Clin Oncol* 1986; 4:958–964.

27. Alonso-Munoz N, Ojeda-Gonzalez M. Randomized trial of tamoxifen versus aminog-lutethimide and versus tamoxifen and aminoglutethimide in advanced postmenopausal breast cancer. *Oncology* 1988; 45:350–353.

28. Lien E, Anker G, Lonning PE, Solheim E, Ueland PM. Decreased serum concentrations of tamoxifen and its metabolites induced by aminoglutethimide. *Cancer Res* 1990; 50:5851–5857.

29. Dowsett M, PC, Johnston SRD, Hoston SJ. Miles DW, Verbeek JA, Smith IE. Pharmacokinetic interaction between letrozole and tamoxifen in postmenopausal patients with advanced breast cancer. *Breast* 1997; 6:245.

29. Lonning P. Aromatase inhibition: past, present and future, in Endocrine Aspects of Breast Cancer. Dowsett M, Parthenon Publishing, Carnforth, UK, 1992, pp 53–76.

30. Dowsett M, Cunningham DC, Stein RC, Evans S, Dehernin L, et al. Dose-related endocrine effects and pharnacokinetics of oral and intramuscular 4-hydroxyandrostenedione in postmenopausal breast cancer patients. *Cancer Res* 1989; 49:1306–1312.

31. Dowsett M, Goss PE, Powles TJ, Hutchison G, Brodie AMH, Jefferate SL, et al. Use of the aromatase inhibitor 4-hydroxyandrostenedione in postmenopausal breast cancer: optimisation of therapeutic dose and route. *Cancer Res* 1987; 47:1957–61.

32. Coombes RC, Goss PE, Dowsett M, Hutchinson G, Cunningham D, Jarman M, Brodie AM. 4-Hydroxyandrostenedione treatment for postmenopausal patients with advanced breast cancer. *Steroids* 1987; 50:245–252.

33. Stein RC, Dowsett M, Coombes RC. Studies of formestane alone and in combination with goserelin in premenopausal breast cancer. *Adv Clin Oncol* 1994; 2:149–154.

34. Jones AL, MacNeill F, Jacobs S, Lonning PE, Dowsett M, Powles TJ. The influence of intramuscular 4-hydroxyandrostenedione on peripheral aromatisation in breast cancer patients. *Eur J Cancer* 1992; 28A:1712–1716.

35. Coombes RC, Stein RC, Dowsett M. Aromatase inhibitors in human breast cancer. *Proc R Society Edinburgh* 1989; 95B:283–291.

36. Hoffken K, Jonat W, Possinger K, Kolbel M, Kunz T, Wagner H, Becher R, et al. Aromatase inhibition with 4-hydroxyandrostenedione in the treatment of postmenopausal patients with advanced breast cancer a phase II study. *J Clin Oncol* 1990; 8:875–880.

37. Pickles T, Perry L, Murray P, Plowman P. 4-hydroxyandrostenedione: further clinical and extended endocrine observations. *Br J Cancer* 1990; 62:309–313.

38. Santen RJ, Manni A, Harvey H, Redmond C. Endocrine treatment of breast cancer in women. *Endoc Rev* 1990; 11:1–45.

39. Goss PE, Garyn KM. Current perspectives of aromatase inhibitors in breast cancer. *J Clin Oncol* 1994; 12:2460–2470.

40. Perez-Carrion R, Alberola C, Calabresi F, Michel RT, Santos R, Delozier T, et al. Comparison of the selective aromatase inhibitor formestane with tamoxifen as first-line hormonal therapy in postmenopausal women with advanced breast cancer. *Ann Oncol* 1994; 9:S19–S24.

41. Geisler J, King N, Anker G, Ornati G, Di Salle E, Lonning PE, et al. In vivo inhibition of whole body aromatisation by exemestane (PNU 155971), a novel steroidal aromatase inhibitor, in postmenopausal breast cancer patients. *Breast Cancer Res Treatment* 1997; 46(1):55.

42. Lonning PE, Paridaens R, Thurlimann B, Piscitelli G, di Salle E. Exemestane experience in breast cancer. *J Steroid Biochem Mol Biol* 1997; 61:151–155.

43. Lonning PE, Jacobs S, Jones A, Haynes B, Powles T, Dowsett M. The influence of CGS 16949A on peripheral aromatisation in breast cancer patients. *Br J Cancer* 1991; 63(5):789–793.

44. Demers LM, LA, Harvey HA, Hanagan J, Mulagha M, Santen RI. The effects of long term fadrozole hydrochloride treatment in patients with advanced stage breast cancer. *J Steroid Biochem Mol Biol* 1993; 44:683–685.

45. Hoffken K. Experience with aromatase inhibitors in the treatment of advanced breast cancer. *Cancer Treatment Rev* 1993; 19(Suppl B):37–44.

46. Bonnefoi WR, Johnston S, Dowsett M, Trunet PF, Houston SJ, da Luz RJ, Rubens RD, et al. Therapeutic effects of the aromatase inhibitor fadrozole hydrochloride in advanced breast cancer. *Br J Cancer* 1996; 73:539–542.

47. Miller AA, Lipton A, Henderson CC, Navari R, Mulagha MT, Cooper J. Fadrozole hydrochloride in postmenopausal patients with advanced breast carcinoma. *Cancer* 1996; 78:789–793.

48. Falkson CI, Falkson HC. A randomised study of CGS 16949A (fadrozole) versus tamoxifen in previously untreated patients with metastatic breast cancer. *Ann Oncol* 1996; 7:465–469.

49. Buzdar AU, Smith R, Vogel C, Bonomi P, Kelter AM, Favis G, et al. Fadrozole HCI (CGS-16949A) versus megestrol acetate treatment of postmenopausal patients with metastatic breast cancer: results of two randomised double blind controlled multiinstitutional trials. *Cancer* 1996a; 77:2503–2513.

50. Thurlimann B, Beretta K, Bacchi M, Castiglione-Certsch M, Goldhirsch A, Jungi WF, et al. First-line fadrozole HCl (CGS 16949A) versus tamoxifen in postmenopausal women with advanced breast cancer. Prospective randomised trial of the Swiss group for Clinical Cancer Research SAKK. *Ann Oncol* 1996; 7:471–479.

51. Demers LM, Melby JC, Wilson TE, Lipton A, Harvey GA, Santen RJ. The effects of CGS 16949A, an aromatase inhibitor on adrenal mineralocorticoid biosynthesis. *J Clin Endocrinol Metab* 1990; 70:1162–1166.

52. Stein RC, Dowsett M, Davenport J, Hedley A, Ford HT, Gazet JC, et al. Preliminary study of the treatment of advanced breast cancer in postmenopausal women with the aromatase inhibitor CGS 16949A. *Cancer Res* 1990; 50:1381–1384.

53. Iveson TJ, Smith IE, Ahern J, Smithers DA, Trunet PF, Dowsett M. Phase I study of the oral nonsteroidal aromatase inhibitor CGS 20267 in postmenopausal patients with breast cancer. *Cancer Res* 1993; 53:266–270.

54. Johnston SRD, Smith IE, Doody D, Jacobs S, Robertshaw H, Dowsett M. Clinical and endocrine effects of the oral aromatase inhibitor vorozole in postmenopausal patients with advanced breast cancer. *Cancer Res* 1994; 54:5875–5881.

55. Juranka PF, Zastaway RL, Ling V. P-glycoprotein multidrug resistance and a super family of membrane-associated transport proteins. *FASEB J* 1989; 3:2583–2592.

55. Yates RA, Dowsett M, Fisher GV, Selen A, Wyld PJ. Arimidex (ZD1033): a selective, potent inhibitor of aromatase in post-menopausal female volunteers. *Br J Cancer* 1996; 73:543–548.

56. Geisler J, King N, Dowsett M, Ottestad L, Lundgren S, Walton P, et al. Influence of Anastozole (Arimidex) a non-steroidal aromatase inhibitor, on in vivo aromatisation and plasma oestrogen levels in postmenopausal women with breast cancer. *Br J Cancer* 1996; 74:1289–1291.

57. Dowsett M, Jones A, Johnston SRD, Jacobs S, Trunet P, Smith IE. In vivo measurement of aromatase inhibition by letrozole (CGS 20267) in postmenopausal patients with breast cancer. *Clin Cancer Res* 1995; 1:1511–1515.

58. Buzdar A, Jonat W, Howell A, Jones SE, Blomqvist C, Vogel CL, Eiermann W, et al. Anastrozole, a potent and selective aromatase inhibitor, versus megestrol acetate in postmenopausal women with advanced breast cancer: results of overview analysis of two phase III trials. *J Clin Oncol* 1996b; 14:2000–2011.

59. Dombernowsky P, Smith I, Falkson G, Leonard R, Panasci L, Bellmunt J, et al. Letrozole, a new oral aromatase inhibitor for advanced breast cancer: double-blind randomized trial showing a dose effect and improved efficacy and tolerability compared with megestrol acetate. *J Clin Oncol* 1998; 16:453–461.

60. Smith I, Dombernowsky P, Falkson G, Leonard R, Panasci L, Bellmunt J, et al. Double-blind trial in postmenapausal (PMP) women with advanced breast cancer (ABC) showing a dose-effect and superiority of 2.5mg letrozole over megestrol acetate. *Eur J Cancer* 1996; 32A:49.

61. Bergh J, Bonneterre J, Illiger HJ, Murray R, Nortier J, Paridaens R, et al. Vorozole (Rivizor™) versus aminoglutethimide (AG) in the treatment of postmenopausal breast cancer relapsing after tamoxifen. *Proc Am Society Clin Oncol* 1997; 16:155a.

62. Marty M, Geschanovich M, Campos B, Romieu G, Lurie H, Bonaventura T, et al. Letrozole, a new potent selective aromatase inhibitor (AI) superior to aminoglutethimide (AG) in postmenopausal women with advanced breast cancer (ABC) previously treated with antiestrogens. *Proc Am Society Clin Oncol* 1997; 16:156a.

63. Buzdar A, Jonat W, Howell A, Yin H, Lee D. Significant improved survival with Arimidex (anastrozole) versus megestrol acetate in postmenopausal advanced breast cancer: updated results of two randomised trials. *Proc Am Society Clin Oncol* 1997; 16:156a.

64. Buzdar AU, Jonat W, Howell A, Jones SE, Blomqvist CP, Vogel CL, et al. Anastrozole versus megestrol acetate in postmenopausal women with advanced breast cancer: Results of a survival update based on a combined analysis of data from two mature phase III trials. *Cancer* (in press).

65. Rose C, Kamby C, Mouridsen HT, Bastholt L, Brinker M, Skovgaard-Poulsen H, Andersen AP, et al. Combined endocrine treatment of postmenopausal patients with advanced breast cancer. A randomized trial of tamoxifen versus tamoxifen plus aminoglutethimide and hydrocortisone. *Breast Cancer Res Treatment* 1986; 7(Suppl):S45–S50.

65a. Dowsett M, Tobias JS, Howell A, Blackman A, Welch H, King N, et al. The effect of anestrogale on the pharnacokinetics of tamoxifen in postmenopausal women with early breast cancer. *Brit J Cancer*

67. Masamura S, Santner SJ, Heitjan DF, Santen RJ. Estrogen deprivation causes estradiol hypersensitivity in human breast cancer cells. *J Clin Endocrinol Metab* 1995; 80:2918–2925.

68. Adams J. Hermaphrodiol: A 'new' estrogen and its role in the etiology of human breast cancer. Commentaries on research in breast disease, vol. 3 (Bulbrook R, Taylor DJ, eds). Alan R. Liss, New York, 1983, pp 133.

69. Rubens RD, Tirson CL, Coleman RE, Knight RK, Tong D, Winter PJ, et al. Prednisolone improves the response to primary endocrine treatment for advanced breast cancer. *Br J Cancer* 1988; 58:626–630.

70. Bates T, Riley DL, Houghton S, Baum M. Breast cancer in elderly women: a Cancer Research Campaign trial comparing treatment with tamoxifen and optimal surgery with tamoxifen alone. *Br J Surg* 1991; 78:591–594.

71. Mustacchi G, Milani S, Pluchinotta A, De Matteus A, Bubagotti A, Berrota A. Tamoxifen or surgery plus tamoxifen as primary treatment for elderly patients with operable breast cancer. *AntiCancer Res* 1994; 14:2197–2200.

72. Fisher B, Gunduz N, Coyle J, Rodock C, Saffer E. Presence of a growth-stimulating factor in serum following tumor removal in mice. *Cancer Res* 1989; 49:1996–2001.

73. Anderson EDC, Anderson E, Hawkins RA, Anderson TJ, Leonard RCF, Chetty U. Primary systemic therapy for operable breast cancer. *Br J Cancer* 1991; 63:561–566.

74. Gazet J-C, Coombes RC, Ford HT, Griffin M, Corbishley C, Nakinde V, Lowndes S, et al. Assessment of the effect of pretreatment with neoadjuvant therapy on primary breast cancer. *Br J Cancer* 1996; 73:758–762.

75. Dixon JM, Love CDB, Tucker S, Bellamy D, Cameron D, Miller WR, Leonard RCF. Letrozole as primary medical therapy for locally advanced and large operable breast cancer. *Breast Cancer Res Treatment* 1997; 46:54.

76. Dixon JM, Love CDB, Tucker S, Bellamy D, Cameron D, Miller WR, Leonard RCF. Letrozole as primary medical therapy for locally advanced breast cancer. *Breast* 1997; 6:245.

77. Wolf DM, Jordan VC. William L. McGuire Memorial Symposium. Drug resistance to tamoxifen during breast cancer therapy. *Breast Cancer Res Treatment* 1993; 27:27–40.

78. Jones AL, Powles T, Law M, Tidy A, Easton D, Coombes RC, et al. Adjuvant aminoglutethimide for postmenopausal patients with primary breast cancer: analysis at 8 years. *J Clin Oncol* 1992; 10:1547–1552.

79. Santen RT, Samojlik E, Wells SA. Resistance of ovary to blockade of aromatisation with aminoglutethimide. *J Clin Endocrinol Metab* 1980; 51:473–477.

80. Harris AL, Dowsett M, Smith IL, Powles TJ. Aminoglutethimide in the treatment of advanced postmenopausal breast cancer. *Cancer Res* 1982; (Suppl)42:3405–3408.

81. Wander HE, Blossey HC, Nagel GA. Aminoglutethimide in the treatment of premenopausal patients with metastatic breast cancer. *Eur J Cancer* 1986; 22:1371–1374.

82. Wouters W, de Coster R, Tuman RW, Bowden CR, Bruynseels J, Vanderpas H, Van Rooy P, et al. Aromatase inhibition by R76713. *J Steroid Biochem* 1989; 34:427–430.

83. Shetty G, Krishnamurthy H, Krishnamurthy HN, Bhatnagar AS, Moudgal RN. Effect of estrogen deprivation on the reproductive physiology of male and female primates. *J Steroid Biochem Mol Biol* 1997; 61:157–166.

84. Miller WR, O'Neill J. The importance of local synthesis of estrogen within the breast. *Steroids* 1987; 50:537–548.

85. Santen RJ, Samojlik E, Worgul TJ. Aminoglutethimide product profile, in *Pharmanual: A Comprehensive Guide to the Therapeutic Use of Aminoglutethimide* (Henderson RSI, ed). Karger, Basel, 1981, pp.101–160.

86. Miller W. Importance of intratumoural aromatase and its susceptibility to inhibitors, in *Aromatase inhibition: then, now and tomorrow.* (Dowsett M, ed). Parthenon Publishing New York, 1994, pp 43–53.

87. Bezwoda WR, MN, Dansey R. Correlation of breast tumour aromatase activity and response to aromatase inhibition with aminoglutethimide. *Oncology* 1987; 44:345–349.

88. Santen RJ, Martel J, Hoahland F, Naftolin F, Roa L, Harada N, Hafer L, et al. Stromal spindle cells contain aromatase in human breast tumors. *J Clin Endocrinol Metab* 1994; 79:627–632.

89. Sasano H, Nagura H, Harada N, Goukom Y, Kimura M. Immunolocalization of aromatase and other steroidogenic enzymes in breast disorders. *Human Pathol* 1994; 25:530–535.

90. Lu Q, Nakmura J, Savinov A, Yue W, Weisz J, Dabbs DJ, et al. Expression of aromatase protein and messenger ribonucleic acid in tumor epithelial cells and evidence of functional significance of locally produced estrogen in human breast cancers. *Endocrinology* 1996; 137:3061–3068.

91. Hamon JT. Loss of hormonal responsiveness in breast cancer, in *Endocrine Management of Cancer: Biological Basis* (Stoll B, ed). Karger, Basel, 1988, pp 61–71.

92. Isaacs J. Clinical heterogeneity in relation to response, in *Endocrine Management of Cancer: Biological Basis* (Stoll B, ed). Karger, Basel, 1988, pp 125–145.

93. Taylor RE, Powles T, Humphreys J, Bettelheim R, Dowsett M, Casey AJ, et al. Effects of endocrine therapy on steroid receptor content of breast cancer. *Br J Cancer* 1982; 45:80–85.

94. Chohan PB, Foster AB, Harland SJ, Jarman M, Leung CS, et al. Metabolism of aminoglutethimide in man; desmolase and aromatase inhibition studies. *R Society Med Int Cong Symp Series* 1982; 53:19–21.

95. Strocchi E, Carnaggi CM, Martoni A, Cellerino R, Miseria S, Malacarne P, Indelli M, et al. Aminoglutethimide in advanced breast cancer: plasma levels and clinical results after low and high doses. *Cancer Chemother Pharmacol* 1991; 27:451–455.

96. Murray FT, Santner S, Samojlik E, Santen R. Serum aminoglutethimide levels: studies of serum half-life, clearance and patient compliance. *J Clin Pharmacol* 1989; 19:704–711.

97. Santens R. Overall experience with aminoglutethimide in the management of advanced breast carcinoma, in *Aminoglutethimide: An Alternative Endocrine Therapy for Breast Carcinoma I.* (Elsdon-Dew RW, Birdwood GFB, eds). Academic Press, London, 1982, pp 3–7.

98. Dowsett M, Harris A, Smith IE, Jeffcoate SL. Endocrine changes associated with relapse in advanced breast cancer patients on aminoglutethimide therapy. *J Clin Endocrinol Metab* 1984; 58:99–104.

99. Murray R, Pitt P. Low-dose aminoglutethimide without steroid replacement in the treatment of postmenopausal women with advanced breast cancer. *Eur J Cancer Clin Oncol* 1985; 21:19–22.

100. Coombes RC, Goss P, Dowsett M, Gazet J-C, Brodie A. 4-Hydroxyandrostenedione treatment of postmenopausal patients with advanced breast cancer. *Lancet* 1984; ii:1237–1239.

101. Bundred NJ, Erenier O, Stewart HJ, Dale BA, Forrest APM. Beneficial response to pituitary ablation following aminoglutethimide. *Br J Surg* 1986; 73:388–389.

103. Kadohama N, Yarborough C, Zhou D, Chen S, Osawa Y. Kinetic properties of aromatase mutants Pro308Phe, Asp309Asn and Asp309Ala and their interactions with aromatase inhibitors. *J Steroid Biochem Mol Biol* 1992; 43:693–701.

103. Miller W. In vitro and in vivo effects of 4-hydroxyandrostenedione on steroid and tumor metabolism, in *4-Hydroxyandrostenedione: A New Approach to Hormone-Dependent Cancer* (DM Coombes RC, ed). Royal Society of Medicine Ltd International Congress and Symposium Series, London, 1992, pp 45–50.

104. Sourdaine P, Parker MG, Telford J, Miller WR. Analysis of the aromatase cytochrome P450 gene in human breast cancers. *J Mol Endocrinol* 1994; 13:331–337.

105. Adams JB, Garda M, Rochefort H. Estrogenic effects of physiological concentrations of 5-androstene-3β,17β-diol and its metabolism in MCF-7 human breast cancer cells. *Cancer Res* 1981; 41:4720–4726.

107. Shearer RJ, Hendry W, Sommerville IF, Ferguson JD. Plasma testosterone. An accurate monitor of hormone treatment in prostatic cancer. *Br J Urol* 1973; 45:668–677.

108. Blackard GE, Byar DP, Jordan WP. Orchidectomy for advanced prostatic carcinoma. *Urology* 1973; 1:553–562.
109. Huggins C. The effect of castration, of estrogen and androgen injection on serum phosphatase in metastatic carcinoma of the prostate. *Cancer* 1941; 1:293–297.
110. Schoonees R, Schalch DS, Reynoso G, Murphy GP. Bilateral adrenalectomy for advanced prostatic carcinoma. *J Urol* 1972; 108:123–125.
111. Robinson MRG, Sheaver RJ, Fergusson JD. Adrenal suppression in the treatment of carcinoma of the prostate. *Br J Urol* 1974; 46:555–559.
112. Robinson M. Aminoglutethimide: medical adrenalectomy in management of carcinoma of the prostate. A review after six years. *Br J Urol* 1980; 52:328–329.
113. Johannessen DC, Lonning PE. Aromatase inhibitors in malignant diseases of aging. *Drugs Aging* 1992; 2(6):530–545.
114. Ponder BAJ, Sheaver RJ, Pococ RD, Miller J, Easton D. Response to aminoglutethimide and cortisone acetate in advanced prostatic carcinoma. *Br J Cancer* 1984; 50:757–763.
115. Plowman PN, Perry LA, Chard T. Androgen suppression by hydrocortisone without aminoglutethimide in orchidectomised men with prostatic cancer. *Br J Urol* 1987; 59:255–257.
116. Dowsett M, Sheaver R, Ponder BAJ, Malone P, Jeffcoate SL. The effects of aminoglutethimide and hydrocortisone, alone and combined, on androgen levels in post-orchidectomy prostatic cancer patients. *Br J Cancer* 1988; 57:190–292.
117. Brodie AMH, Son C, King DA, Meyer KM, Inkster SE. Lack of evidence for aromatase in human prostatic tissues: effects of 4-hydroxyandrostenedione and other inhibitors on androgen metabolism. *Cancer Res* 1989; 49:6551–6555.
118. Bashirelahi N, Sidh SM, Sanefuji H. Androgen, estrogen and their distribution in epithelial and stromal cells of human prostate, in *Steroid Receptors, Metabolism and Prostatic Cancer* (De Voogt S, eds). Excerpta Medica, Amsterdam, 1990, pp 240–255.
119. Shearer RJ, Davies JH, Dowsett M, Malone PR, Hedley A. Aromatase inhibition in advanced prostatic cancer: preliminary communication. *Br J Cancer* 1990; 62:275–276.
120. Pirke KM, Doerr P. Age related changes and interrelationship between plasma testosterone, estradiol and testosterone binding globulin in normal adult males. *Acta Endocrinol* 1973; 74:792–800.
121. Seppel U. Correlation among prostate stroma, plasma estrogen levels and urinary estrogen excretion in patients with benign prostatic hypertrophy. *J Clin Endocrinol Metab* 1978; 47:1230–1235.
122. Ranniko S, Adlercreutz H. Plasma estradiol, free testosterone, sex hormone binding globulin and prolactin in benign prostatic hyperplasia and prostate cancer. *Prostate* 1983; 4:223–229.
123. Habernicht UF, Schwarz K, Schweikert HU, Neumann F, El Etreby MF. Development of a model for the induction of estrogen-related prostatic hyperplasia in the dog and its response to the aromatase inhibitor 4-hydroxy-4-androstene-3,17-dione: preliminary results. *Prostate* 1986; 8:181–194.
124. Habernicht UF, Schwarz K, Neumann F, El Etreby MF. Induction of estrogen-related hyperplastic changes in the prostate of the cynomolgus monkey *(Macaca fascicularis)* by androstenedione and its antagonism by the aromatase inhibitor 1-methyl-androsta-l,4-diene-3,17-dione. *Prostate* 1987; 11:313–326.
125. Habernicht UF, El Etreby F, Lewis R, Ghoniem G, Roberts J. Induction of metachromasia in experimentally induced hyperplastic/hypertrophic changes in the prostate of the cynomolgus monkey *(Macaca fascicularis). J Urol* 1989; 142:1624–1626.
126. Moore RA, McLellan AM. A histological study of the effect of sex hormones on the human prostate. *J Urol* 1938; 40:641–657.
127. Khanna Om P. Effect of nonautonomic drugs on the vesical neck, in *Benign Prostatic Hypertrophy* (Hinman F, ed). Springer-Verlag, New York, 1983, pp 384–404.

128. Habernicht U-F, Tunn UW, Senge T, Schroder FH, Schweikert HU, Bartsch G, El Etreby MF. Management of Benign Prostatic Hyperplasia with particular emphasis on aromatase inhibitors. *J Steroid Biochem Mol Biol* 1993; 44:557–563.

129. Schweikert HU, Tunn UW. Effects of the aromatase inhibitor testolactone on human benign prostatic hyperplasia. *Steroids* 1987; 50:191–200.

130. Schweikert HU, Tunn UW, Habenicht UF, Amold J, Senge T, Schulze H, et al. Effects of estrogen deprivation on human benign prostatic hyperplasia. *J Steroid Biochem Mol Biol* 1993; 44:573–576.

131. Gingell JC, Knogagel H, Kurth KH, Tunn UW. Placebo controlled double-blind study to test the efficacy of the aromatase inhibitor atamestane in patients with benign prostatic hyperplasia not requiring operation. *J Urol* 1995; 154:402–403.

132. Radlmaier A, Erkenberg HU, Fletcher MS, Fourcade RO, Reis-Santos JM, van Aubel OG, Bono AV. Estrogen reduction by aromatase inhibition for benign prostatic hyperplasia: results of a double-blind, placebo-controlled, randomized clinical trial using two doses of the aromatase inhibitor atamestane. *Prostate* 1996; 29(4):199–208.

133. Pollow K, Lubbert H, Boquoi E, Kreuyzer G, Pollow B. Characterisation and comparison of receptors for 17β-estradlol and progesterone in human proliferative endometrium and endometrial carcinoma. *Endocrinology* 1975; 96:319–328.

134. Yamamoto T, Kitawaki J, Urabe M, Honjo H, Tamura T, Noguchi T, et al. Estrogen productivity of endometrium and endometrial cancer tissue; influence of aromatase on proliferation of endometrial cancer cells. *J Steroid Biochem Mol Biol* 1993; 44:463–468.

135. Quinn MA, Murray R, Pepperell RJ. Tamoxifen and aminoglutethimide in the management of patients with advanced endometrial carcinoma not responsive to medroxyprogesterone. *Aust N Zeal J Obstet Gynaecol* 1981; 21:226–229.

136. Yamamoto T, Tamura T, Kitiwaki J, Okada H. Evidence for estrogen synthesis in adenomyotic tissues. *Am J Obstet Gynecol* 1993; 69:734–738.

137. Yano S, IY, Nakao K. Studies on the effect of the new non-steroidal aromatase inhibitor fadrozole hydrochloride in an endometriosis model in rats. *Arzneimittelforschung* 1996; 46:92–195.

138. Takayama K, Zeitoun K, Gunby RT, Sasano H, Carr BR, Bolun SE. Treatment of severe postmenopausal endometriosis with an aromatase inhibitor. *Fertil Steril* 1998; 69:709–713.

139. Santen RJ, Santner S, Harvey HA, Lipton A, Simmons M, et al. Marked heterogeneity of aromatase activity in human malignant melanoma tissue. *Eur J Cancer Clin Oncol* 1988; 24:1811–1816.

140. Harvey H, Lipton A, Simmons M, Santen R, Bartholomew M. Chemotherapy and aromatase inhibition in metastatic malignant melanoma. *Proc Am Society Clin Oncol* 1988; 7:A978.

141. Block S, Bonneterre J, Adenis A, Pion JM, Demaille A. Aminoglutethimide in malignant melanoma. A phase II study. *Am J Clin Oncol* 1992; 15(3):260–261.

142. Hemsell DL, Edman CD, Marks IF, Siiteri PK, MacDonald PC. Massive extraglandular aromatization of plasma androstenedione resulting in feminization of a prepubertal boy. *J Clin Invest* 1977; 60:455–464.

143. Berkovitz GD, Guerami A, Brown TR, MacDonald PC, Migeon CJ. Farr gynaecomastia with increased extraglandular aromatization of plasma C19-steroids. *J Clin Invest* 1985; 75:1763–2769.

144. Bulun SE, Noble LS, Takayama K, Dodson MM, Agarwal V, Fisher C, et al. Endocrine disorders associated with inappropriately high aromatase expression. *J Steroid Biochem Mol Biol* 1997; 61:133–139.

145. Bulun S. Endocrinopathies associated with excessive aromatase expression. Program and Abstracts, 4th International Aromatase Conference, p S-6.

146. Feinlieb M. Breast cancer and artificial menopause: a cohort study. *J Nat Cancer Inst* 1968; 41:315–329.

147. Thomas HV, Key T, Allen DS, Moore JW, Dowsett M, Fentiman IS, et al. A prospective study of endogenous serum hormone concentration and breast cancer risk in post-menopausal women on the island of Guernsey. *Br J Cancer* 1997; 76(3):401–405.
148. Nissen-Meyer, R. Primary breast cancer: the effect of primary ovarian irradiation *Ann Oncol* 1991; 2:34–346.
149. Cuzik J, Baum M. Tamoxifen and contralateral breast cancer. *Lancet* 1985; 2:28.
150. Powles TJ, Hardy J, Ashley SE, Cosgrove D, Davey JH, Dowsett M, McKinna JA, et al. Chemoprevention of breast cancer. *Breast Cancer Res Treatment* 1989; 14:23–31.
151. Gunson DE, Steele RE, Chau RY Prevention of tumours in female rats by fadrozole, an aromatase inhibitor. *Br J Cancer* 1995; 72:72–75.
152. Durgam VR, Tekmal RR. The nature and expression of int-5, a novel MMTV integration locus gene in carcinogen-induced tumors. *Cancer Lett* 1994; 87:179–286.
153. Siegelmann-Danieli N, Zidan J, McGlynn KA, Buetow KH. DNA-based variation at the aromatase gene (CYP1B) and its role in breast cancer susceptibility. *Proc Am Society Clin Oncol* 1996; 15:23.
166. Boccuzi G, Brignardello E, Dimonaco D, Forte C, Leonardi L, Pizzini A. Influence of dehydroepiandrosterone and 5-en-androstene-3-beta, 17-beta-diol on the growth of MCF-7 human breast cancer cells induced by 17-beta estcadiol. *Anticancer Res* 1992; 12:799–803.

13 LH-RH Agonists for the Treatment of Breast Cancer

Development and Current Status

Roger W. Blamey

1. INTRODUCTION

In a momentous discovery arising out of his research, in 1896 Beatson showed that the growth of some breast cancers could be interrupted by oophorectomy *(1)*. He operated on three women, one of whom clearly responded, achieving a remission of 42-mo duration. Interestingly, the response rate in many series since that time has remained close to one in three.

From: *Hormone Therapy in Breast and Prostate Cancer*
Edited by: V. C. Jordan and B. J. A. Furr © Humana Press Inc., Totowa, NJ

Oophorectomy or ovarian irradiation went in and out of fashion, but by the 1960s it was accepted as the standard treatment for premenopausal women with advanced breast cancer.

The use of ovarian ablation as adjuvant systemic therapy was investigated in trials begun by Paterson in 1948 *(2)* and by Nissen-Meyer in 1957 *(3)*. Meta-analysis by the Early Breast Cancer Trialists' Collaborative Group (EBCTCG) has demonstrated that adjuvant systemic treatment by ovarian removal, ablation or suppression in women aged less than 50 years, brings about an overall significant improvement in long-term survival *(4)*.

Although neither the surgical nor radiotherapeutic methods are considered major invasive procedures, they do have complications. In addition, ovarian irradiation may take 6 wk or more to suppress estrogen production and suppression is inconsistent *(5)*. Both oophorectomy and ovarian irradiation are irreversible and induce a permanent menopausal state with the associated long-term pharmacological effects of estrogen withdrawal, whether or not a patient responds to treatment. This can have considerable impact on patient acceptability, bearing in mind that the typical response rate is approx only one in three. It was this latter issue that largely fueled attempts to find both a predictor for response, provided by estrogen-receptor (ER) analysis and an alternative medical therapy.

AstraZeneca Pharmaceuticals (then ICI) began a search for a pharmaceutical method of ovarian suppression. A number of analogues of luteinizing hormone-releasing hormone (LH-RH) were synthesized. The most promising, selected from tests on animals, was ICI 118630, later known as "Zoladex" (goserelin acetate). Many of the initial studies, including a Phase I study of pharmacological and clinical efficacy in advanced breast cancer *(6)*, were carried out as combined work between the Tenovus Institute, Cardiff and the Professorial Unit of Surgery at Nottingham City Hospital.

2. CLINICAL PHARMACOLOGY/MODE OF ACTION

Following a single daily (500 or 1000 µg) injection, Zoladex was found initially to stimulate increases in plasma concentrations of both luteinizing hormone (LH) and follicle-stimulating hormone (FSH) but on continued treatment, rapid, very effective declines in LH, FSH, estradiol, and progesterone were produced. Plasma estradiol concentrations were reduced to the levels found in oophorectomized or postmenopausal women *(6)*.

A monthly biodegradable depot preparation of Zoladex (3.6 mg) later became available and tests in 24 assessable patients with advanced breast cancer confirmed its ovarian-suppressive activity *(7)*.

Zoladex acts on the anterior pituitary gland by a process known as 'receptor down-regulation' *(8)*. The normal stimulus for the release of gonadotrophins, FSH and LH, from the pituitary gland is pulsatile secretion of LH-RH by the hypothalamus. In the premenopausal female, gonadotrophins induce the secre-

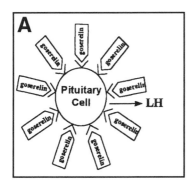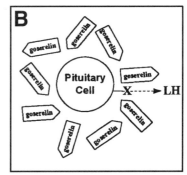

Fig. 1. (A) Hypersecretion of LH following acute administration of 3.6 mg Zoladex. **(B)** Hyposecretion of LH following chronic administration of 3.6 mg Zoladex.

tion of estrogens from the ovary, the most important of which is estradiol. Following initial administration of 3.6 mg Zoladex, all the LH-RH receptors on the surface of the pituitary cell become occupied by goserelin (Fig. 1A). This results in a transient increase in serum LH, but the occupied LH-RH receptors form clusters and gradually internalize into the cell. New receptors are re-synthesized but become rapidly occupied and internalize due to the goserelin, which is continually released from the Zoladex 3.6 mg depot. Hence, on chronic administration, the continuous presence of the LH-RH agonist prevents a sufficient quantum of LH-RH receptors from being present on the cell surface to allow synthesis and secretion of LH. Consequently, the production and secretion of estrogens is suppressed to castrate or postmenopausal levels (Fig. 1B).

3. EARLY TESTS OF CLINICAL EFFECTS

Zoladex was initially administered in Nottingham to patients with either distant metastases or locally advanced breast cancer as a 500 µg (*n* = 5) or 1000 µg (*n* = 22) daily subcutaneous injection. A further 26 patients then received the 3.6 mg Zoladex depot formulation by monthly subcutaneous injection *(6)*. No patient had received either prior endocrine or cytotoxic therapy.

Forty-five of a total of 53 patients were assessable for response to treatment. There were 14 objective responders and 3 women were judged to have stable disease (no evidence of progression over 6 mo therapy), leaving 28 patients who progressed. As expected, ER status was the main determinant of response: 13 of the 14 responders were either ER-positive (*n* = 10) or ER-unknown (*n* = 3); only 1 of 19 ER-negative tumors responded.

Surgical oophorectomy (the standard treatment of the day) on progression was a requirement of the study and was performed on 26 patients: 4 subsequently showed a response having failed to respond to Zoladex. In one, serum estradiol had not been suppressed to castrate levels by daily injection of Zoladex. The other three patients underwent early oophorectomy because of the trial protocol, after only 1, 2, and 3 mo of Zoladex therapy; this is an insufficient time to allow proper assessment of response.

After these 26 patients had undergone oophorectomy as a second-line treatment, it became clear from plasma estrogen concentrations that Zoladex was in fact performing well in suppressing ovarian function, particularly as the depot preparation. It also showed that subsequent oophorectomy was an unnecessary procedure, producing neither further fall in estradiol concentration nor further response, after adequate Zoladex therapy. The use of oophorectomy on progression following Zoladex therapy was then discontinued.

The overall response rate to Zoladex in the 45 assessable patients was 31%, highly comparable to that expected from oophorectomy in young women or tamoxifen in older women *(7,9–13)*, with a response rate in ER-positive tumors of over 50%.

4. EFFECTS OF ZOLADEX ON OVARIAN HISTOLOGY

The histology of 39 ovaries *(14)* from 23 patients treated with Zoladex as primary therapy who underwent oophorectomy after disease progression was compared with that of 68 ovaries from 34 patients treated with oophorectomy as primary therapy in a trial *(14)* in premenopausal women with advanced breast cancer. Both treatment groups showed similar follicular-phase development. Only 3/23 of the Zoladex group against 19/34 of the primary oophorectomy group showed evidence of luteinization. Follicular cysts were seen significantly more often in Zoladex patients.

Zoladex appears to arrest the development of follicles with formation of follicular cysts but, despite low FSH levels, folliculogenesis is not inhibited.

5. CLINICAL EXPERIENCE OF 3.6 MG ZOLADEX DEPOT IN THE TREATMENT OF ADVANCED BREAST CANCER

Zoladex is the most extensively tested LH-RH analogue in advanced breast cancer *(7,15)*. Between 1982 and 1988, 333 pre- and perimenopausal women with histologically confirmed, locally advanced (stage III) or metastatic (stage IV) breast cancer were entered into a series of 29 open, noncomparative clinical trials in centers throughout Europe to assess the efficacy and/or tolerability of 3.6 mg Zoladex depot as first-line therapy. The trials followed a standard design that facilitated pooling of the data.

Of the 333 patients studied, 228 were finally eligible for efficacy evaluation: 83 patients (36.4%) showed a complete or partial response to Zoladex, the median time to response amongst these patients being 12 wk (range 4–49 wk). A further 49.6% of patients were categorized as "no change" (absence of objective progression, with insufficient evidence of a partial response). A subjective response (i.e., a decrease in symptoms) was observed in 68% of patients who were symptomatic on entry, with a median time to subjective response of 8 wk (range 1 to 52 wk) (7).

In responding patients, the duration of response ranged from 4 to >160 wk, with a median duration of 44 wk, indicating that Zoladex is associated with durable responses in advanced breast-cancer patients. Importantly, responses to Zoladex were seen in all age groups studied and in all breast-tumor types. Higher response rates were seen in those patients with ER-positive and/or well-differentiated tumors.

Clinical responses were observed both in patients initially presenting with advanced disease and in those who developed recurrent disease following a disease-free interval since first diagnosis. Responses were seen whether or not patients had received previous adjuvant therapy and, interestingly, in the small group of patients who had received prior endocrine therapy for advanced disease. Responses were observed at all sites of metastases including major viscera, such as lung and liver (7).

At the time of data cut-off for the survival analysis, 153/228 evaluable patients had died (67.1%) and the data were, therefore, considered mature. The median overall survival time was 26.5 mo (range 0.8–69.0 mo), with some 20% of patients still alive at 5 yr of follow-up (16,17). This compares favorably with the reported survival times for other endocrine therapies in the treatment of advanced breast cancer in premenopausal patients, such as oophorectomy (9) or tamoxifen (10,11). Best objective response was the strongest predictor of lengthy survival, along with ER status, and this finding exemplifies the observation that, despite the introduction of cytotoxic therapies, length of survival depends on response to first-line endocrine therapy (18,19).

Treatment in this study was well-tolerated, with no withdrawals due to adverse reactions. Menopausal side effects were the most common (e.g., hot flashes 76%; loss of libido 47%) (7).

These studies demonstrate that Zoladex provides an effective medical alternative to conventional ovarian ablation in the management of advanced breast cancer in pre/peri-menopausal women.

6. DIRECT COMPARISON WITH SURGICAL OVARIAN ABLATION

In the largest randomized trial of surgical ovarian ablation vs medical ovarian suppression to date, the Southwest Oncology Group (SWOG), the North Central Cancer Treatment Group (NCCTG), and the Eastern Co-operative Oncology Group (ECOG) compared Zoladex with surgical oophorectomy (20). Based on the hypothesis that medical treatment with Zoladex would be preferred if it were shown to be equivalent—or, at most, only slightly less effective than surgery—with an acceptable tolerability profile, 136 evaluable premenopausal patients with ER-positive and/or progesterone receptor (PR)-positive advanced breast cancer were randomized to treatment either with oophorectomy or with 3.6 mg Zoladex every 4 wk.

The study was originally designed as an equivalence trial, with 80% power to rule out a 50% improvement in survival due to oophorectomy. Due to slow recruitment, the study was terminated early, resulting in a final power of 60% for the alternative hypothesis of equivalent survival.

Objective response was difficult to assess for the group as a whole, because a large number of patients had bone-only or nonassessable disease. In those patients whose disease was measurable, the overall response rate was 9/29 (31%) for Zoladex and 8/30 (27%) for oophorectomy. Only two responses were recorded in patients with assessable bone disease, both on Zoladex.

Survival duration was considered a more accurate indicator of benefit than objective response for patients in this study. There were no significant differences between treatments in terms of either failure-free survival (FFS) or overall survival (OS).

7. USE OF ZOLADEX IN COMBINATION WITH TAMOXIFEN

Suppression of ovarian function is the systemic therapy of choice in a premenopausal woman and tamoxifen ('Nolvadex'), an antiestrogen, is the established agent in postmenopausal women. Since Zoladex therapy effectively renders the woman postmenopausal, it seemed logical to determine whether the use of a combination of these two agents might be superior to use of Zoladex alone.

In a pilot study at Nottingham City Hospital *(21)*, 50 pre-menopausal women were treated with the combination of Zoladex plus tamoxifen as first-line therapy for advanced disease. The combination was confirmed to be endocrinologically sound *(22)*. Serum gonadotrophin, estradiol, and progesterone concentrations were reduced by the combination treatment as successfully as with Zoladex therapy alone.

The response rate (CR + PR) was 18%, with stable disease (≥ 6 mo) in a further 30% Patients with both objective response and stable disease had an excellent duration of disease control.

Following a successful pilot study in Nottingham *(23)*, a larger randomized trial (ICI 2302) was initiated *(24)*. 318 pre- and perimenopausal women randomized to either Zoladex alone or Zoladex plus tamoxifen as first-line treatment for advanced breast cancer. Treatment groups were comparable at entry for menopausal status (pre- or peri-), age, weight, disease-free interval, hormone-receptor status, histological grade and site (tissue) of disease.

There were no significant differences in response rate (31% for Zoladex vs 35% for the combination) but a significant advantage in time to progression was observed in favor of combination treatment.

The side-effect profile was very similar in both study arms: the reported adverse events were essentially those of the menopause and no additional safety issues associated with the combination were identified.

8. EFFECT ON SKELETAL DISEASE

A separate analysis of patients with skeletal metastases only at entry to the study ($n = 115$) was also performed. This was one of only three subgroup analyses carried out, the others being hormone-receptor status and analysis by response.

There were significant differences in favor of combination therapy in response rate *(24)* and in time to progression and survival.

9. META-ANALYSIS: LH-RH AGONIST PLUS TAMOXIFEN VS LH-RH AGONIST ALONE

Three other smaller trials have compared the combination of an LH-RH agonist plus tamoxifen with an LH-RH agonist alone in pre- and perimenopausal women with advanced breast cancer: the EORTC 10881 study *(25)*, an Italian trial *(26)* and a Japanese trial (unpublished results).

To make an adequate summary of the results of these four randomized trials and to combine the results to increase the power of the statistical comparisons, the study co-ordinators decided to perform a meta-analysis, which was carried out by the EORTC Data Centre *(15)*. A total of 506 patients were included, 399 (79%) received Zoladex as the LH-RH agonist and the remainder (in the EORTC trial) buserelin.

The meta-analysis showed the combination of LH-RH agonist plus tamoxifen to be superior to LH-RH agonist alone in the treatment of advanced breast cancer in pre- and perimenopausal women. The combination treatment demonstrated significant advantage in all three clinical endpoints studied: overall survival, progression-free survival, and objective response (Fig. 1). Combination treatment was associated with a greatly increased duration of response, with a median of 602 d compared with 350 d in those receiving LH-RH agonist alone.

Subgroup analyses for ER status, disease-free interval, and bone as dominant site of metastasis show that within each of the subgroups there is a trend for longer overall survival in favor of combination treatment, consistent with the overall conclusion *(15)*.

A further advantage of the use of combination therapy is that the ovarian-stimulating effect of tamoxifen, resulting in ovarian-cyst formation, is resolved by co-treatment with Zoladex *(27)*. There may also be reduced loss of bone as a result of Zoladex treatment by co-administration of tamoxifen.

10. A NEW COMBINATION: "TOTAL ESTROGEN BLOCKADE?"

As a result of the meta-analysis, it is clear that there is advantage to using this combination of agents, each of which have different modes of action: Zoladex lowers circulating estrogen, rendering the woman postmenopausal, allowing tamoxifen, the agent of choice in postmenopausal women, to block at the receptor level the action of the residual estrogen.

Further endocrine agents with different modes of action are the new-generation aromatase inhibitors such as Arimidex (anastrozole). Arimidex is a well-tolerated, selective, oral aromatase inhibitor that reduces serum estradiol towards the limit of detection in postmenopausal women *(28)*. It is of proven efficacy in post-menopausal women with advanced breast cancer, both as first-line endocrine treat-ment *(29)* in comparison with tamoxifen and as second line after tamoxifen *(30)* in comparison with megestrol. Arimidex is being tested in combination with tamox-ifen as adjuvant treatment for early breast cancer in postmenopausal women *(31)*.

In premenopausal women, it should be possible to induce "total estrogen block-ade" by lowering serum estradiol to the postmenopausal range by ovarian suppres-sion with Zoladex, further reducing estrogen by inhibition of aromatase with Arimidex and then adding tamoxifen to block the action of any small amount of residual estrogen or any dietary estrogen at the receptor level. A trial to test this hypothesis has been proposed (ANZAD: Arimidex, Nolvadex, and Zoladex in Advanced Disease) in women with hormone receptor-positive tumors *(32)*.

11. ZOLADEX AS ADJUVANT THERAPY

Ovarian ablation is the oldest adjuvant systemic therapy tested in a number of clinical trials and the EBCTCG Overview meta-analysis clearly substanti-ated its efficacy *(4)*. The magnitude of effect appears similar to that of tamox-ifen in postmenopausal women *(33)* or of cytotoxic chemotherapy in premenopausal women *(34)*.

With the proven ability of Zoladex, both to inhibit ovarian function and to induce responses in breast cancer, there was every reason to expect that Zoladex has the same adjuvant effect as ovarian suppression *(35)*.

Several large randomized trials involving over 6,000 women have evaluated the role of Zoladex in this setting. The results of these were presented at the American Society of Clinical Oncology (1999), the 6th Nottingham Interna-tional Breast Cancer Conference (1999), and the 2nd European Breast Cancer Conference (2001).

The ZIPP Trial *(36)*, carried out in Sweden, the UK, and Italy, randomized patients to Zoladex vs no extra therapy following what was defined as "standard" treatment for primary breast cancer (over 40% of cases had received adjuvant chemotherapy as part of their standard treatment). Significantly fewer events were reported at a mean of 5 yr in the patients randomized to receive Zoladex in addition to standard therapy. This relative risk reduction (RR = 0.77) is of the same order as that found in the EBCTCG analysis *(4)* of the effects of adjuvant ovarian ablation or removal, indicating that Zoladex given for 2 yr appears as efficient as other means of permanent ovarian suppression.

The Eastern Co-operative Oncology Group INT-0101 Study *(37)* showed that the addition of Zoladex plus tamoxifen significantly improved the recurrence-free survival, in women also given cytotoxic therapy with cyclophosphamide, Adriamycin and 5-fluororacil (CAF), whereas Zoladex alone did not do so. This was a further demonstration of the effectiveness of the combination of the two hormonal agents.

The Italian GROCTA-2 *(38)*, the Austrian AC05 *(39)*, and the Zebra (Zoladex Early Breast Cancer Research Association) *(40)* trials directly compared the hormonal regime of Zoladex plus tamoxifen with the cytotoxic regime cyclophosphamide, methotrexate and 5-fluororacil (CMF) in premenopausal women with ER-positive tumors. The Italian trial demonstrated overall parity in survival and disease-free survival; the Austrian trial showed advantage, (significant in the latter) for the hormonal regime. The Zebra trial emphasized the importance of ER status: in ER-positive tumors, there was again equivalence between Zoladex and CMF, there was no evidence of a Zoladex effect in ER-negative tumors.

In advising individual women on their absolute chance of gain from adjuvant systemic therapy, the Nottingham Prognostic Index *(41)* may be used to give the predicted survival without adjuvant therapy of groups of women with tumors of differing prognostic factors. The relative risk reduction given by an adjuvant therapy, as demonstrated in the EBCTCG overview *(4)*, is then applied to each group, allowing calculation of the absolute extra number predicted to be alive in each prognostic group at a particular time interval. For example from Table 1, 14 more women per 100 treated who are in the poor prognostic group (PPG) are alive at 10 yr as a result of adjuvant ovarian ablation or suppression, in addition to the 18 predicted to be alive without therapy. However, only 1 more woman per 100 treated in the excellent prognostic group would be alive as a result of such therapy in addition to the 91% alive without treatment.

Since the beneficial effect of ovarian suppression is presumably gained only in the ER-positive cases (around 60% of tumors in women under 50 and 70% in women over 50) the absolute gains are even more pronounced in these patients. Table 2 shows the calculated benefits from hormonal therapies for ER-positive tumours in both women aged <50 (for ovarian ablation or suppression) and aged 50–60 (from tamoxifen). The magnitude of effect of the hormonal therapies is seen to be the same in young women treated by ovarian suppression as in older women treated without tamoxifen.

Table 1
Calculation of Overall Effect on 10-Yr Survival of Ovarian Suppression
in Six Prognostic Groups, Applying Relative Risk Reduction Found
in EBCTCG Overview

	% Alive in each prognostic group		
Prognostic group	Without therapy	With therapy	% Extra alive in group
EPG	90.9	92.1	1.2
GPG	80.6	83.7	3.1
MPI I	71.1	75.9	4.8
MPG II	58.5	65.6	7.1
MPG III	39.8	50.3	10.5
PPG	18.3	32.7	14.4

In this and later tables EPG, excellent; GPC, good; MPG I, II, and II, moderate I, II, and III; PPG, poor; Nottingham Prognostic Groups.

Table 2
Comparison of Calculated Effects on 10-Yr
Survival of Endocrine Treatments in Women Aged
45 (Ovarian Ablation, Removal, or Suppression)
and 55 (Tamoxifen) with ER-positive Tumors

	% Extra alive in each prognostic group	
Prognostic group	Aged 45 o^x	Aged 55 Tam
EPG	1.4	1.3
GPG	3.8	3.5
MPG I	6.0	5.5
MPG II	8.9	8.1
MPG III	13.1	12.0
PPG	18.1	18.7

CMF has an overall benefit similar to that of ovarian ablation (Table 3). Since CMF also brings about a chemical ovarian ablation in 65–75% of women treated (37,38,42,43) it is certain that part of its adjuvant effect must be from ovarian suppression. Subset analysis in the Austrian (39) and the Zebra (40) trials and evidence summarized in two reviews (42,43) give further support to this conclusion, since deaths and recurrences in women given CMF were significantly fewer in those rendered amenorrhoeic by the therapy. Another study (43) showed that the effect of chemotherapy in young women rendered amenorrhoeic was significant only in ER-positive tumors. It is, therefore, reasonable to assume that the magnitude of the effect pro-

Table 3
Calculation of Overall Effect on 10-Yr Survival of Polychemotherapy

| Prognostic group | % Alive in each prognostic group | | % Extra alive in group |
	Without therapy	With therapy	
EPG	90.9	92.2	1.3
GPG	80.6	83.9	3.3
MPII	71.1	76.2	5.1
MPG II	58.5	66.1	7.6
MPG III	39.8	51.0	11.2
PPG	18.3	33.8	15.5

Table 4
Calculation of Effect on 10-Yr Survival of Polychemotherapy After Subtraction of 75%
of the Overall Effect of Ovarian Suppression (Table 1) from the Overall Effect
of Polychemotherapy (Table 2) in Women Aged 45 (="True Cytotoxic Effect")

| Prognostic group | % Alive without therapy | % Extra alive in each prognostic group | | | | | |
		Overall from polychemo-therapy		Pure cytotoxic component		Ovarian ablative component
EPG	90.9	1.3	=	0.5	+	0.8
GPG	80.6	3.3	=	1.1	+	2.2
MPG I	71.1	5.1	=	1.7	+	3.4
MPG II	58.5	7.6	=	2.6	+	5.0
MPG III	39.8	11.2	=	3.9	+	7.3
PPG	18.3	15.5	=	5.4	+	10.1

duced on ER-postive tumors by the hormonal side effect of CMF is equivalent to 65–75% of the effect produced by ovarian suppression alone. This assumption allows calculation of the separate effects on survival produced by CMF: that from its effect on the ovaries and that produced by the pure cytotoxic action on the tumor. By subtraction of 75% of the overall effect achievable by ovarian ablation from the overall benefit from CMF the pure cytotoxic effect on the tumor is revealed. In the PPG, 15 more women are seen to be alive from CMF therapy but of these 10 would have also been alive from ovarian-suppressive therapy alone; therefore only 5 would be alive because of a pure cytotoxic effect (Table 4).

That this is indeed likely to be the magnitude of the pure cytotoxic effect in premenopausal women is verified by the calculated pure cytotoxic effect in young women being the same as the overall effect of CMF in

Table 5
Comparison of Pure Cytotoxic Effect
of Polychemotherapy on Women Aged 45
with Overall Effect of Polychemotherapy
in Women Aged 55

| Prognostic group | % Extra alive in each prognostic group | |
	Aged 45 pure cytotoxic effect	Aged 55 overall effect
EPG	0.5	0.5
GPG	1.1	1.2
MPG I	1.7	1.9
MPG II	2.6	2.8
MPG III	3.9	4.2
PPG	5.4	5.8

postmenopausal women, in whom there is no ovarian-suppressive effect to subtract (Table 5).

It has been claimed that cytotoxic agents have a greater effect in young women and hormone treatments in older, and many units at present use adjuvant cytotoxic therapy for all premenopausal women with invasive cancers. The trials have confirmed the theoretical calculations: hormonal therapy has a powerful overall adjuvant effect on ER-positive tumors. In contrast, much of the effect of cytotoxic therapy on ER-positive tumors is brought about by its ovarian-suppressive action and this part could be gained by ovarian-suppressive therapies alone.

As has been demonstrated it is now possible to predict the chance of benefit from adjuvant ovarian suppression for the individual women with an ER-positive tumor, depending on the prognosis and the receptor status (Tables 1–5). Along with this the side effects of Zoladex and of CMF have to be considered. The GROCTA-2 (38) study documented the side effects well; as expected menopausal symptoms dominated the recipients of Zoladex and Tamoxifen and the usual side effects of cytotoxic therapy (nausea, leucopenia, infections) those of CMF.

However the Zebra study (40) demonstrated that 70% of the women treated with CMF became permanently amenorrhoeic, whereas the majority of women treated with Zoladex returned to cycling. The menopausal side effects after two years therapy were therefore reversed, a trend followed in the Quality of Life and Bone Density sub-protocols.

These considerations must result in a change in the way in which young women are treated (Tables 2, 6).

Table 6
Recommendations at
Nottingham City Hospital for
Adjuvant Therapy by Prognostic
Group in Women Aged 45 with
ER-positive Tumors

Prognostic group	
EPG	Nil
GPG	HT
MPG I	HT
MPG II	HT
MPG III	HT
PPG	HT+CT

The adjuvant therapy of choice in premenopausal women with ER-positive tumors is now Zoladex plus tamoxifen. Since adjuvant hormone therapy does not have high toxicity, it should probably be given to all except the excellent prognostic group. In women with ER-negative tumors, the calculated extra gain from the pure cytotoxic effect of CMF is disappointingly small and only in those women with poor prognoses does the gain appear enough to offset the side effects; in women with ER-positive tumors and in the poor prognostic group, the additional effect of cytotoxic to hormonal therapy may be considered.

12. CONCLUSION

To obtain an objective response to first-line hormonal therapy is of the utmost importance to a woman with advanced breast cancer. Zoladex is an established agent for ovarian suppression in premenopausal women with advanced breast cancer and has the advantages of being noninvasive and of being more reliable in controlling circulating oestradiol than ovarian ablation by radiotherapy. Zoladex therapy can be discontinued if there is no response, so sparing women menopausal side-effects.

The meta-analysis of LH-RH agonist vs LH-RH agonist plus tamoxifen indicates that the combination treatment provides significant additional benefit, particularly in terms of the clinically valuable duration of response.

The trials of Zoladex-containing hormonal regimes against CMF as an adjuvant therapy indicate overall parity of response in ER-positive tumors but far fewer side-effects. A major part of the effect of CMF in ER-positive tumors is achieved through its ovarian-suppressive side effect and this hormonal effect is considerably stronger than the pure cytoxic effect on the tumor. Hormonal therapy with Zoladex-containing regimes should now replace cytotoxic therapy as the adjuvant therapy of choice for women with ER-positive tumors.

REFERENCES

1. Beatson GT. On the treatment of inoperable cases of carcinoma of the mamma: suggestions for a new method of treatment with illustrative cases. *Lancet* 1896; ii:104–107.
2. Paterson R, Russell MH. Clinical trials in malignant disease: part II. Breast cancer: value of irradiation of the ovaries. *J Fac Radiol* 1959; 10:103–133.
3. Nissen-Meyer R. Primary breast cancer: the effect of primary ovarian irradiation. *Ann Oncol* 1991; 2:343–346.
4. Early Breast Cancer Trialists' Collaborative Group. Ovarian ablation in early breast cancer: overview of the randomised trials. *Lancet* 1996; 348:1189–1196.
5. Stein JJ. Surgical or irradiation castration for patients with advanced breast cancer. *Cancer* 1969; 24:1350–1354.
6. Williams MR, Walker KJ, Blamey RW, et al. The use of an LH-RH agonist (ICI 118630, 'Zoladex') in advanced premenopausal breast cancer. *Br J Cancer* 1986; 53:629–636.
7. Blamey RW, Jonat W, Kaufmann M, et al. Goserelin depot in the treatment of premenopausal advanced breast cancer. *Eur J Cancer* 1992; 28A:810–814.
8. Furr BJA. Pharmacology of luteinising hormone-releasing hormone (LHRH) analogue, 'Zoladex'. *Horm Res* 1989; 32(Suppl 1):86–92.
9. Veronesi U, Cascinelli N, Greco M, et al. A reappraisal of oophorectomy in carcinoma of the breast. *Ann Surg* 1981; 205:18–21.
10. Buchanan RB, Blamey RW, Durrant KR, et al. A randomised comparison of tamoxifen with surgical oophorectomy in premenopausal patients with advanced breast cancer. *J Clin Oncol* 1986; 4:1326–1330.
11. Ingle JN, Krook JE, Green SJ, et al. Randomised trial of bilateral oophorectomy versus tamoxifen in premenopausal women with metastatic breast cancer. *J Clin Oncol* 1986; 4:178–185.
12. Frachia AA, Farrow JH, DePalo AJ, et al. Castration for primary inoperable or recurrent breast carcinoma. *Surg Gynecol Obstet* 1969; 128:1226–1234.
13. Lewison EF. Prophylactic versus therapeutic castration in the total treatment of breast cancer. A collective review. *Obstet Gynecol Surv* 1962; 17:769–802.
14. Williamson K, Robertson JFR, Blamey RW. Effect of LHRH agonist, Zoladex on ovarian histology. *Br J Surg* 1988; 75:595–596.
15. Klijn JGM, Blamey RW, Boccardo F, et al. A new standard treatment for advanced premenopausal breast cancer: A meta-analysis of the Combined Hormonal Agent Trialists' Group (CHAT). *Eur J Cancer* 1998; 34:(Suppl 5): S90 Abs 405.
16. Blamey RW, Jonat W, Kaufmann M, et al. Survival data relating to the use of goserelin depot in the treatment of premenopausal advanced breast cancer. *Eur J Cancer* 1993; 29A:1498.
17. Blamey RW. The introduction of the LHRH agonist, goserelin ('Zoladex') into clinical practice. *Endocr Rel Cancer* 1997; 4:229–232.
18. Williams MR, Todd JH, Blamey RW, et al Survival patterns in hormone treated advanced breast cancer. *Br J Surg* 1986; 75:752–755.
19. Robertson JFR, Nicholson RI, Blamey RW, et al. Confirmation of a prognostic index or metastatic breast cancer. *Breast Cancer Res Treatment* 1992; 22:221–227.
20. Taylor CW, Green S, Dalton WS, et al. Multicenter randomised clinical trial of goserelin versus surgical ovariectomy in premenopausal patients with receptor-positive metastatic breast cancer: an Intergroup Study. *J Clin Oncol* 1998; 16:994–999.
21. Dixon AR, Jackson L, Robertson JFR, Blamey RW, et al. Combined goserelin and tamoxifen in premenopausal advanced breast cancer *Eur J Cancer* 1991; 24:806–807.

22. Robertson, JFR, Walker, KJ, Nicholson RI, Blamey RW, et al. Combined and endocrine effects of LHRH agonist, Zoladex and tamoxifen (Nolvadex) therapy in premenopausal women with breast cancer. *Br J Surg* 1989; 76:1262–1265.

23. Nicholson RI, Walker KJ, Blamey R, et al. 'Zoladex' plus tamoxifen versus 'Zoladex' alone in pre- and peri-menopausal metastatic breast cancer. *J Steroid Biochem Mol Biol* 1990; 37:989–995.

24. Jonat W, Kaufmann M, Blamey RW, et al. A randomised study to compare the effect of the luteinising hormone releasing hormone (LHRH) analogue goserelin with or without tamoxifen in pre and perimenopausal patients with advanced breast cancer. *Eur J Cancer* 1995; 31A:137–142.

25. Klijn JGM, Beex L, Mauriac L, et al. Combined treatment with the LHRH-agonist buserelin (LHRH-A) and tamoxifen (TAM) vs single treatment with each drug alone in premenopausal metastatic breast cancer. Final results of EORTC study 10881. *Ann Oncol* 1998; 9(Suppl 4):11(Abs 540).

26. Boccardo F, Rubagotti A, Perrotta A, et al. Ovarian ablation versus goserelin with or without tamoxifen in pre- perimenopausal patients with advanced breast cancer: results of a multicentric Italian study. *Ann Oncol* 1994; 5:337–342.

27. Cohen I, Tepper R, Figer A, et al. Successful co-treatment with LHRH agonist for ovarian over-stimulation and cystic formation in premenopausal tamoxifen exposure. *Cancer Res Treatment* 1999; 55:199–125.

28. Plourde PV, Dyroff M, Dowsett M, et al. 'Arimidex': A new, oral, once-a-day aromatase inhibitor. *J Steroid Biochem Mol Biol* 1995; 53:175–179.

29. Thuerliman BJK, Nabholtz JM, Bannetone J, Robertson JFR, et al. on behalf of Arimidex Study Group. Preliminary results of two comparative multicentre clinical trials comparing the efficacy and tolerability of Arimidex (anastrazole) and tamoxifen (TAM) in postmenopausal women with advanced breast cancer. *Breast* 1999; 8:214(Abs).

30. Buzdar AU, Jonat W, Howell A, et al. Anastrozole versus megestrol acetate in the treatment of postmenopausal women with advanced breast carcinoma. Results of a survival update based on a combined analysis of data from two mature phase III trials. *Cancer* 1998; 83:1142–1152.

31. Houghton J, Baum M, ATAC Study-Group. 'Arimidex', tamoxifen alone or in combination (ATAC) adjuvant trial in post-menopausal breast cancer. *Eur J Cancer* 1998; 34 (Suppl 5): S83(Abs 385).

32. Blamey RW. The role of selective non-steroidal aromatase inhibitors in future treatment strategies. *Oncology* 1997; 54 (Suppl 2):27–31.

33. Early Breast Cancer Trialists' Collaborative Group. Tamoxifen for early breast cancer; an overview of the randomised trials. *Lancet* 1998; 351:1451–1467.

34. Early Breast Cancer Trialists' Collaborative Group. Polychemotherapy for early breast cancer; an overview of the randomised trials. *Lancet* 1998; 352:930–942.

35. Jonat W. Luteinizing hormone-releasing hormone analogues: the rationale for adjuvant use in premenopausal women with early breast cancer *Br J Cancer* 1978; 78 (Suppl 4):5–8.

36. Baum M, Rutgers E for ZIPP trial. Zoladex and tamoxifen as adjuvant therapy in premenopausal breast cancer: a randomised trial *Breast* 1999; 8:233.

37. Davidson NE, O'Neill A for ECOG, SWOG and CACGB. Effect of chemohormonal therapy in premenopausal node positive, receptor positive breast cancer (INT-0101) *Breast,* 1999; 8:232.

38. Boccardo P, Rubagotti A for Italian Breast Cancer Adjuvant Study Group. CMF vs tamoxifen plus ovarian stimulation as adjuvant treatment of ER positive pre-menopausal breast cancer. *Breast* 1999; 8:233.

39. Jakesz R, Gnant M for ABCSG. Combination goserelin and tamoxifen is more effective than CMF in premenopausal patients with hormone responsive tumours (Abstract).

40. Jonat W. *Eur J Cancer* 2000; 36 Suppl. 5:567.
41. Blamey RW The design and clinical use of the Nottingham Prognostic Index in breast cancer *Breast* 1996; 5:156–157.
42. Mastro LD Venturini M, Sertoli R, Rosso R. Amenorrhea induced by adjuvant chemotherapy in early breast cancer patients: prognostic role and clinical implications *Breast Cancer Res Treatment* 1997; 43:183–190.
43. Sacks NPM, A'Hern RP, Baum M. How much of the effect of chemotherapy is due to hormonal manipulation, in *Medical Radiology. Non-Disseminated Breast Cancer* (Fletcher GH, & Levitt SH, eds). Springer-Verlag, Berlin, 1993.
44. Brincker H, Rose C, Rank F. Evidence of a castration-mediated effect of adjuvant cytotoxic chemotherapy in premenopausal breast cancer *J Clin Oncol* 1987; 5:1771–1778.

IV ANDROGENS AND ANDROGEN WITHDRAWAL

14 Molecular Action of Androgens

Shutsung Liao, Junichi Fukuchi, and Yung-Hsi Kao

CONTENTS

1. HISTORICAL INTRODUCTION

1.1. Discovery of Androgens

Around 200 BC in China, crystals, obtained by sublimation of extracts of male sexual and accessory organs, were used for treatment of patients who lacked "maleness" activity. These crystals may have been pure androgens. By 700–1000 AD, the concept of "Nai Tang" (inner elixir) and "Wai Tang" (outer elixir), which resemble "endocrinology" and "pharmacology" today, formed the conceptual basis for Chinese medicine. Unfortunately, utilization of these great discoveries was hampered by monopolistic secrecy and lack of scientific follow-up, as for many Chinese medicines. In the United States and Europe, male hormones were isolated and their structures were determined in the 1920s. Many of the physiological functions of androgens were identified during the following three decades. Pure androgenic steroids were used in hospitals for certain medical treatments in the 1930s. In the 1940s, Charles Huggins of the University of Chicago initiated hormonal therapy of cancer,

From: *Hormone Therapy in Breast and Prostate Cancer*
Edited by: V. C. Jordan and B. J. A. Furr © Humana Press Inc., Totowa, NJ

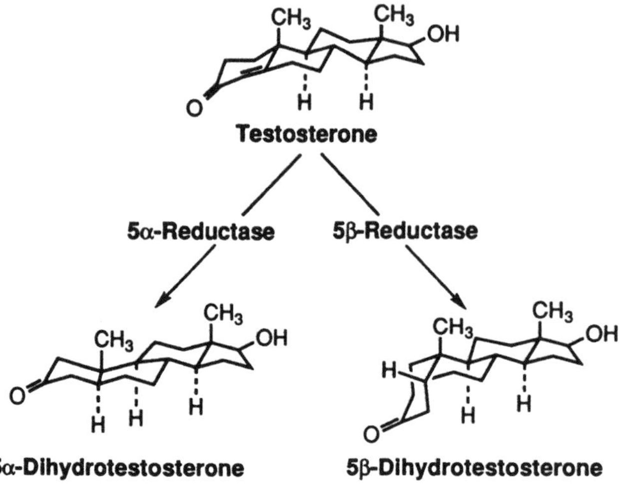

Fig. 1. Enzymatic conversion of testosterone to 5α- and 5β-dihydrotestosterone.

demonstrating that prostate cancer could be treated by castration and estrogen administration *(1)*.

1.2. Differential Functions of Androstanes

The major blood androgen, testosterone, is produced by the testis, but adrenals and ovaries also produce small amounts of testosterone in males and females. Dehydroepiandrosterone and androstenedione secreted by adrenals and ovaries can be converted to testosterone by peripheral enzymatic conversion. Testosterone is converted by 5α- or 5β-reductase to 5α- or 5β-dihydrotestosterone, which are isomeric androstanes differing in molecular configuration about carbon 5 (Fig. 1). Many androgens are derivatives of 5α-androstanes, whereas 5β-androstanes are not androgenic. In vivo, 5α- and 5β-androstanes are not interconverted. Testosterone and androgenic 5α-androstanes can enhance erythropoietic activity by stimulating erythropoietin production in kidney, while nonandrogenic 5β-androstanes can promote erythropoiesis by stimulating heme biosynthesis in liver and through other unknown mechanisms. It is now clear that 5α-DHT is the key active androgen in many peripheral target organs, including prostate and skin. Both testosterone and 5α-DHT appear to play important roles during developmental stages of androgen-regulated organs. Testosterone also has additional role in regulating certain functions of brain and testis as well as muscle growth in adults. Some of these activities may be dependent on estrogens synthesized by aromatization of the A-ring of testosterone.

1.3. Hormone-Gene Theory and Androgen Receptor

In the early 1960s, we showed that androgens could rapidly enhance the RNA-synthesizing activity in the cell nuclei *(2)* and increase the level of mRNA associated with prostate-cell nuclei and ribosomes *(3,4)*. These observations supported the "Hormone-Gene" theory that tied the molecular action of steroid hormones to the regulation of gene expression.

Discovery of the estrogen receptor (ER) by Elwood Jensen at the University of Chicago in the late 1950s was based on the observation that the major ovarian estrogen, 17β-estradiol, without metabolic conversion, could be retained by target organs, such as the uterus *(5)*. Discovery of the androgen receptor (AR) took a different course. In our laboratory *(6)* and in the laboratory of Jean Wilson and Nicholas Bruchovsky *(7)*, it was found, in 1967, that testosterone was retained in the form of 5α-dihydrotestosterone (5α-DHT) in prostate-cell nuclei where androgen was believed to modulate gene expression. Since this nuclear retention was dependent on a protein *(8)* that could specifically bind 5α-DHT and other potent androgens but not nonandrogenic steroids *(9)*, the protein was identified as AR.

AR, like receptors for other steroid hormones, is a member of the nuclear-receptor superfamily, which acts as a ligand-inducible transcription factor by recognizing androgen-response elements (ARE) of target genes to modulate expression of genes involved in development, differentiation, and regulation of target organs.

2. 5α-REDUCTASES

2.1. Structure and Mutation

5α-Reductase catalyzes the conversion of testosterone to 5α-DHT in the presence of NADPH (Fig. 2). In human, monkeys, and rodents, there are two isozymes of 5α-reductase, type 1 and type 2, expressed from different genes *(10)*. They are hydrophobic proteins of approx 30,000 daltons and share 50% identity in their amino acid sequences. About three dozen different mutations in the 5α-reductase type 2 gene have been described in individuals with a diagnosis of 5α-reductase deficiency. These mutations lead to a form of male pseudohermaphroditism. The level of testosterone in these patients is adequate for development of the epididymis, vas deferens, and seminal vesicle from the Wolffian ducts, but is inadequate for virilization of the urogenital sinus and development of the prostate and external genitalia. A male pattern of musculoskeletal development also takes place during puberty, but growth of beard and other body hair, development of acne, and male-pattern baldness are often lacking in these individuals. Some of these mutations result in a total lack of steroid 5α-reductase activity, while others decrease the efficiency of the enzyme by lowering the enzyme's affinity for either testosterone or NADPH.

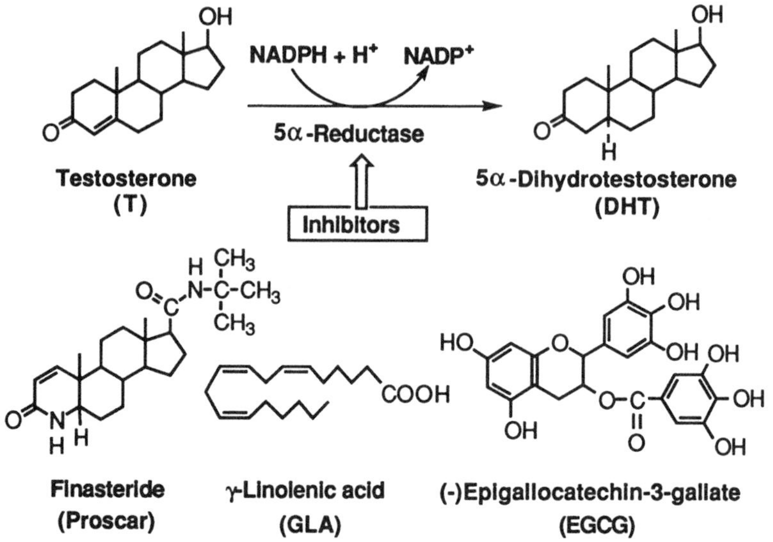

Fig. 2. 5α-Reductase-catalyzed formation of 5α-dihydrotestosterone from testosterone and three different forms of 5α-reductase inhibitors.

No mutations in the steroid 5α-reductase type 1 gene have been linked to the syndrome of 5α-reductase deficiency. Testosterone is the direct precursor for the enzymatic synthesis of both 17β-estradiol and 5α-dihydrotestosterone. If steroid 5α-reductase is absent, more testosterone may be converted to estradiol. The buildup of toxic levels of estradiol may lead to fetal death *(11)*.

2.2. 5α-Reductase Inhibitors

Antiandrogens that inhibit androgen binding to AR can be beneficial for treatment of many androgen-dependent diseases, but there can be undesirable side effects. Inhibitors of 5α-reductase may have unique advantages, since they can selectively suppress 5α-DHT-dependent abnormalities, such as prostate cancer, benign prostate hyperplasia (BPH), acne, baldness, female hirsutism, skin aging, and androgen-dependent breast tumor and hepatoma without significantly affecting physiological processes believed to be controlled by testosterone, such as libido, spermatogenesis, sexual behavior, and smooth-muscle growth *(12,13)*.

A number of natural and synthetic compounds that are inhibitors of 5α-reductase have been identified (Fig. 2). Among them, a class of 4-aza-steroids has been extensively studied. A synthetic 4-aza-steroid, finasteride (17β-(N-tert-butylcarbamoyl)-4-aza-5α-androst-1-en-3-one), is now prescribed under the tradename Proscar for the treatment of BPH. In about 20–30% of BPH patients, finasteride appears to be effective in shrinking prostates of large size

HUMAN ANDROGEN RECEPTOR

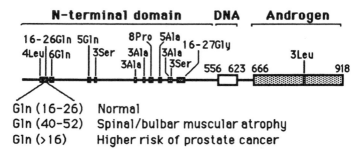

Gln (16–26)   Normal
Gln (40–52)   Spinal/bulbar muscular atrophy
Gln (>16)   Higher risk of prostate cancer

Fig. 3. Schematic diagram of the structure of human androgen receptor with N-terminal, DNA-binding, and androgen-binding domains. The position of oligo- and poly amino acid stretches are indicated. AR having a long polyglutamine stretch (40–52 Gln) in the N-terminal domain has been related to Kennedy's disease, while a shorter stretch (>16 Gln) in this domain may indicate high risk of prostate cancer.

and composed of a large percentage of epithelial cells *(14)*. Prostates composed mostly of stromal cells or of small to moderate size are less responsive to finasteride treatment. Finasteride is also being tested in clinical trials as a chemopreventative for prostate cancer and as a therapeutic agent for treatment of some forms of alopecia.

A variety of compounds found in the diet are also potent inhibitors of 5α-reductase. Some of these phytochemicals include unsaturated fatty acids *(15)*, flavanoids *(16)*, and catechin gallates *(17)* (Fig. 2). Topical administration of γ-linolenic acids has been shown to suppress androgen-dependent growth of hamster flank organs *(18)*.

3. ANDROGEN RECEPTOR

3.1. Structure

Rat and human (h) ARs have about 900–920 amino acids with a molecular mass of about 98 kDa *(19,20)* (Fig. 3). The exact size of ARs may vary because of variations in the length of polyglycine and polyglutamine stretches in the amino-terminal region of the receptor. AR mRNA is transcribed from a single gene present on the q11–12 region of the X-chromosome *(21)* and the eight exons of the gene cover more than 90 kb of DNA *(22)*. ARs, like other steroid receptors, are comprised of four functional domains *(23)* (Fig. 3):

1. The amino-terminal domain of the AR makes up more than half of the receptor and a single exon encodes most of this domain. This domain is poorly conserved among all members of the steroid hormone-receptor family in both the sequence and length. A striking feature of this domain in hAR is the presence of

two homopolymeric stretches (16–27 residues each) of glycine and glutamine. These polyamino acids may be important for regulation of AR activity.

2. The DNA-binding domain consists of about 70 amino acids and is located next to the amino-terminal domain (Fig. 3). Steroid receptors as a group have high amino acid-sequence similarity (56–79% identity) in this DNA-binding domain. Sulfurs of eight cysteines in this domain coordinate two Zn^{2+} ions in a tetrahedral configuration forming motifs that are called "zinc fingers." After binding of an androgen, the receptors interact as homodimers with a specific palindromic sequences of DNA (ARE) in genes that AR regulates in the cell nucleus. These DNA sequence are called hormone-response elements (HRE) and have the consensus sequence 5'-AGNACANNNTGTNCT-3' (24). Since this HRE sequence is also recognized by receptors for progestins, glucocorticoids, and mineralocorticoids, additional factors may be required for AR-specific gene activation.

3. A hinge domain with about 30 amino acids is located between the DNA-binding domain and androgen-binding domain at the carboxyl-terminus of the AR. A nuclear-localization signal is present in this domain, although other domains may have sequences that are important for nuclear localization of AR.

4. The androgen-binding domain has about 300 amino acids that recognize androgenic molecules. Since deletion of as much as 90% of the amino acids from the androgen-binding domain produces an AR that does not bind steroids, but will constitutively activate transcription at levels of 40–100% of the full-length ARs, it is assumed that a region in the steroid-binding domain inhibits the transcriptional properties of the AR, but this inhibition can be relieved by steroid binding. Recent studies have suggested that hormone binding may induce conformational changes of receptor domains and promote association of nuclear receptors with various protein factors that are involved in regulation of transcription (see Subheading 3.3.).

3.2. AR Gene Mutation

Several hundred AR gene mutations have been documented. The majority of these mutations occur in the DNA- and androgen-binding domains. More than 90% of these mutations are due to a single base (point) mutation, while a minority of cases involves complete and partial gene deletion as well as small insertions. These mutations produce premature termination codons and amino acid substitutions, resulting in ARs that cannot interact with androgens properly, and therefore, lead to androgen insensitivity (25–28).

AR mutations have also been detected in some human prostate cancers (29,30). One mutation in the androgen-binding domain changes the ligand specificity of AR so that estrogens and progestins as well as some antiandrogens, such as hydroxyflutamide, act like androgens and activate the mutated AR and promote prostate-cancer growth (31,32).

In the amino terminal domain of AR, expansion of the poly (Gln) stretch from the normal length of 16–26 to 40–50 residues (Fig. 3) has been related to the rare X-chromosome-linked disease, spinal and bulbar muscular atrophy (Kennedy disease) *(33)*. Recently, a higher risk of prostate-cancer incidence was linked to individuals with AR having a poly (Gln) stretch shorter than 16 residues *(34,35)*. It is important to note that individuals with complete deletions of the AR gene have complete androgen insensitivity, but are otherwise healthy and do not exhibit symptoms of muscular atrophy or prostate cancer.

3.3. AR-Associated Proteins

The first steroid receptor-associated protein that received attention was a heat-shock protein (HSP90) *(36)*. It was suggested that heat-shock protein may assist in maintaining a steroid-receptor conformation necessary for ligand-binding. Since nuclear receptors are ligand (hormone)-activated transcription factors that regulate the expression of genes, many other nuclear proteins are expected to interact with and regulate the functions of nuclear receptor. Nuclear receptor-associated proteins may be involved in recruiting transcriptional factors to the promotor, stabilization of transcriptional machinery, or providing specificity needed for hormone-receptor function. Some of these proteins are known as nuclear transcriptional coactivators or corepressors.

A number of protein-protein interactions involving AR and other steroid receptors have been described *(37)*. Many of these interactions occur with several different nuclear receptors. A coactivator specific for AR (ARA70) has been described *(38)*. A section of the N-terminal domain of AR has been shown to interact with the general transcriptional factor TFIIF and the TATA-box binding protein (TBP), supporting the contention that AR is involved in recruitment of protein factors to the transcriptional machinery *(39)*. The hormone-binding domain of ARs and other steroid receptors contain "leucine zipper"-like structures that may be important for receptor dimerization or receptor binding of other proteins (such as Jun, fos, or cyclic AMP response element-binding protein) and play a key role in controlling gene expression, positively or negatively. Some nuclear proteins contain leucine-rich motifs that interact with liganded nuclear receptors *(40,41)*. It has been suggested that a ligand-induced switch of heterodimeric nuclear receptors from repressor to activator may involve the exchange of complexes containing histone deacetylases with those that have histone acetylase activity *(42,43)*.

4. ANDROGEN RECEPTOR AND ANDROGEN-RELATED PROGRESSION AND SUPPRESSION OF PROSTATE CANCER

4.1. Progression of Androgen-Dependent Prostate-Cancer Cells

The development and growth of prostate cancer is dependent on androgen initially, making it vulnerable to androgen ablation and antiandrogen therapies. However, prostate cancer gradually loses androgen dependency and tumor

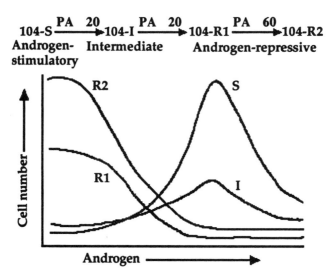

Fig. 4. Representative androgen responses of human prostate cancer LNCaP cells in culture. LNCaP 104-S cells (S) exhibited biphasic androgen responses (proliferative stimulation at low concentrations and inhibition by higher concentrations of androgen). After these cells were cultured in an androgen-depleted medium for 20 passages, the growth of cells (LNCaP-104-I) was less dependent on androgen. After an additional 60 passages, the cells (LNCaP 104-R1 and 104-R2) grew very well in the absence of androgen but became very sensitive to proliferative repression by low concentrations of androgen.

cells that are resistant to endocrine therapy ultimately proliferate. There is no effective method for treatment of androgen-independent prostate cancer. For better understanding of the mechanism involved in the progression of androgen-dependent prostate-cancer cells to androgen-independent prostate-cancer cells, we established a clonal androgen-dependent, human prostate-cancer LNCaP 104-S cell line. LNCaP 104-S cells were then allowed to go through passages in androgen-depleted culture medium and their changes in androgen-dependency and other cellular properties were analyzed *(44)* (Fig. 4). After more than a year of passaging in androgen-depleted culture medium, androgen-dependent LNCaP 104-S cells progressed to LNCaP 104-R2 cells that can grow well in the absence of androgen but are proliferatively repressed by 0.1 nM or lower concentrations of androgen *(44)*.

4.2. Androgen-Specific Suppression of the Growth of Androgen-Independent Prostate Tumor

Androgen-dependent LNCaP 104-S cells can grow well in normal but not in castrated athymic mice *(45)*. In contrast, LNCaP 104-R2 cells can grow well in castrated athymic mice but not in intact athymic mice. Administration of testosterone propionate to castrated athymic mice can prevent the initial growth or cause regression of large LNCaP 104-R2 tumors. Tumor are suppressed with testosterone, testosterone propionate, and 5α-DHT, but not with nonandrogenic 5β-DHT, estradiol, or medroxyprogesterone acetate. The androgenic effect was clearly not due to a general toxicity of androgen because androgen stimulated the growth of male accessory organs, such as seminal vesicle, and LNCaP 104-S tumors in the same animals. In castrated mice with LNCaP 104-R2 tumors, testosterone propionate administration increased expression of prostate-specific antigen (PSA) suggesting that AR was functional. After this initial increase, the blood level of PSA decreased as LNCaP 104-R2 tumors regressed *(45)*.

Another androgen-repressed prostate-cancer cell line, ARCaP, was established recently by Zhau et al. *(46)*. ARCaP cells were obtained from the ascites fluid of a patient with advanced metastatic cancer. Both androgen and estrogen suppressed the growth of ARCaP cells in culture or in athymic mice. Unlike LNCaP-104R2 cells, ARCaP cells express low levels of mRNAs for AR and PSA and the expression of PSA is also repressed by androgen. Whereas androgen repression of LNCaP 104-R2 tumors is apparently dependent on functional AR, androgen and estrogen repression of ARCaP tumors may be dependent on another mechanism.

4.3. Stimulation of the Growth of Androgen-Independent Tumors by Finasteride and Antiandrogens

5α-Reductase inhibitors, such as finasteride, can prevent testosterone action that is dependent on conversion of testosterone to 5α-DHT. As expected, finasteride inhibited testosterone-dependent growth of male accessory organs and LNCaP 104-S tumors whose growth is dependent on 5α-DHT. However, if LNCaP 104-R2 tumors were allowed to grow in castrated mice and then testosterone was given to the mice to suppress the tumor growth, additional administration of finasteride was able to inhibit testosterone suppression and stimulated the growth of the LNCaP 104-R2 tumors (Fig. 5). Finasteride did not affect the growth of human prostate PC-3 tumors that lack AR expression or human breast MCF-7 tumors in female athymic mice *(45)*. These observations indicated that the stimulation of the tumor growth by finasteride was due to its inhibition of the formation of 5α-DHT that interacted with AR to exert tumor suppression. In line with this view, antiandrogens such as Casodex *(47)* that prevent 5α-DHT binding to AR also stimulated the growth of LNCaP 104-R2 tumor under androgen suppression. Casodex administration also allows the LNCaP 104-R tumors to grow in normal nude mice as fast as tumors in castrated mice.

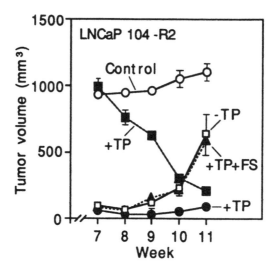

Fig. 5. Testosterone-dependent suppression and finasteride-dependent stimulation of the growth of LNCaP 104-R2 tumors in castrated male athymic mice *(43)*. The tumors grew well in control mice for 7 wk (○), but after these mice were treated with testosterone propionate (TP), the size of tumors was reduced by about 80% in 4 wk (■). If TP was given at the 4th wk, the tumor growth was prevented (●). Removal of TP (□) or administration of finasteride (▲) at the 7th wk resulted in the regrowth of the tumors.

4.4. Androgen Receptor and Reversible Progression

AR is clearly involved in both the androgen stimulation of androgen-dependent growth of LNCaP 104-S tumor and the suppression of androgen-independent LNCaP 104-R2 tumors. We have found that, in culture or in athymic mice, the cellular AR level in LNCaP 104-R2 cells is more than 10 times that in the LNCaP 104-S cells. Such an increase in AR level is not totally surprising since LNCaP 104-R2 cells are produced after a long period of culture in androgen-depleted medium and the AR mRNA level in prostate cells can be negatively regulated by androgen *(19)*. In fact, high levels of AR have been found in prostate cancer patients after the failure of hormonal therapy *(48)*. The molecular process involved in growth stimulation and suppression in the two types of cells is not clear.

We have observed that LNCaP 104-R2 can adapt to androgen in culture or in athymic mice and this adaptation may be related to the reduction of the AR level in LNCaP 104-R2 cells. It appears that the AR level is a determining factor that reversibly changes the nature of androgenic responses between androgen-stimulated growth and suppressed growth (Fig. 6). Whether the reversible nature of prostate cancer can be utilized to establish a new androgen-intermittent therapy needs further evaluation. Additional studies are also needed to

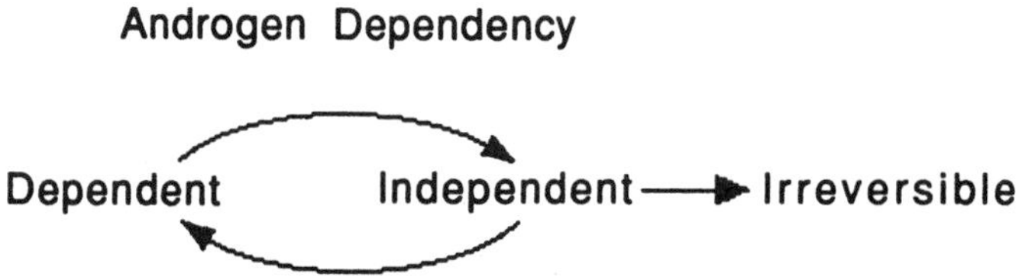

Androgen Dependency

Dependent   Independent ──▶ Irreversible

Fig. 6. Androgen-dependent human prostate cancer, LNCaP 104-S, cells can progress to androgen-independent LNCaP 104-R1 and R2 cells, which may adapt to androgen in cultures or in mice and become androgen-dependent cells again. These cells may, through unknown pathways, become AR-negative cells that can not be stimulated or suppressed by androgen.

understand how AR-positive, androgen-independent prostate tumors can progress to AR-negative, prostate tumors that are both androgen-independent and androgen-insensitive.

5. SUMMARY

Basic research that led to the discovery of the role of 5α-DHT and AR in androgen action, and the subsequent structural delineation of AR and AR genes, has made it possible to unlock the molecular mechanisms of androgen action and provide a better understanding of many medical abnormalities related to androgen action and dysfunction. The molecular basis of many androgen-insensitivity syndromes are now better understood and new potentially effective therapeutic agents based on inhibition of 5α-reductases and AR function have emerged for treatment of various medical problems, such as baldness, acne, BPH, and prostate cancer. Findings that agents that can control androgen action are in the natural environment as components in the diets or as pollutants, will continue to broaden our attention. The fact that androgens, 5α-reductase inhibitors, and antiandrogens can work both in a positive or negative manner, dependent on the cellular expression and mutation of AR or 5α-reductase genes, cancer-cell progression, and other conditions, suggests that medical uses of these agents need careful evaluation. Yet, these seemingly unexpected findings are important in drawing a true picture that can guide us to a more profound understanding of the molecular action of androgen and the methods for its regulation.

ACKNOWLEDGMENT

The research from the authors' laboratory was supported by Grants CA 58073 and DK 41670 from the U. S. National Institute of Health.

REFERENCES

1. Huggins C, Stevens RE, Hodges CV. Studies on prostatic cancer. II. The effects of castration on advanced carcinoma of the prostate gland. *Arch Surg* 1941; 43:209–223.
2. Liao S, Leininger KR, Sagher D, Barton RW. Rapid effect of testosterone on ribonucleic acid polymerase activity of rat ventral prostate. *Endocrinology* 1965; 77:763–765.
3. Liao S, Williams-Ashman HG. An effect of testosterone on amino acid incorporation by prostatic ribonucleoprotein particles. Proc Natl Acad Sci USA 1962; 48:1956–1964.
4. Liao S. Influence of testosterone on template activity of prostatic ribonucleic acids. *J Biol Chem* 1965; 240:1236–1243.
5. Jensen EV, Jacobson HI. Basic guide to the mechanism of estrogen action *Recent Prog Hormone Res* 1962; 18:387–414.
6. Anderson KM, Liao S. Selective retention of dihydrotestosterone by prostatic nuclei. *Nature* 1968; 219:277–279.
7. Bruchovsky N, Wilson JD. The conversion of testosterone to 5α-androstan-17β-ol-3-one by rat prostate in vivo and in vitro. *J Biol Chem* 1968; 243:2012–2021.
8. Fang S, Liao S. Androgen receptors: steroid- and tissue-specific retention of a 17β-hydroxy-5α-androstan-3-one protein complex by the cell nuclei of ventral prostate. *J Biol Chem* 1971; 246:16–24.
9. Liao S, Liang T, Fang S, Castaneda E, Shao TC. Steroid structure and androgenic activity: specificities involved in the receptor binding and nuclear retention of various androgens. *J Biol Chem* 1973; 248:6154–6162.
10. Russell DW, Wilson JD. Steroid 5α-reductase: two genes/two enzymes. *Ann Rev Biochem* 1994; 63:25–61.
11. Mahendroo MS, Cala KM, Landrum CP, Russell DW. Fetal death in mice lacking 5α-reductase type 1 caused by estrogen excess. *Mol Endocrinol* 1997; 11:917–927.
12. Metcalf BW, Levy MA, Holt DA. Inhibitors of steroid 5α-reductase in benign prostatic hyperplasia, male pattern baldness and acne. *Trends Pharmacol* 1989; 10:491–495.
13. Randall VA. Role of 5α-reductase in health and disease. *Bailliere's Clin Endocrinol Metab* 1994; 8:405–431.
14. Stoner E, Group TFS. The clinical effects of a 5α-reductase inhibitor, finasteride, on benign prostatic hyperplasia. *J Urol* 1992; 147:1298–1302.
15. Liang T, Liao S. Inhibition of steroid 5α-reductase by specific aliphatic unsaturated fatty acids. *Biochem J* 1992; 285:557–562.
16. Evans BAJ, Griffiths K, Morton MS. Inhibition of 5 alpha-reductase in genital skin fibroblasts and prostate tissue by dietary lignans and, isoflavonoids. *J Endocrinol* 1995; 147:295–302.
17. Liao S, Hiipakka RA. Selective inhibition of steroid 5α-reductase isozymes by tea epicatechin-3-gallate and epigallocatechin-3-gallate. *Biochem Biophys Res Comm* 1995; 214:833–838.
18. Liang T, Liao S. Growth suppression of hamster flank organs by topical application of γ-linolenic and other fatty acid inhibitors of 5α-reductase. *J Invest Dermatol* 1997; 109:152–157.
19. Chang C, Kokontis J, Liao S. Structural analysis of complementary DNA and amino acid sequences of human and rat androgen receptors. *Proc Natl Acad Sci USA* 1988; 85:7211–7215.
20. Lubahn DB, Joseph DR, Sar M, Tan J, Higgs HN, Larson RE, et al. The human androgen receptor: complementary deoxyribonucleic acid cloning, sequence analysis and gene expression in the prostate. *Mol Endocrinol* 1988; 2:1265–1275.
21. Brown CJ, Goss SJ, Lubahn DB, Joseph DR, Wilson EM, French FS, Willard HF. Androgen receptor locus on the human X chromosome: regional localization to Xq11–12 and description of a DNA polymorphism. *Am J Hum Genet* 1989; 44:264–269.

22. Kuiper GGJM, Faber PW, van Rooij HCJ, van der Korput JAGM, Ris-Stalpers C, Klassen P, et al. Structural organization of the human androgen receptor gene. *J Mol Endocrinol* 1989; 2:R1–R4.

23. Liao S, Kokontis J, Sai T, Hiipakka RA. Androgen receptors: structures, mutations, antibodies and cellular dynamics. *J Steroid Biochem* 1989; 34:41–51.

24. Roche PJ, Hoare SA, Parker MG. A consensus DNA-binding site for the androgen receptor. *Mol Endocrinol* 1992; 6:2229–2235.

25. Sai T, Seino S, Chang C, Trifiro M, Pinsky L, Mhatre A, et al. An exonic point mutation of the androgen receptor gene in a family with complete androgen insensitivity. *Am J Hum Genet* 1990; 46:1095–1100.

26. Ris-Stalpers C, Trifiro MA, Kuiper GGJM, Jenster G, Romalo G, Sai T, et al. Substitution of aspartic acid-686 by histidine or asparagine in the human androgen receptor leads to a functionally inactive protein with altered hormone-binding characteristics. *Mol Endocrinol* 1991; 5:1562–1569.

27. Hiipakka RA, Liao S. Androgen physiology: androgen receptors and action, in *Endocrinology, Third edition* (DeGroot LI, ed). Saunders Co., Philadelphia, PA, 1995, pp 2336–2351.

28. Quigley CA, De Bellis A, Marschke KB, el-Awady MK, Wilson EM, French FS. Androgen receptor defects: historical, clinical, and molecular perspectives. [published erratum appears in *Endocr Rev* 1995; 16: 546] *Endocr Rev* 1995; 16:271–321.

29. Newmark JR, Hardy DO, Tonb DC, Carter BS, Epstein JI, Isaacs WB, et al. Androgen receptor gene mutations in human prostate cancer. *Proc Natl Acad Sci USA* 1992; 89:6319–6323.

30. Taplin M-E, Bubley GJ, Shuster TD, Frantz ME, Spooner AE, Ogata GK, et al. Mutation of the androgen-receptor gene in metastatic androgen-dependent prostate cancer. *N Engl J Med* 1995; 332:1393–1398.

31. Veldscholte J, Ris-Stalpers C, Kuiper GGJM, Jenster G, Berrevoets C, Claassen E, et al. A mutation in the ligand binding domain of the androgen receptor of human LNCaP cells affects steroid binding characteristics and response to anti-androgens. *Biochem Biophys Res Comm* 1990; 173:534–540.

32. Kokontis J, Ito K, Hiipakka RA, Liao S. Expression and function of normal and LNCaP androgen receptors in androgen-insensitive human prostatic cancer cells: altered hormone and antihormone specificity in gene transactivation. *Receptor* 1991; 1:271–279.

33. La Spada AR, Wilson EM, Lubahn DB, Harding AE, Fischbeck KH. Androgen receptor gene mutations in X-linked spinal and bulbar muscular atrophy. *Nature* 1991; 352:77–79.

34. Giovannucci E, Stampfer MJ, Krithivas K, Brown M, Brufsky A, Talcott J, et al. The CAG repeat within the androgen receptor gene and its relationship to prostate cancer. *Proc Natl Acad Sci USA* 1997; 94:3320–3323.

35. Stanford JL, Just JJ, Gibbs M, Wicklund KG, Neal CL, Blumenstein BA, Ostrander EA. Polymorphic repeats in the androgen receptor gene: molecular markers of prostate cancer risk. *Cancer Res* 1997; 57:1194–1198.

36. Smith DF, Toft DO. Steroid receptors and their associated proteins. *Mol Endocrinology* 1993; 7:4–11.

37. Shibata H, Spencer TE, Onate SA, Jenster G, Tsai SY, Tsai MJ, O'Malley BW. Role of co-activators and co-repressors in the mechanism of steroid/thyroid receptor action. *Recent Prog Horm Res* 1997; 52:141–164.

38. Yeh S, Chang C. Cloning and characterization of a specific coactivator, ARA70, for the androgen receptor gene. *Proc Natl Acad Sci USA* 1996; 93:5517–5521.

39. McEwen IJ, Gustafsson J-A. Interaction of the human androgen receptor transactivation function with the general transcription factor TFIIF. *Proc Natl Acad Sci USA* 1997; 94:8485–8490.

40. Heery DM, Kalkoven E, Hoare S, Parker MG. A signature motif in transcriptional co-activators mediates binding to coactivators. *Nature* 1997; 387:733–684.

41. Torchia J, Rose DW, Inostroza J, Kamei Y, Westin S, Glass CK, Rosenfield MG. The transcriptional co-activator p/CIP binds CBP and mediates nuclear-receptor function. *Nature* 1997; 387:677–684.

42. Ogryzko VV, Schiltz RL, Russanova V, Howard BH, Nakatani Y. The transcriptional coactivator p300 and CBP are histone acetyltransferases. *Cell* 1996; 87:953–960.

43. Heinzel T, Lavinsky RM, Mullen T-M, Söderström M, Laherty CD, Torchia J, et al. A complex containing N-CoR, mSin3 and histone deacetylase mediates transcriptional repression. *Nature* 1997; 387:43–48.

44. Kokontis J, Takakura K, Hay N, Liao S. Increased androgen receptor activity and altered c-*myc* expression in prostate cancer cells after long-term androgen. *Cancer Res* 1994; 54:1566–1573.

45. Umekita Y, Hiipakka RA, Kokontis JM, Liao S. Human prostate tumor growth in athymic mice: inhibition by androgens and stimulation by a 5α-reductase inhibitor. *Proc Natl Acad Sci USA* 1996; 93:11802–11807.

46. Zhau HY, Chang SM, Chen BQ, Wang Y, Zhang H, Kao C, et al. Androgen-repressed phenotype in human prostate cancer. *Proc Natl Acad Sci USA* 1996; 93:15152–15157.

47. Furr BJA. Casodex: preclinical studies and controversies, in *Annals of the New York Academy of Sciences: Steroid Receptors and Antihormones* (Henderson D, Philibert D, Roy AK, eds. Teutsch G, eds). New York Academy of Sciences, New York, NY, 1995, pp 79–96.

48. Hobisch A, Culig Z, Radmeyer C, Bartsch G, Klocker H, Hittmair A. Distant metastases from prostatic carcinoma express androgen receptor protein. *Cancer Res* 1995; 55:3068–3072.

15 Steroidal Antiandrogens

Fritz H. Schröder and Albert Radlmaier

Contents

Introduction
Clinical Applications of CPA
References

1. INTRODUCTION

The era of antiandrogens started in 1962 with a steroidal compound. At that time an attempt was made to find progestogens for the indication of imminent abortion. Since most progestogens exerted androgenic activity, and consequently presented a risk for masculinisation of female fetuses, suitable candidates were investigated for their androgenic potential. It turned out that a derivative of hydroxyprogesterone, cyproterone acetate (CPA), was devoid of intrinsic androgenicity, but caused feminization of male rat fetuses, comparable to the clinical feature of testicular feminization (1). Further experiments revealed the underlying mechanism, and showed that it consisted of a direct inhibition of the action of androgens at the target organ. The inhibition is a result of interaction at the level of the androgen receptor (AR), where CPA competes with the endogenous ligand (2). This competitive blockade at the AR is the characteristic property of an antiandrogen. All subsequently developed antiandrogens have this basic mechanism of action in common.

1.1. Relevant Compounds

After discovering the antiandrogenicity of cyproterone acetate, the next step was to find out whether structural changes in the molecule would result in more potent antiandrogenic compounds. These attempts, however, proved to be unsuccessful (3). No steroidal substance surpassed the antiandrogenic potency of CPA. Figure 1 shows an example of how different modifications of

From: *Hormone Therapy in Breast and Prostate Cancer*
Edited by: V. C. Jordan and B. J. A. Furr © Humana Press Inc., Totowa, NJ

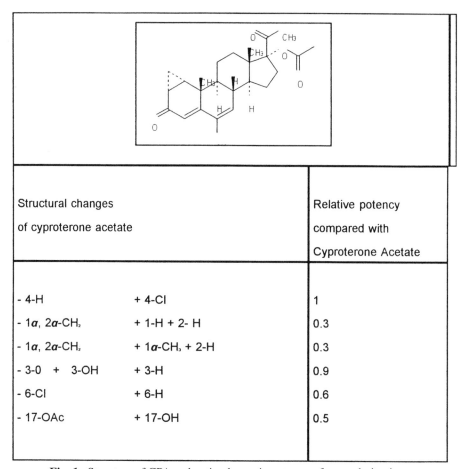

Structural changes of cyproterone acetate		Relative potency compared with Cyproterone Acetate
- 4-H	+ 4-Cl	1
- 1α, 2α-CH₂	+ 1-H + 2- H	0.3
- 1α, 2α-CH₂	+ 1α-CH₃ + 2-H	0.3
- 3-0 + 3-OH	+ 3-H	0.9
- 6-Cl	+ 6-H	0.6
- 17-OAc	+ 17-OH	0.5

Fig. 1. Structure of CPA and antiandrogenic potency of some derivatives.

the structure can alter antiandrogenic efficacy. Besides having antiandrogenic activity, CPA also has a strong progestational component. The progestational effect is linked to the presence of the acetyl group at position C17 of the steroid. Consequently, the free alcohol of CPA, cyproterone, which lacks the acetyl group, is devoid of progestational properties. However, it still exerts antiandrogenic activity, although less pronounced than CPA. Consequently, cyproterone was the first compound falling into the nowadays well-known class of pure antiandrogens.

Currently, there are four steroidal antiandrogens available in clinical practice, CPA, chlormadinone acetate (CMA), megestrol acetate, and dienogest, all of which are also potent progestogens. CPA and CMA are

Table 1
Steroidal Antiandrogens with relevance for Tumor Therapy

Substance	approved indications	manufacturer
Cyproterone acetate	prostate cancer hypersexuality androgenisation female acne* HRT*	Schering AG
Megestrol acetate	endometrial cancer breast cancer	Bristol Myers
Chlormadinone acetate	prostate cancer BPH	Teikoku
Zanoterone = WIN 49596	development discontinued	Sterling-Winthrop
Osaterone acetate = TZP 4238	in clinical development for BPH and prostate cancer	Teikoku

* low dose in combination with ethinylestradiol

used as classical antiandrogens in the therapy of androgen-dependent diseases, with prostate cancer being the most important one. Megestrol acetate, however, is used exclusively as a progestogen in the treatment of breast cancer and endometrial cancer. Dienogest is not used in oncology, but as a progestogenic compound in an oral contraceptive pill and will not be discussed further here.

Two other steroidal antiandrogens worth mentioning are osaterone acetate (TZP-4238) and zanoterone (WIN 49596) (Table 1). These substances were recently brought from research into clinical development. Osaterone acetate has a similar pharmacological profile to the marketed compounds *(4)*. It is currently in clinical development in Japan for prostate cancer and benign prostatic hyperplasia (BPH). Zanoterone is a pure antiandrogen *(5)* whose use in the treatment of BPH has been investigated in a Phase II study. This development was discontinued, however, due to insufficient clinical efficacy *(6)*.

1.2. Pharmacology

Preclinical pharmacological studies are useful and valuable within the framework of a compound-finding program and in helping to decide which compounds should undergo clinical development. However, it should be kept in mind that preclinical comparisons of compounds that have already been approved are of limited value. The possible drawbacks and pitfalls of comparing the relative potencies of antiandrogens in preclinical studies have been highlighted in a recent publication *(7)*. Special attention was drawn to the problems regarding in vitro studies on binding affinity to the androgen receptor.

The basic prerequisites for a substance that acts by competitive inhibition are as follows:

1. High affinity for the receptor;
2. Long-lasting binding to the receptor; and
3. Ability to achieve a continuous competitively high concentration at the target site (thus enabling sufficient displacement of the natural ligand from the receptor).

Consequently, the ideal antiandrogen should show strong potency in each of these factors. In reality, the compounds currently available present a mixed picture with relative strengths in one area and relative weaknesses in others. However, the low potency in each of the aforementioned factors can be counterbalanced by giving higher doses and/or adjusting the dosing schedule. Ultimately, the decisive question is whether the dosage needed to achieve clinically relevant androgen deprivation is tolerable and/or whether the necessary dosing interval is convenient and practicable.

In general, steroidal antiandrogens have a higher binding affinity to the AR than to nonsteroidal antiandrogens. An exception to this is zanoterone, which binds with lower affinity than flutamide and bicalutamide. Relative binding affinity (RBA) for the canine prostate AR measured 18 h post incubation (binding of the potent synthetic androgen R 1881/methyltrienolone = 100) was found to be 2.87 for CPA, 0.48 for bicalutamide, 0.36 for hydroxyflutamide (active metabolite of flutamide), and 0.07 for zanoterone *(8)*. For the rat prostate AR, RBA was reported after an 18-h incubation to be 1.7 for CPA, 0.43 for bicalutamide, 0.13 for hydroxyflutamide, and 0.05 for zanoterone *(9)*. The RBA of megestrol acetate is more or less comparable to that of CPA [10]. A comparison between CMA and osaterone acetate (OSA) revealed a 2–3 times higher binding affinity for OSA *(11)*. Experiments on RBAs after short-term and long-term incubation indicate that dissociation from the receptor occurs early in zanoterone and hydroxyflutamide, whereas for CPA and bicalutamide binding to the receptor is longer *(9)*.

Experience, however, shows that the results from in vitro-binding studies do not necessarily correctly predict the antiandrogenic efficacy *(12)* in in vivo-models. Furthermore, in an in vivo situation, relative antiandrogenic potency may differ depending on whether the experiment is performed in intact or in castrated animals.

Antiandrogens interrupt the negative feedback loop that controls androgen production. This interruption causes a counterregulatory increase in androgen concentration, which can diminish the efficacy of the antiandrogen. Due to their progestational property, the available steroidal antiandrogens exert antigonadotropic activity. Therefore, in intact males they induce a pharmacodynamic response different from that of pure antiandrogens. The antigonadotropic activity prevents counterregulation, and even decreases peripheral testosterone concentrations. This difference between pure antiandrogens and antiandrogens with antigonadotropic effect is of relevance for therapeutic use.

In males the antiandrogenic activity partially neutralizes the antigonadotropic effect at the hypothalamic-pituitary level; this does not occur in the female. The antigonadotropic potency of CPA and CMA has been studied in rats of both sexes. In male animals, the depression of testicular weight served as test model, whereas inhibition of ovulation was used in female rats *(13)*. As could be expected, the antigonadotropic effect was more pronounced in females than in males. In this female rat model, the central inhibitory activity of CPA was slightly less pronounced than that of CMA. This indicates that the inherent ratio of antiandrogenic to progestogenic property shows a more pronounced dominance of the antiandrogenic activity of CPA than for CMA. A comparative characterization of CMA and OSA indicated that OSA is more potent as an antiandrogen, whereas it is weaker with regard to the antigonadotropic potency *(4)*. The relative antiandrogenic potency assessed by the inhibition of prostatic regrowth in castrated, testosterone-substituted rats was examined for CPA, CMA, OSA, and flutamide

(11). CPA and OSA were significantly more potent than CMA, exerting seven-fold (CPA) and eight-fold (OSA) higher activity; flutamide was the most potent substance (10-fold). A slightly different experimental setting using the prevention of prostatic involution after castration by testosterone showed flutamide to be most potent, followed by CPA and megestrol acetate *(14)*. However, if this experiment is performed in intact rats the order of antiandrogenic potency is CPA > Megestrol acetate > flutamide. This proves the importance of the antigonadotropic effect in preventing the counterregulatory increase of endogenous androgens.

The available information suggests the ranking of the steroidal antiandrogens to be as follows with respect to antiandrogenic potency: OSA ≥ CPA > megestrol acetate > zanoterone > CMA; and with respect to antigonadotropic potency: CMA ≥ CPA > megestrol acetate > OSA > zanoterone (no effect).

It is well-established that under special conditions antiandrogens might act as agonists. Experiments with the androgen-dependent, prostate-cancer cell line, LNCaP, first revealed this phenomenon *(15)*. This unwanted event is the consequence of a mutation in the AR. In prostate-cancer therapy, clinical responses were seen in a subgroup of patients with progression of disease during antiandrogenic therapy, after cessation of antiandrogens or estrogens. It seems that mutated receptors can be activated by classical ligands for hormone receptors, including antiandrogens (steroidal as well as nonsteroidal), estrogens, progestogens, and also by growth factors (e.g., insulin-like growth factor 1 [IGF = 1], keratinocyte growth factor, epidermal growth factor [EGF] *(16)*. This implies that AR contributes not only to the growth of androgen-dependent prostate cancer but also to the growth of androgen-independent prostate cancer. This suggests that new therapeutic modalities that not only block, but also eliminate AR may provide a promising approach towards more effective therapy *(17)*.

1.3. Preclinical Safety

Toxicological studies showed that progestational steroids are relatively nontoxic. The lethal dose in acute toxicity studies is in excess of 1 g/kg. Thus, the ingestion of high multiples of the therapeutic dose in men is likely to present no acute toxic risk. Established tests for mutagenicity and carcinogenicity do not indicate such side effects for steroidal antiandrogens. There is, obviously, a teratogenic potential due to the possibility of feminization of male fetuses. This possible side effect is of relevance for substances that are used in indications that include females of childbearing age within the patient population. This is the case for CPA, which is approved for treatment of hirsutism and acne in women.

When given over long time periods to rodents, steroidal compounds can induce liver tumors. This was considered as being a species-specific effect with no relevance for risk assessment in humans. This opinion was challenged when newly developed, sophisticated techniques demonstrated that CPA caused the formation of DNA adducts in hepatocytes of rats *(18)*. It was speculated that a direct relationship between DNA-adduct formation and the development of benign and malignant liver tumors might exist. A further finding that DNA adducts could also be demonstrated in hepatocytes of humans treated with CPA aroused the suspicion that the substance could be carcinogenic in the human liver. This uncertainty prompted a large number of preclinical and clinical investigations focusing on the question of liver carcinogenicity. DNA-adduct formation is not specific for CPA, but occurs with estradiol and other steroidal antiandrogens (CMA, megestrol acetate) *(19)*, or nonsteroidal compounds such as, e.g., the antiestrogen tamoxifen *(20)*. An epidemiological surveillance was, therefore, initiated in the patient population with the highest theoretical likelihood of developing liver tumors, since they had received high doses of CPA for long periods of time (up to 10 yr or more). The results of this program led to the conclusion that CPA does not increase the risk for the development of liver tumors in men *(21)*.

1.4. Pharmacokinetics

All currently available steroidal antiandrogens are active when given orally. Peak plasma levels were achieved for CPA within 3–4 h after administration. The terminal half-life in plasma is about 38 h. Excretion of CPA and its metabolites is about 70% in feces, mainly in the form of glucuronidated metabolites and about 30% in urine, preferentially in nonconjugated metabolites *(22)*.

For megestrol acetate, the peak concentration in plasma after oral administration occurs within 2–3 h. Plasma half-life is 15–20 h. It is mainly excreted in urine (about 60–80%) and to a minor extent in feces (about 10–30%). The primary route of excretion is renal, accounting for 60–80%, the remaining 10–30% is in the bile. In urine, both conjugated and nonconjugated metabolites occur, whereas in feces, glucuronide-conjugated metabolites are prevalent *(23)*.

The peak concentration in plasma of chlormadinone acetate was reported to occur within 2 h after oral intake *(24)*; the terminal half-life is rather long (about 80 h) *(25)*. Excretion is via the urine and feces in the form of glucuronidated metabolites.

After a single dose in male volunteers, zanoterone demonstrated peak plasma concentrations 2.6–4.4 h after dosing. The plasma half-life was approx 3 d, thus enabling a once-daily administration *(26)*.

2. CLINICAL APPLICATIONS OF CPA

Among the steroidal antiandrogens, CPA is the best established compound in clinical use. The discussion of the clinical effectiveness of steroidal antiandrogens will, therefore, be limited to CPA in prostate cancer. A considerable volume of early Phase II information, but only a modest amount of data resulting from Phase III studies, is available. After the identification of significant side effects of diethylstilbestrol (DES), this treatment has become uncommon. CPA remains the most appropriate compound for primary treatment of prostate cancer that can be applied per os. Next to the oral application, which is preferred by a considerable number of patients, CPA has the advantage of a very rapid onset of action. Potentially, CPA has the capability of counteracting both testicular and adrenal androgens. Walsh et al. *(27)* have shown that the effect of adrenal androgens on the rat ventral prostate is counteracted effectively by CPA. As for any other antiandrogen, the proper dosage is difficult to determine. The only direct and proper parameter is the target-cell response, which is obviously difficult to study in humans. Several approaches have been used, which have resulted in an approximation to the human dosage of 4 mg/kg/d. For a man weighing 75 kg, therefore, the appropriate dosage would be 300 mg/d. The issue of determining the proper dosage of CPA has been reviewed by Schröder *(28)*. The recommended dosages in monotherapy are 200–300 mg, if used in total androgen-blockade regimens 100–200 mg/d are recommended. CPA is available in most countries of the world and is considered standard management of prostate cancer in all clinical settings in which endocrine treatment is applied.

2.1. CPA as Monotherapy

CPA became available for clinical trials in the early 1960s and registration in countries around the world started in the year of 1972 for treatment of sexual deviations. Early clinical trials in prostate cancer were carried out in Europe and in the United States, and showed that CPA was effective with respect to the primary tumor as a target, relief of symptoms of metastatic disease, and in lowering the tumor-marker substances, acid and alkaline phosphatases *(29–32)*. This happened at the time when diethylstilbestrol, often given orally in very high dosages, was standard treatment; castration or the combination of castration with diethylstilbestrol were alternatives. With the description of the severe side effects of the standard dosage of 5 mg DES applied in the first large randomized studies of the Veterans Administration Cooperative Research Group (VACURG) *(33),* the issue of side effects and the establishment of similar or equal effectiveness of therapeutic options gained paramount importance.

2.1.1. RANDOMIZED STUDIES

For the reasons mentioned earlier, it is not surprising that, besides effectiveness, the pattern of side effects was of great interest within the protocols designed for the conduct of randomized studies in the 1970s and 1980s. The first randomized study was conducted by an international cooperative group headed by Jacobi from the Department of Urology at the University of Mainz *(34)*. This study randomized previously untreated locally advanced nonmetastatic and metastatic prostate-cancer patients to treatment with either CPA 300 mg intramuscularly per week vs estradiol undecylate 100 mg intramuscularly per month. The duration of the trial was fixed to 6 mo, and the endpoints were endocrine parameters, local and distant response, marker response, as well as progression. Side effects were evaluated. Two comprehensive reports on this study are available. One reporting on 42 patients contributed by the institution of the study coordinator and a second one on 191 patients, the contribution of the international study group as a whole *(34,35)*. The criteria of response were improvement, no change, or deterioration. Percentages allotted to these parameters amounted to 48, 44, and 8% for CPA and to 52, 41, and 7% for estradiol undecylate, respectively. Overall, side effects were seen in 94% in the estradiol group and in 37% in the CPA group. The differences between the two treatments mainly amounted to gynecomastia, breast tenderness, and leg edema. Two patients in each treatment group died of cardiovascular disease. Considering the limited duration of time, time to progression, cancer-related survival, and overall survival were not used as endpoints. The end conclusion of the study was that with relation to the response parameters used (local tumor progression, improvement of urine flow, histological regression, improvement of bone scans, relief of ureteral obstruction, and marker-substance decrease) both treatments were equally effective. While the study group considered CPA an "acceptable alternative" for standard estrogen treatment, the side-effect profile of CPA was considerably more favorable.

In 1976, the EORTC Genitourinary Group initiated a study comparing oral CPA at a dosage of 250 mg/d to medroxyprogesterone acetate (MPA) at a loading dose of 500 mg intramuscularly 3 times weekly for 8 wk followed by 100 mg orally twice daily vs 3 mg of diethylstilbestrol given in 3 doses of 1 mg per os daily (Protocol 30761). Of 236 patients entered, 210 were eligible, 75 received CPA, 71 MPA, and 64 DES. Response, time to progression, survival, and toxicity were assessed. The final result was published in 1986 by Pavone-Macaluso et al. *(36)*. As far as time to progression is concerned, overall diethylstilbestrol and CPA did not differ but were significantly better than MPA. This difference was not reproduced in the M0 patients. Survival data did not show differences between DES and CPA while survival on MPA was significantly shorter (Fig. 2). In this study, performance status and the presence or absence of metastases were the most important prognostic factors. The paper includes a careful comparison of patient characteristics at entry, which did not

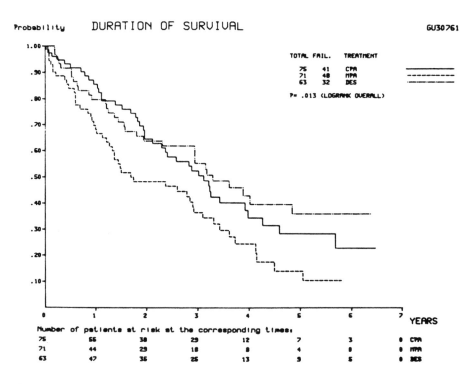

Fig. 2. Kaplan-Meier projections of overall survival per treatment arm, CPA, MPA, and DES. CPA vs DES: n.s., DES/CPA vs MPA: $p \leq 0.036$. Adapted with permission from ref. *(36)*.

show major differences between the treatment groups. An important lesson from this study was that complete response of metastatic disease is rare; it was only seen in 3–5% of cases. The side effects are subject to a separate report and will be discussed in Subheading 2.6. *(37)*.

In 1989, the EORTC Genitourinary Group initiated a direct comparison of flutamide 750 mg/d with CPA 300 mg/d in previously untreated patients with metastatic prostate cancer and favorable prognostic factors. This selection criterion required that there was no pain due to metastatic disease, and that at least two of the three following factors were present:

1. WHO performance status is 0;
2. Normal alkaline phosphatase level; and
3. Classification smaller than T4.

This study, EORTC Protocol 30892, recruited 310 patients between September 1990 and April 1996. The final evaluation is still pending but an assessment of side effects at the time of closure of the protocol (April 1, 1996) has recently been published *(38)* and yields, important information with respect to the effect of both drugs on libido, potency, and sexual performance. These data will be reviewed in Subheading 2.6.

A preliminary report on a study comparing CPA to goserelin and diethyl-stilbestrol was published in 1990 *(39,40)*. In a subgroup of patients who had no contraindications for DES treatment, this study shows a longer median survival time for goserelin acetate and DES in comparison to CPA. Numbers are, however, small ($n = 33$ DES; $n = 35$ CPA; $n = 69$ goserelin) and a final report on this study is not available. In the larger study population (CPA $n = 71$; goserelin $n = 152$) comprising patients with contraindications for DES, and patients who have been included by urologists declining to use DES, median survival is not different between CPA and goserelin.

Another study conducted by the British Prostate Group compared three treatment arms, CPA (300 mg/d), goserelin (monthly depot), and the combination of both drugs until clinical progression *(41)*. The study showed a similar response rate for the three treatment arms, however, median time to progression was shorter for CPA monotherapy. This difference is most likely a manifestation of lower compliance. Oral treatment depends on patient's reliability for regular drug intake, whereas the regimens using luteinizing hormone-releasing hormone (LH-RH) agonist depots are under complete control of the treating physician.

2.2. CPA in Combination Treatment

As mentioned earlier, CPA has a double mechanism of action: in standard dosages it lowers plasma testosterone by 70–75%, whereas orchidectomy or estrogen therapy achieves an 85% decrease *(42)*. This leads to decreased levels of 5α-dihydrotestosterone in the prostate, which is counteracted by competitive binding of CPA to the androgen receptor *(43)*. De Jong et al. *(44)* showed that, in BPH tissue of men pretreated with CPA prior to transurethral prostatic surgery, molar CPA levels exceed DHT levels by about 30-fold if calculated per gram of wet weight and about twofold in the nuclei. The completeness of androgen blockade can only be judged by target-tissue response, which in almost all monotherapy studies cited earlier was comparable to other standard forms of treatment. Potentially, if the dosage used is high enough, CPA has the capability of blocking androgens of testicular and adrenal origin. Thus, its use should lead to what has been termed "total androgen blockade" by Labrie et al. *(45)*.

2.3.1. CPA AND TOTAL ANDROGEN BLOCKADE

Two smaller studies and three major studies have been conducted using CPA as an antiandrogen in combination with castration or an LH-RH analog. These studies have been subject to a recent meta-analysis of the Prostate Cancer Trialists' Collaborative Group *(46)*. These studies included a total of 1159 patients; the results of one study *(41)* were not available for inclusion. The meta-analysis, which included the remaining 810 patients, did not show any differences in 5-yr overall survival. This was in line with the overall result of the meta-analysis, which included 5710 patients of whom 3283 had died, which produced a 3.5% advantage for total androgen blockade, which was statistically not significant.

Protocol 30805 of the EORTC compared in a randomized prospective study castration to castration plus CPA and to 1 mg DES/d in patients with metastatic disease. No differences in time to progression and overall survival were seen in the final analysis of the trial *(47)*. This is of particular interest since it is well-known that 1 mg DES does not suppress plasma testosterone to castration levels. Protocol 30843 of the EORTC was again a three-arm study comparing short-term vs long-term addition of CPA to the LH-RH agonist buserelin in comparison with orchidectomy in metastatic prostate cancer. Again, no difference in time to progression and survival was seen *(48)*. The third large study utilizing CPA was the aforementioned trial conducted by the British Prostate Group *(41)*. The combination of CPA plus LHRH agonist did not result in a prolonged median time to progression as compared to LH-RH agonist alone. It can be concluded that CPA did not prolong time to progression or improve overall survival in any of the prospective randomized studies comparing total androgen blockade to standard forms of treatment. The data are in line with the results of a meta-analysis of all available studies. CPA, like all other available antiandrogens, therefore, cannot be recommended for continuous long-term use in total androgen blockade regimens.

2.3.2. FLARE PREVENTION

The phenomenon of disease "flare" was first described by Waxman et al. *(49)* as an exacerbation of symptoms and markers accompanying the initial rise of plasma testosterone with the use of LH-RH agonists as monotherapy in the treatment of metastatic prostate cancer. Schröder et al. *(50)* in a study of the LH-RH agonist buserelin, suspected that early progression, due to flare, was associated with death in 3 of 58 prostate-cancer patients. In a recent literature review, it is estimated that at least 15 patients died of flare due to the initial rise of plasma testosterone with the use of an LH-RH agonist as monotherapy *(51)*. Klijn et al. showed in 1985 that 3 times 50 mg of CPA given during the initial period of treatment with the LHRH agonist buserelin does not prevent the initial surge of plasma testosterone, but does lead to an immediate lowering of the activity of acid and alkaline phosphatase in plasma *(52)*. These markers are thought to correlate with tumor mass. None of the patients treated in this way experienced symptoms of disease exacerbation. The effect of different antiandrogens in preventing the flare phenomenon was later investigated by Boccon-Gibod et al. *(53)*, Waxman et al. *(54)*, and Kuhn et al. *(55)*. It was shown that CPA given at least 1 wk prior to the initiation of LH-RH agonist, application leads to a blunting of the rise of plasma testosterone and to the prevention of clinical and biochemical flare. A decrease of plasma testosterone is not achieved by nonsteroidal antiandrogens, but they will, however, prevent clinical and biochemical flare if used prior to the application of LH-RH agonists. The information given by Klijn et al. *(52)* is one of the best pieces of evidence showing that 150 mg of CPA/d initiated together with the LH-RH agonist effectively counteracts androgens at the target cell, even if concentrations are supraphysiological.

2.3.3. PREVENTION OF HOT FLUSHES

Hot flushes are characterized by a sudden sensation of heat often originating in the chest, and then spreading to other parts of the body leading to sweating, mostly in the area of the forehead, chest, and back. Hot flushes occur in women during menopause and are very common after castration or with the use of an LH-RH agonist. Hot flushes are probably due to the lack of the normal stimulatory effect of circulating androgens on hypothalamic opioids, which is missing with these forms of endocrine treatment, and which leads to a sudden release of norepinephrine, which interferes with thermoregulatory mechanisms in the hypothalamus *(57)*. Hot flushes rarely occur under CPA, and can be prevented by low dosages of CPA in men having undergone castration or being treated with LH-RH agonists. This was shown in a crossover study by Eaton and McGuire *(58)* of 12 patients with troublesome hot flushes, who were alternatively treated with CPA 300 mg/d and placebo. There was a significant reduction in the mean daily number of hot flushes during 21-d treatment from an average of 9.4 under placebo to 2.3 under CPA. This observation has been confirmed in other trials and in routine clinical practice.

2.3.4. CPA COMBINED WITH DIETHYLSTILBESTROL

CPA, as mentioned earlier, leads to an incomplete suppression of plasma testosterone levels, which decrease by about 70% and remain at about three times castration values. In a very systematic approach to the problem, Rennie et al. *(59)* investigated and compared 12 different procedures of androgen deprivation. These authors found that the combination of CPA with an extremely low dose (0.1 mg/d) of DES led to a very effective withdrawal of androgens in terms of plasma testosterone and tissue dihydrotestosterone. The same group later showed that 200 mg of CPA, and even 100 mg/day, was sufficient to achieve a similar endocrine response, which was correlated to very favorable clinical responses in a Phase II situation *(60,61)*. The approach has many potential advantages, and, from an endocrinological point of view, is very logical: this regimen combines the testosterone-reducing effects of two compounds, therefore, only small amounts of estrogen are required to bring down plasma testosterone to approximately castrate levels. Once castrate levels have been achieved, only low doses of CPA are necessary to counteract remaining androgens, mainly of adrenal origin. The regimen was shown to be associated with few side effects and a very low cost. The combination of low-dose CPA with low-dose DES was never studied in a Phase III situation in comparison to standard management. Considering the endocrine results and the observations in patients treated with this regimen *(60)*, this combination treatment is very likely to be competitive with other standard forms of therapy.

2.4. Intermittent Endocrine Treatment

The endocrine effects of CPA are reversible. With the discontinuation of CPA treatment, testosterone levels return to normal usually within 8 wk and within 14 wk at most *(61)*. This reversibility makes CPA a suitable agent in neoadjuvant- and adjuvant-treatment regimens as well as within the concept of intermittent endocrine therapy, which was introduced primarily through experiments relating to the Shionogi androgen-dependent breast-cancer line *(62)*, and which was clinically tested in an initial Phase II study reported by Goldenberg et al. *(63)*. Akakura and his colleagues *(62)* transplanted Shionogi tumor material into male mice, and applied castration when the tumor had grown to a mass of about 3 g. After regression to about 30% of the original weight, the tumor tissue of the intermittent androgen-suppression group was retransplanted into intact mice and the process of castration and regression was repeated. The control group consisted of a group of mice transplanted with the tumor in whom castration was applied as a continuous form of endocrine treatment. In these experiments, and also in similar experiments conducted by Gleave et al. *(64)*, using LNCaP sublines, the progression to endocrine independence was markedly delayed with intermittent treatment. The authors, however, did not control for the possibility that the retransplantation of the tumor tissue in itself and in endocrinologically intact animals might have an impact on the time to progression to endocrine independence. However, even with these doubts about the capability of intermittent treatment to delay progression to endocrine-independence, the concept remains attractive. Phase III trials are underway in Europe and in the United States, which compare intermittent treatment to continuous treatment. Obvious advantages in quality of life are expected to result from the intermittent treatment schemes. Whether intermittent treatment will be associated with a prolongation or shortening of time to progression, time to cancer death, and overall survival, is an open question at this time. One of the pitfalls of the regimen is that it can only be applied to those patients who show an initial rather complete response of serum prostate-specific antigen (PSA). If one assumes that a disadvantage with respect to overall survival would result,

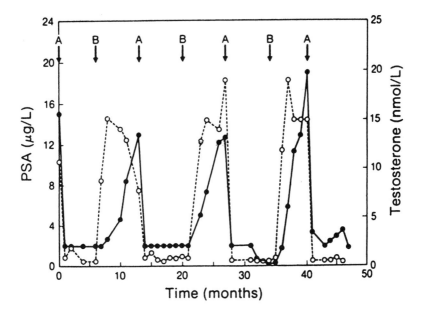

Fig. 3. Example of intermittent endocrine treatment in a single patient. 0, plasma testos-terone: ..., serum PSA. Treatment intervals 6, 7, 7, 7 mo, no treatment intervals 7, 7, 6 mo. Adapted with permission from ref. *(62)*.

the treatment may still be valuable. During a recent symposium of the European School of Urology, 160 participants were asked the questions:

1. Would you trade survival time for intact libido and potency?
2. If you are ready to trade survival time for libido and potency, how much time of your life would you be ready to give up: 3 mo, 6 mo, 9 mo, or 12 mo and more?

About half of the participants answered positively, and those who were ready to trade survival time against intact libido and potency, all were ready to give a year or more.

Although intermittent endocrine treatment at this time is experimental, the completion of Phase III studies is to be expected. The idea, however, is gaining acceptance and its use with appropriate procedures of complete information to the patient cannot be prevented.

An example of the effect of intermittent treatment on peripheral testosterone and PSA levels is given in Fig. 3.

2.5. Second-Line Endocrine Treatment

There is strong evidence in the literature that hormone-independent prostate cancer can be stimulated by androgens. The available evidence has resulted from experiments attempting synchronization of hormone-independent cell populations by intermittent stimulation with androgens *(65)*, and attempts to stimulate the uptake of radioactive strontium in patients with hormone-unresponsive prostate cancer by androgens *(66)*. Older literature, describing the effect of adrenalectomy, hypophysectomy, aminoglutethimide, and of other means of suppressing remaining androgenic activity in patients progressing under first-line endocrine therapy, has been summarized by Schröder *(67)*. Bilateral adrenalectomy in 116 cases found by review of the literature showed objective and subjective responses in 34 and 74% of cases with a duration of 2.5 and 4.0 mo on average. Aminoglutethimide studied in 84 patients gave objective and subjective responses in 25 and 57%, with durations of 3–25 mo and 2 wk to 2 yr, respectively.

With the increasing acceptance worldwide of the low value of total androgen blockade as a first-line treatment, the option of using antiandrogens in second-line endocrine treatment gains renewed importance. Smith and coworkers *(31)* treated 35 patients with prior relapse or nonresponse to estrogen treatment with 300 mg CPA/d orally. Bone pain was reduced in 12 of 19, and performance was improved in 5 of 13 patients. The size of the prostate seemed to be further reduced in 12 of 28 of these cases. The responses apparently were of short duration. The issue of second-line endocrine treatment by means of antiandrogens, and especially of CPA, is grossly understudied. Appropriate Phase III studies should be designed. Potential agents for comparison might be prednisone, aminoglutethimide, with or without prednisone, or chemotherapeutic agents, respectively, signal transduction inhibitors, matrix metalloproteinase inhibitors (MMPs), or inhibitors of angiogenesis, which may turn out to be effective in this disease.

2.6. Side Effects of CPA

The endocrine-related effects of CPA and its side effects have been extensively evaluated in Phase II and Phase III trials.

2.6.1. ENDOCRINE-RELATED EFFECT

In the past it was thought that virtually all patients using CPA at standard dosages lose libido and become impotent. In a recent Phase III evaluation of potency and sexual performance, which compares the effects of CPA to the pure antiandrogen flutamide *(38)*, it was shown that about 20% of those patients who were sexually active at entry remained so under treatment. There was no difference between the two treatment groups. This finding is compatible with an evaluation of the effect of surgical castration, in which a persistence of libido and potency was also reported in 21% of cases *(68)*. Some patients under treatment with CPA feel rather tired and lethargic. This side

Table 2
CV side effects (30761)

EORTC 30761 – CARDIOVASCULAR TOXICITY (CPA, N = 82, MPA, N = 73, DES, N = 114)			
	CPA %	MPA %	DES %
No toxicity	90.5	81.7	65.8
Edema	2.4	6.1	11.0
ECG changes	1.2	6.1	8.2
Myocard infarct	3.6	0	1.4
Thrombo-embolism	2.4	6.1	8.2
p-values: DES vs MPA = 0.025 DES vs CPA = 0.001			

After de Voogt et al [37]

Table 3
EORTC 30892: Side effects (March 1996)

	Flutamide (n=130)		CPA (n=134)		
	n	%	n	%	p-value
Painful gynaecomastia	59	45.4	10	7.5	0.001
Diarrhea	30	23.1	13	9.7	0.000
Nausea	25	19.2	8	6.0	0.002
Liver function deterioration	13	10.0	6	4.5	0.045
Thrombosis, embolus	0		6	4.5	0.011

CPA, cyproterone acetate

Other side effects not differing between treatment arms: myocardial infarction, cerebrovascular accident, gynaecomastia not painful, hot flushes, dizziness, others

effect is reversible with discontinuation of treatment. Gynecomastia and painful gynecomastia under CPA are infrequent. Gynecomastia or painful gynecomastia were described in 13% *(35)*, 7.5% *(38)*, and 6% *(37)*.

2.6.1.1. Other Side Effects. In the EORTC studies evidence is presented, showing that CPA at standard dosage has significantly fewer cardiovascular side effects than 3 mg of DES *(37)*. A summary of these findings is given in Table 2. In absence of an untreated control group, it will remain unknown what the incidence of cardiovascular events would have been without any form of endocrine treatment. It is possible that the data collected in the CPA arm of the

EORTC studies are compatible with the natural prevalence of cardiovascular and thromboembolic events in this population.

Table 3 gives a summary of the side effects encountered in EORTC protocol 30892 *(38)* in comparison with the side effects of flutamide. It must, however, be taken into consideration that in this study patients with recent active cardiovascular disease were not eligible for recruitment.

Severe damage and acute hepatitis-like syndromes with CPA are rare and mostly reversible. The issue of the clinical significance of DNA adduct formation has already been reviewed in Subheading 1.3.

2.7. Conclusions

CPA used in monotherapy is a valid alternative to other forms of endocrine treatment of prostate cancer. It has been shown to be equally effective to regimens of estrogen treatment in randomized prospective comparisons in nonmetastatic and metastatic patients.

In combination regimens aiming at total androgen blockade superiority of combinations with castration and LH-RH agonists above standard treatment could not be shown.

With the discontinuation of the use of oral estrogen treatment for prostate cancer, CPA remains the most appropriate substance for oral administration, a form of application preferred by many patients. CPA has been conclusively shown to suppress the clinical and biochemical flare phenomenon that arises during the initial phase of treatment with an LH-RH agonist. Also, hot flushes occurring after castration or during treatment with LH-RH agonists are alleviated by CPA. CPA is suitable for second-line endocrine treatment, but its effectiveness in this situation has not been sufficiently studied.

The endocrine effects of CPA are reversible. This makes the drug suitable for adjuvant- and neoadjuvant-treatment regimens as well as for intermittent endocrine treatment.

The side effects of CPA mainly relate to its endocrine effects; the possibility of modest cardiovascular and thromboembolic side effects mainly in men with prior cardiovascular problems; and to incidental, mostly reversible liver-function deterioration.

REFERENCES

1. Hamada H, Neumann F, Junkman K. Intrauterine antimaskuline Beeinflussung von Rattenfeten durch ein stark gestagen wirksames Steroid. *Acta Endocrinologica* (Copenhagen) 1963; 44:380–388.
2. Junkmann K, Neumann F. Zum Wirkungsmechanismus von an Feten antimaskulin wirksamen Gestagenen. *Acta Endocrinologica* (Copenhagen) 1964; 90:139–154.
3. Neumann F. Pharmacology and clinical uses of cyproterone acetate, in *Pharmacology and Clinical Uses of Inhibitors of Hormone Secretion and Action* (Furr BJA, Wakeling AE, eds). Baillière Tindall, 1987, pp 132–159.

4. Prous J, Mealy N, Castaner J. Osaterone acetate. Treatment of benign prostatic hyperplasia, androgen receptor antagonist. *Drugs of the Future* 1993; 18:516–519.

5. Snyder BW, Winneker RC, Batzold FH. Endocrine profile of WIN 49596 in the rat: a novel androgen receptor antagonist. *J Steroid Biochem* 1989; 33:1127–1132.

6. Berger BM, Naadimuthu A, Boddy A, et al. The effect of Zanoterone, a steroidal androgen receptor antagonist, in men with benign prostatic hyperplasia. *J Urology* 1995; 154:1060–1064.

7. Furr BJA. Relative potencies of flutamide and 'Casodex.' *Endocr-Rel Cancer* 1997; 4:197–202.

8. Juniewicz PE, McCarthy M, Lemp BM, et al. The effect of the steroidal androgen receptor antagonist Win 49,596, on the prostate and testis of beagle dogs. *Endocrinology* 1990; 126:2625–2634.

9. Winneker RC, Wagner MM, Batzold FH. Studies on the mechanism of action of WIN 49596: a steroidal androgen receptor antagonist. *J Steroid Biochem* 1989; 33:1133–1138.

10. Gaillard-Moguilewsky M. Pharmacology of antiandrogens and value of combining androgen suppression with antiandrogen therapy. *Urology* 1991; 37(Suppl):5–12.

11. Kondo Y, Homma Y, Aso Y, et al. Relative potency of antiandrogens with reference to intracellular testosterone in the rat prostate. *Prostate* 1996; 29:146–152.

12. Wakeling AE, Furr BJA, Glen AT, et al. Receptor binding and biological activity of steroidal and nonsteroidal antiandrogens. *J Steroid Biochem* 1981; 15:355–359.

13. Neumann F, Gräf K-J, Hasan SH, et al. Central actions of antiandrogens, in *Androgens and Antiandrogens* (Martini L, Motta M, eds). Raven Press, 1977, New York pp 163–177.

14. El Etreby MF, Habenicht U-F, Louton T, et al. Effect of cyproterone acetate in comparison to flutamide and megestrol acetate on the ventral prostate, seminal vesicle and adrenal glands of adult male rats. *Prostate* 1987; 11:361–375.

15. Wilding G, Chen M, Gelmann EP. Aberrant response in vitro of hormone-responsive prostate cancer cells to antiandrogens. *Prostate* 1989; 14:103–115.

16. Culig Z, Hobisch A, Cronauer MV, et al. Androgen receptor activation in prostatic tumor cell lines by insulin-like growth factor-I, keratinocyte growth factor, and epidermal growth factor. *Cancer Res* 1994; 54:5474–5478.

17. Parczyk K, Schneider MR. The future of antihormone therapy: innovations based on an established principle. *J Cancer Res Clin Oncol* 1996; 12:2383–396.

18. Topinka J, Andrae U, Schwarz LR, et al. Cyproterone acetate generates DNA-adducts in rat liver and in primary rat hepatocyte cultures. *Carcinogenesis* 1993; 14:423–427.

19. Feser W, Kerdar RS, Blode H, et al. Formation of DNA-adducts by selected sex steroids in rat liver. *Human Exp Toxico* 1996; 15:556–562.

20. Han X, Liehr JG. Induction of covalent DNA adducts in rodents by tamoxifen. *Cancer Res* 1992; 52:1360–1363.

21. Heinemann LAJ, Will-Shahab L, van Kesteren P, et al. Safety of cyproterone acetate: report of active surveillance. *Pharmacoepidemiol Drug Safety* 1997; 6:169–178.

22. Neumann F. Pharmacology of cyproterone acetate: a short review, in *Antiandrogens in Prostate Cancer* (ESO Monographs), (Denis L, ed). Springer-Verlag, Berlin, 1996; pp 31–44.

23. Canetta R, Florentine S, Hunter H, et al. Megestrol acetate. *Cancer Treatment Rev* 1983; 10:141–157.

24. Nash JF, Bopp RJ, Shreve RW, et al. A study of chlormadinone acetate concentrations in human plasma following the oral administration of tablets. *Curr Ther Res* 1971; 13:407–411.

25. Dugwekar YG, Narula RK, Laumas KR. Disappearance of $1\alpha^3$H chlormadinone acetate from the plasma of women. *Contraception* 1973; 7:27–45.

26. Berger R, Roemeling R, Weiss R, et al. Single dose safety, tolerance and pharmacokinetics of WIN 49596, a novel steroidal androgen receptor antagonist, in young and elderly volunteers. *J Clin Pharmacol* 1991; 41:867.

27. Harper ME, Pike, A, Peeling, WB, Griffiths, K. Steroids of adrenal origin metabolized by human prostatic tissue both in vivo and in vitro. *J Endocr* 1974; 60:117–125.

28. Schröder, FH. Cyproterone acetate: Mechanism of action and clinical effectiveness in prostate cancer treatment. *Cancer* 1993; (Suppl) 72(12):3810–3815.

29. Scott WW, Schirmer, HKA. A new progestational steroid effective in the treatment of prostatic cancer. *Transact Am Assoc Genito-Urinary Surg* 1966; 58:54–60.

30. Geller J, Vazakas, G, Fruchtman, B. The effect of cyproterone acetate on advanced carcinoma of the prostate. *Surg Gynecol Obstet* 1968; 127:748–758.

31. Smith RB, Walsh, PC, Goodwin, WE. Cyproterone acetate in the treatment of advanced carcinoma of the prostate. *J Urol* 1973; 110:106–108.

32. Wein AJ, Murphy, JJ. Experience in the treatment of prostatic carcinoma with cyproterone acetate. *J Urol* 1980; 109:68–70.

33. Mellinger GT, as member of the Veterans Administration Co-operative Urological Research Group. Treatment and survival of patients with cancer of the prostate. *SGO* 1967; 124:1011–1017.

34. Jacobi GH, Altwein, JE, Kurth, KH, Basting, R, Hohenfellner, R. Treatment of advanced prostatic cancer with parenteral cyproterone acetate: a phase III randomised trial. *Br J Urol* 1980; 52:208–215.

35. Jacobi GH. Intramuscular cyproterone acetate treatment for advanced prostatic carcinoma: results of the first multicentric randomized trial. Proceedings Androgens and Antiandrogens, International Symposium, Utrecht, 1982; pp 161–169.

36. Pavone-Macaluso M, de Voogt HJ, Viggiano G, Barasolo E, Lardennois B, de Pauw M Sylvester, R. Comparison of diethylstilbestrol, cyproterone acetate and medroxyprogesterone acetate in the treatment of advanced prostatic cancer: final analysis of a randomized phase III trial of the European Organization for Research on Treatment of Cancer Urological Group. *J. Urol.* 1986; 136:624–631.

37. de Voogt, HJ, Smith, Ph H, Pavone-Macaluso, M, de Pauw M, Suciu, S, Members of the EORTC GU Group. Cardiovascular side effects of Diethylstilbestrol, Cyproterone acetate, Medroxyprogesterone acetate and Estramustine phosphate used for the treatment of advanced prostatic cancer: results from European Organization for Research on Treatment of Cancer trials 30761 and 30762. *J Urol* 1986; 135:303–307.

38. Schröder FH, Whelan, P, Kurth, KH, Sylvester, R, Pauw, M de, and members of the EORTC Genitourinary Group. Antiandrogens as monotherapy for metastatic prostate cancer: a preliminary report on EORTC protocol 30892, in *Recent Advances in Prostate Cancer and BPH, Proceedings of the IV Congress on Progress and Controversies in Oncological Urology* (PACIOU IV, Rotterdam, The Netherlands, April 11–13, 1996) (Schröder FH, ed). Parthenon Publishing, New York, 1997, pp 141–146.

39. Moffat LEF. Comparison of Zoladex, diethylstilbestrol and cyproterone acetate treatment in advanced prostate cancer. *Eur Urol* 1990; 18(Suppl)3:26–27.

40. Osborne DR, Moffat, LEF, Kaisary A, et al. A comparison of Zoladex, cyproterone acetate and stilboestrol in the treatment of patients with advanced prostatic carcinoma, in *Recent Advances in Urological Cancers: Diagnosis and Treatment* Murphy G, Khoury S, Chatelain C, Denis L, eds. Paris, Alan R. Liss, New York, NY, 1990, June 27–29. pp 53–55.

41. Thorpe SC, Azmatullah S, Fellows GJ, et al. A prospective, randomised study to compare goserelin acetate (Zoladex®) versus cyproterone acetate (Cyprostat®) versus a combination of the two in the treatment of metastatic prostatic carcinoma. *Eur Urol* 1996; 29:47–54.

42. Varenhorst E, Wallentin L, Carlström K. The effects of orchiectomy, estrogens, and cyproterone acetate on plasma testosterone, LH and FSH concentrations in patients with carcinoma of the prostate. *Scand J Urol Nephrol* 1982; 16:31–36.

43. Brinkmann AO, Lindh LM, Breedveld Dl, Mulder E, Molen HJ van der. Cyproterone acetate prevents translocation of the androgen receptor in the rat prostate. *Mol Cell Endocrinol* 1983; 32:117–129.

44. de Jong FH, Reuvers PJ, Bolt-de Vries J, Mulder E, Blom JHM, Schröder, FH. Androgens and androgen-receptors in prostate tissue from patients with benign prostatic hyperplasia: effects of cyproterone acetate. *J Steroid Biochem Mol Biol* 1992; 42(1):49–55.

45. Labrie F, Dupont A, Belanger A, Lacoursiere Y, Raynaud JP, Husson JM, et al. New approaches in the treatment of prostate cancer: complete instead of partial withdrawal of androgens. *Prostate* 1983; 4:579–594.

46. Prostate Cancer Trialists' Collaborative Group. Maximum androgen blockade in advanced prostate cancer: an overview of 22 randomised trials with 3283 deaths in 5710 patients. *Lancet* 1995; 346 (8970):265–269.

47. Robinson MRG, Smith PH, Richards B, Newling DWW, Pauw M de, Sylvester R. The final analysis of the EORTC Genito-Urinary Group Phase III clinical trial (Protocol 30805) comparing orchidectomy, orchidectomy plus cyproterone acetate and low dose stilboestrol in the management of metastatic carcinoma of the prostate. *Eur Urol* 1995; 28:273–283.

48. Klijn JGM, de Voogt HJ, Studer UE, Schröder FH, Sylvester R, de M Pauw. Short-term versus long-term addition of cyproterone acetate to buserelin therapy in comparison with orchidectomy in the treatment of metastatic prostate cancer. *Cancer* 1993; 72:3858–3869.

49. Waxman J, Man A, Hendry WF, Whitfield HN, Besser GM. Short reports. Importance of early tumor exacerbation in patients treated with long acting analogues of gonadotrophin releasing hormone for advanced prostatic cancer. *BMJ* 1985; 291:1387–1388.

50. Schröder FH, Lock MTWT, Chadha DR, Debruyne FMJ, Karthaus HFM, de Jong FH, et al. Metastatic cancer of the prostate managed with Buserelin versus Buserelin plus Cyproterone acetate. *J Urol* 1987; 137:912–918.

51. Thompson IM, Zeidman EJ, Rodriguez FR. Sudden death due to disease flare with luteinizing hormone-releasing agonist therapy for carcinoma of the prostate. *J Urol* 1990; 144:1479–1480.

52. Klijn JGM, de Voogt HJ, Schröder FH, de Jong FH. Combined treatment with Buserelin and Cyproterone acetate in metastatic prostatic carcinoma. *Lancet II,* August 31, 1985; 493:(Letter to the Editor).

53. Boccon-Gibod L, Laudat MH, Dugue MA, Steg A. Cyproterone acetate lead-in prevents initial rise of serum testosterone induced by luteinizing hormone-releasing hormone analogs in the treatment of metastatic carcinoma of the prostate. *Eur Urol* 1986; 12:400–402.

54. Waxman J, Williams G, Sandow J, et al. The clinical and endocrine assessment of three different antiandrogen regimens combined with a very long-acting gonadotrophin-releasing hormone analogue. *Am J Clin Oncol* 1988; 11:(Suppl), S152–S155.

55. Kuhn JHM, Billebaud T, Navratil H, et al. Prevention of transient adverse effects of a gonadotropin releasing hormone analog (buserelin) in metastatic prostatic carcinoma by administration of an antiandrogen (Nilutamide). *N Engl J Med* 1989; 321:413–418.

56. Frodin T, Alund G, Varenhorst E. Measurement of skin blood-flow and water evaporation as a means of objectively assessing hot flushes after orchiectomy in patients with prostatic cancer. *Prostate* 1985; 7:203–208.

57. Radlmaier A, Bormacher K, Neumann F. Hot flushes: mechanism and prevention, in *EORTC Genitourinary Group Monograph 8: Treatment of Prostatic Cancer: Facts and Controversies Schröder T.H. ed.,* Wiley-Liss, New York, NY, 1990, pp 131–140.

58. Eaton AC, McGuire N. Cyproterone acetate in treatment of post-orchidectomy hot flushes. *Lancet* 1983; 2(8363):1336–1337.

59. Rennie PS, Bruchovsky N, Goldenberg SL, Lawson D, Fletcher T, Foekens JA. Relative effectiveness of alternative androgen withdrawal therapies in initiating regression of rat prostate. *J Urol* 1988; 139:1337–1342.
60. Goldenberg SL, Bruchovsky N, Rennie PS, Coppin CM. The combination of cyproterone acetate and low dose diethylstilbestrol in the treatment of advanced prostatic carcinoma. *J Urol* 1988; 140:1460–1465.
61. Goldenberg SL, Bruchovsky N. Use of cyproterone acetate in prostate cancer. *Urol Clin North Am* 1991; 18(1):111–122.
62. Akakura K, Bruchovsky N, Goldenberg SL, Rennie PS, Buckley AR, Sullivan LD. Effects of intermittent androgen suppression on androgen-dependent tumors. *Cancer* 1993; 71:2782–2790.
63. Goldenberg SL, Bruchovsky N, Gleave ME, Sullivan LD, Akakura K. Intermittent androgen suppression in the treatment of prostate cancer: a preliminary report. *Urology* 1995; 45(5):839–845.
64. Gleave M, Bruchovsky N, Goldenberg SL, Rennie P. Intermittent androgen suppression: rationale and clinical experience, in *Recent Advances in Prostate Cancer and BPH, Proceedings of the IV Congress on Progress and Controversies in Oncological Urology* (PACIOU IV, Rotterdam, The Netherlands, April 11–13, 1996) (Schröder FH, ed. Parthenon Publishing, New York, L. 1997, pp 109–120.
65. Manni A, Santen RJ, Boucher AE, Lipton A, Harvey H, Simmonds M, et al. Androgen depletion and repletion as a means of potentiating the effects of cytotoxic chemotherapy in advanced prostate cancer. *J Steroid Biochem* 1987; 27(1–3):551–556.
66. Fowler JE, Whitmore WF. The response of metastatic adenocarcinoma of the prostate to exogenous testosterone. *J Urol* 1981; 126:372–375.
67. Schröder FH. Total androgen suppression in the management of prostatic cancer. A critical review, in *Progress in Clinical and Biological Research, vol 185A. EORTC GU Group Monograph 2. Part A. Therapeutic Principles in Metastatic Prostatic Cancer.* (Schröder FH, Richards B, eds). Alan R. Liss, New York, 1985, pp 307–317.
68. Ellis WJ, Grayhack JT. Sexual function in aging males after orchiectomy and estrogen therapy. *J Urol* 1963; 89(6):895–899.

16 Nonsteroidal Antiandrogens

Geert J. C. M. Kolvenbag and Barrington J. A. Furr

CONTENTS

1. INTRODUCTION

Antiandrogens offer treatment options for patients with early and advanced prostate cancer, either as a single agent or as part of a combination with surgical or medical castration. They are most frequently used as a component of combined androgen blockade (CAB) in locally advanced or metastatic disease. The antiandrogens are classified by their chemical structure as either steroidal compounds, typified by cyproterone acetate, or nonsteroidal compounds, which are discussed here. Three nonsteroidal antiandrogens (NSAAs) are currently available: flutamide, nilutamide, and bicalutamide (Fig. 1). Flutamide has been in clinical use for more than 20 years. It is a pro-drug and is converted in the liver to the active metabolite 2-hydroxyflutamide *(1)*. Nilutamide has been marketed in several European countries for a number of years, and more recently in the USA. Bicalutamide, the most recent addition to this therapeutic group, has also been approved in Europe and the USA. In contrast to

From: *Hormone Therapy in Breast and Prostate Cancer*
Edited by: V. C. Jordan and B. J. A. Furr © Humana Press Inc., Totowa, NJ

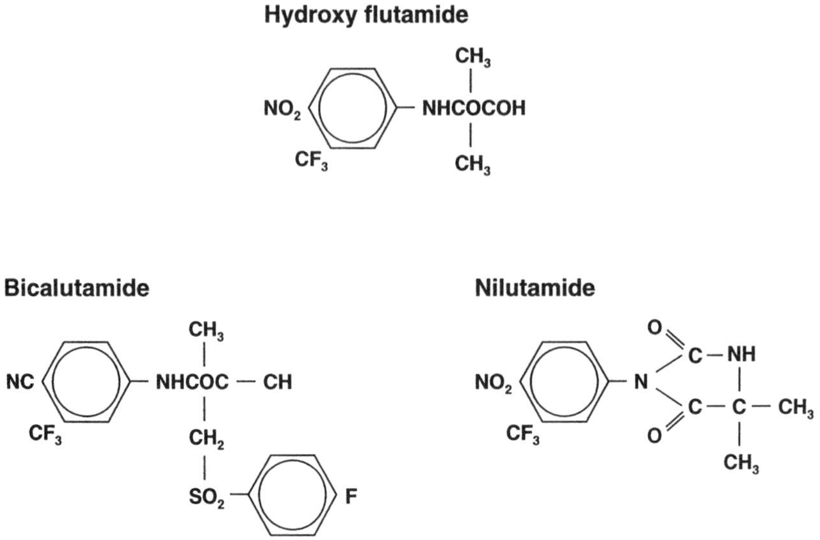

Hydroxy flutamide

Bicalutamide

Nilutamide

Fig. 1. Structure of the nonsteroidal antiandrogens.

flutamide, bicalutamide and nilutamide do not require metabolic conversion to exert a therapeutic effect. Bicalutamide is a racemic compound and only the R-enantiomer displays antiandrogenic activity *(2)*.

2. PRECLINICAL DATA

The androgen-responsive nature of prostate cancer was established by Huggins and colleagues in the early 1940s *(3)*. The principal androgenic hormone in the normal prostate is 5α-dihydrotestosterone (DHT), which is formed locally from testosterone. Various androgen-responsive genes are modulated by the complex formed by the interaction of DHT with the nuclear androgen receptor (AR). The NSAAs are competitive inhibitors at this receptor and antagonize the stimulatory effects of androgens on the cells of the prostate gland. All three NSAAs are pure antiandrogens; that is, they do not interact with other steroidal receptors *(4–6)*. The precise molecular mode of action of the NSAAs at the AR has yet to be established conclusively. Bicalutamide has been shown to be a poor penetrator of the blood-brain barrier (BBB) in experimental animals and exhibits peripheral selectivity *(7,8)*. In contrast, flutamide and nilutamide also act centrally to inhibit the negative feedback of androgen activity, thereby increasing luteinizing hormone and testosterone concentrations *(9)*. However, bicalutamide is not peripherally selective in humans *(10)*.

In vitro receptor-binding studies reveal that the affinity of the NSAAs for the rat and human AR is 2% or less of that of the natural-ligand DHT. Most

Table 1
Relative Binding Affinity of the Nonsteroidal Antiandrogens
for Prostate Androgen Receptors

| | | Relative binding affinity | |
| | | Bicalutamide: | Bicalutamide: |
Study	Species	2-hydroxyflutamide	nilutamide
Furr et al. 1987 (7)	Rat	4.0	ND
Winneker et al. 1989 (13)	Rat	3.3	ND
Teutsch et al. 1994 (12)	Rat	2.3	2.3
Luo et al. 1996 (14)	Rat	1.3	5.2
Kemppainen and Wilson 1996 (15)	Human	~3.0	ND
Ayub and Levell 1989 (4)	Human	2.5	1.6
Luo et al. 1996 (14)	Human	1.0	2.1

ND, not determined.

comparative studies indicate that 2-hydroxyflutamide and nilutamide have comparable affinity for rat and human prostatic tissue in vitro (4,11,12), which is lower than that of bicalutamide (Table 1). Differences in test results between laboratories (4,7,12–15) may be due to variability in conditions, including drug losses due to nonspecific binding, and the use of commercial or self-synthesized compound (16,17). Most published data also show that bicalutamide is more potent than flutamide in androgen-dependent tissues in vivo (7,18–21). No similar comparative studies have been reported that involved nilutamide.

The NSAAs are active in a number of in vitro murine and human tumor models (5,22–24). In contrast, in the human LNCaP cell line, in which the AR is mutated, nilutamide and 2-hydroxyflutamide demonstrate agonist activity, whereas bicalutamide has definite antagonistic properties (15,25–28). Although the clinical significance of these observations is still unclear, AR mutations with similar in vitro functional properties as the LNCaP receptor have been found in patients with relapse following first-line NSAA therapy (29–31). In vivo, bicalutamide was as effective as castration in preventing tumor growth in the Dunning R3327H model in intact and castrated rats (32) and was more effective than flutamide (6). Nilutamide has been shown to reduce the incidence and development of the SC115 tumor in intact mice (5).

In summary, all the NSAAs have a lower affinity for the AR than natural androgens: bicalutamide has greater affinity than 2-hydroxyflutamide and nilutamide. The NSAAs are effective in several in vitro tumor models, but in some models flutamide and nilutamide show agonist activity. This has not been observed with bicalutamide to date. The preclinical data reviewed here suggest differences between the NSAAs with respect to dosing and potential efficacy.

However, their therapeutic dose and clinical effectiveness can only be truly defined in clinical trials.

3. DOSING CONSIDERATIONS

The clinically used doses of flutamide (750 mg/d) and nilutamide (300 mg/d) appear to be empirical because we were unable to discover any published dose-finding studies from US and European clinical trials. A Japanese Phase II study of four dosing regimens of flutamide (90, 375, 750, and 1125 mg/d) showed similar objective response rates at the three higher doses (46–48%), whereas no response was seen at the low dose of 90 mg/d *(33)*. However, side effects were dose-related.

In contrast, dose-ranging studies with bicalutamide have been conducted using both prostatic acid phosphatase (PAP) and prostate-specific antigen (PSA) as tumor markers. The definition of an objective response used in the initial evaluation of bicalutamide, a fall of at least 50% in the serum PAP, was based on the PAP response to the dose of goserelin needed to cause medical castration. The PAP decrement was dose-dependent in the bicalutamide 10–50 mg dosage range, with a response rate of 53 and 83% after 8 wk treatment at the 30 and 50 mg dosage levels, respectively. Tolerability at both doses was acceptable and bicalutamide 50 mg was selected for further study as a component of CAB and for monotherapy *(34)*.

Further studies conducted after PSA became widely accepted as an endpoint have consistently indicated that the biochemical response to bicalutamide in terms of PSA reduction is also dose-related up to doses of 200 mg, with the PSA decrement after 3 mo of bicalutamide 150 mg/d being comparable with that after surgical castration *(35)*.

As discussed later, bicalutamide 50 mg is as effective as flutamide 750 mg as a component of CAB, with both treatments producing a median decline in PSA after 3 mo of 99% *(36)*. However, as the median PSA fall during the initial evaluation of bicalutamide 50 mg monotherapy was 86–88% compared with 96–97% for castration *(37)*, monotherapy studies with bicalutamide have now been undertaken at the higher dose of 150 mg/d.

The significant pharmacokinetic differences between the NSAAs have implications for dosing and therefore compliance, an important consideration in an elderly population. The half-life ($t_{1/2}$) of flutamide after a single dose is 4.3–6.6 h *(38)* and, consequently, flutamide is administered via a three times per day regimen. Although the $t_{1/2}$ of nilutamide is 23–87 h (mean 56 h) *(39)*, suggesting that once-daily dosing would be appropriate, a three times per day regimen has been employed in most clinical trials. Bicalutamide has a $t_{1/2}$ of about 6 d on single dosing and 7–10 d after multiple dosing *(40)* and can therefore be administered as a single daily dose. Furthermore, plasma bicalutamide

Table 2
Studies Showing Superior Survival with Combined Androgen Blockade
in Metastatic Prostate Cancer

Study	Treatment groups	No. of patients	Follow-up (mo)	Time to progression	Overall survival
Crawford et al. 1989 (44)	Leuprolide + flutamide Leuprolide + placebo	603	42	16.5 vs 13.9 mo ($p = 0.039$)	35.5 vs 28.3 mo ($p = 0.035$)
Denis et al. 1993 (45)	Goserelin + flutamide Orchiectomy	327	60	71 vs 46 wk ($p = 0.002$)	34.4 vs 27.1 mo ($p = 0.02$)
Dijkman et al. 1997 (46)	Orchiectomy + nilutamide Orchiectomy + placebo	457	82–102	21.2 vs 14.7 mo ($p = 0.0024$)	27.3 vs 23.6 mo ($p = 0.0326$)

concentrations show minimal diurnal variation, so consistent androgen receptor blockade is maintained throughout the dosing interval.

All three NSAAs undergo hepatic metabolism and conjugation before renal elimination (38,39,41); however, dosage modification in the presence of mild to moderate hepatic impairment or renal dysfunction is not necessary.

4. NSAAS AS A COMPONENT OF CAB

Testicular ablation has been the cornerstone of management for advanced prostate cancer since the seminal work of Huggins and colleagues (3) demonstrating the hormone-dependence of this tumor. Castration can now be achieved either surgically or using the luteinizing hormone-releasing hormone (LH-RH) agonists (42). However, although castration almost completely suppresses testicular androgens, secretion of androgens by the adrenal gland is unaltered. It has been hypothesized that the tumor relapse, which generally occurs around 18 mo after castration, may be due to residual stimulation by the adrenal androgens. CAB, the addition of an antiandrogen to castration, has been advocated as a means of prolonging the interval to disease progression and patient survival. The first studies with CAB used the steroidal compound cyproterone acetate (43). Since then, there has been a plethora of studies comparing CAB with conventional therapy, using both steroidal antiandrogens and the NSAAs, flutamide and nilutamide.

Mature data from three large, randomized double-blind trials show a consistent survival benefit with CAB (Table 2) (44–46). In the first of these studies, the combination of leuprolide plus flutamide was compared with leuprolide in a placebo-controlled manner *(44)*. After a median of 42 mo follow-up, the median progression-free survival in the CAB arm was significantly prolonged by 2.6 mo ($p = 0.039$) and the overall median survival by 7.2 mo ($p = 0.035$). Positive results were also reported from an European Organization for Research and Treatment of Cancer (EORTC) study comparing goserelin plus flutamide with orchiectomy *(45);* CAB increased the time to first progression (objective or subjective) by 25 wk ($p = 0.002$), overall survival by 7.3 mo ($p = 0.02$), and time to death from cancer by 15.1 mo. More recently, Dijkman et al. *(46)* have reported that at 8.5 yr follow-up, the addition of nilutamide to orchiectomy prolonged the progression-free interval by 44% ($p = 0.002$), time to death from cancer by 24% ($p = 0.013$), and overall survival by 16% ($p = 0.033$). In this study, normalization of the PSA within 3 mo (CAB, 59%; orchiectomy, 28%) was associated with a more favorable outcome irrespective of treatment group.

Most of the other published CAB studies show a small, but non-significant, benefit for the combined approach, with none finding castration superior to CAB. A large Southwest Oncology Group (SWOG) trial (INT-0105) designed to answer many of the outstanding issues concerning CAB was initiated in 1989. Patients with metastatic (M1) disease ($n = 1347$) were randomly assigned to either orchiectomy plus flutamide or orchiectomy plus placebo, and the trial had the statistical power to detect a 25% improvement in the median survival time achieved with orchiectomy. The first analysis of this study *(47),* failed to show any significant improvement in either progression-free or overall survival with CAB, despite a significant increase in the PSA normalization rate at 3 mo (80 vs 68%; $p = 0.001$).

Several meta-analyses of the CAB studies, using varying study selection criteria, have produced conflicting results *(48–51)*. It seems most likely that, overall, the benefits of CAB are more modest than originally anticipated. This modest advantage of CAB has been confirmed by the latest meta-analysis of 27 randomized trials, which also suggests that results of studies that included cyproterone acetate were less favorable than those with NSAAs *(52)*. It is clear, however, that those who gain most may be patients with minimal disease at treatment onset. In two of the three studies demonstrating overall survival gains with CAB, outcome in minimal disease was markedly improved in the CAB arm compared with castration, whereas between-group differences in patients with extensive metastases were not significant *(44,45)*. In the US study, CAB increased median progression-free survival of patients with minimal disease (defined as metastases in the pelvis/axial skeleton only and/or soft-tissue nodes) by 29 mo and overall survival by 19 mo compared with LH-RH agonist monotherapy. In the European study the death hazard ratio for CAB in the minimal disease subgroup (defined as <5 bony metastases) was 0.6. A few other studies reporting no overall survival benefit with CAB also suggest that outcome is influenced by the extent of disease *(53,54)*. However, in the 283 men with minimal disease evaluated in the INT-

0105 study, the addition of flutamide to orchiectomy did not significantly improve either time to progression or death *(47)*.

Recently an exploratory analysis by Sarosdy et al. suggested that the duration of NSAA use as part of CAB may affect survival. Patients receiving more than 120 d of NSAA therapy had a longer survival than those receiving less than 120 d of NSAA therapy as part of CAB (median survival 1035 and 302 d, respectively; $p = 0.0001$) *(55)*.

Only one head-to-head, double-blind comparison of NSAAs (bicalutamide and flutamide) has been carried out in the CAB setting. After a median of 160 wk follow-up in 813 men with M1 disease, time to progression, and overall survival were longer in the bicalutamide arm, but the difference was not significant *(56)*. Earlier results from this study revealed that PSA response, subjective response, and quality of life were also comparable *(36)*. However, an exploratory analysis of this study revealed that patients with minimal disease in the bicalutamide group were 25% less likely to experience disease progression or to die than in the flutamide arm *(57)*.

A therapeutic response to the withdrawal of antiandrogens after relapse on CAB has recently been described. The PSA declines shortly after withdrawal, and is often associated with improvements in measurable disease, bone scan, and cancer-related symptoms. This phenomenon was initially reported in patients withdrawn from flutamide *(58–62)*, but has now been reported following both nilutamide and bicalutamide withdrawal *(63–65)*. The duration of response is generally short (<6 mo), but has been prolonged by the addition of aminoglutethimide *(59,61)*. An observational study initiated as part of the double-blind trial of bicalutamide and flutamide showed that 50% of men withdrawn from flutamide ($n = 8$) and 29% of the men withdrawn from bicalutamide ($n = 14$) had a favorable PSA response, although the time course differed due, at least partly, to the differences in $t_{1/2}$ *(66)*. Further studies are needed to identify factors predictive of a withdrawal response and to clarify the underlying mechanism.

5. MONOTHERAPY IN CLINICAL STUDIES

The profile of patients with advanced prostate cancer has changed dramatically in the past few years due to increased awareness of the disease and the expansion in PSA screening. Thus, many of the prostate cancer patients seen today are middle-aged men with a life expectancy of at least 5–10 yr and are naturally reluctant to undergo castration. NSAA monotherapy, which maintains serum testosterone levels and therefore theoretically preserves sexual potency, is one alternative.

The dose employed in most monotherapy studies of flutamide is that used for CAB (250 mg three times/d). Jacobo and colleagues *(68)* administered a higher dose (1500 mg/d) to four patients, but found that this conferred no advantage with respect to progression compared with 750 mg/d, while Sogani and colleagues *(69)* reported transaminase elevations with 1500 mg/d, which resolved at the lower dose. Several small noncomparative studies of flutamide monotherapy carried out in the 1980s reported response rates of 20–70%, with median survival of 12–30 mo *(70–76)*. However, none of these studies used PSA monitoring to assess response. Sexual potency was retained in 80–100% of patients.

A number of Phase III studies of flutamide monotherapy have also been conducted *(68,77–81)*. Many of these lacked the power to detect a significant difference, the endpoints used were often inadequate and follow-up was too short. The more recent and larger studies are summarized in Table 3. Pavone-Macaluso *(79)* and Boccon-Gibod and colleagues *(81)* reported survival equivalence between flutamide monotherapy and conventional therapy (CAB and orchiectomy, respectively); however, in one recent study flutamide was inferior to medical castration using diethylstilbestrol *(80)*.

Bicalutamide has been more extensively studied as monotherapy than the other NSAAs. Three early studies used the dosage recommended for CAB (50 mg/d) *(86–88)* and an overview analysis of these studies, involving more than 1000 patients, showed a median difference in survival of approx 3 mo favoring castration *(37)*. However, as dose-finding studies have shown that the PSA response is dose-dependent *(35)*, higher doses (100 and 150 mg/d) have since been compared with castration (medical or surgical) in previously untreated patients with M0 or M1 disease in two large international studies. The 150 mg dose was chosen for further study based on the early PSA response. The data from the M0 and M1 subgroups has been analyzed separately because there was a qualitative interaction between outcome and disease stage *(82)*. At a median 100 wk follow-up, with 43% deaths in M1 patients, there was a significant survival advantage of 6 wk favoring castration (Table 3), while quality of life and symptomatic response favored bicalutamide *(82)*. However, for the M0 patients bicalutamide was not significantly different from castration for survival outcome at a median of 6.3 yr follow-up with 56% deaths (Table 3) *(83)*. Significant quality of life advantages for bicalutamide over castration with respect to sexual interest (p = 0.029) and physical capacity (p = 0.046) were also apparent in these patients. Furthermore, there is an indication that bone mineral density in patients treated with bicalutamide is similar to that of age-matched controls. This is in contrast to patients treated with castration who showed a loss of bone-mineral density. Analyses of two smaller European studies comparing bicalutamide 150 mg monotherapy with CAB did not reveal any significant survival difference between the treatment groups, but bicalutamide was better-tolerated than CAB and quality of life benefits associated with bicalutamide therapy were confirmed *(84,85)*.

Table 3

Recent Phase III Studies of Nonsteroidal Antiandrogens as Monotherapy in Advanced Prostate Cancer

Study	Comparator	Patient population (disease stage; no. of patients)	Median follow-up	Median time to progression	Median survival
Flutamide 250 mg tds					
Boccon-Gibod et al. 1997 (81)	Orchiectomy	D2; n = 104	36 mo	Flutamide: 396 d Orchiectomy: 370 d	NS
Pavone-Macaluso 1994 (79)	CAB	C/D; n = 319	2 yr	ND	NS (about 44% at 2 yr)
Chang et al. 1996 (80)	DES 3 mg/d	D2; n = 80	48 mo	Flutamide: 9.7 mo DES: 26.4 mo	Flutamide: 28.5 mo DES: 43.2 mo
Bicalutamide 50 mg/d					
Bales and Chodak 1996 (37)	LH-RHa or orchiectomy	D2; n = 1196	17 mo	Bicalutamide: 46% progressed during follow-up Castration: 35% progressed	Bicalutamide: 765 d Castration: 862 d
Bicalutamide 150 mg/d					
Tyrrell et al. 1998 (82)	LH-RHa or orchiectomy	M1; n = 903	100 wk	Castration > bicalutamide (hazard ratio = 1.44)	Castration > bicalutamide (hazard ratio = 1.3)
Iversen et al. 2000 (83)	Goserelin acetate or orchiectomy	M0; n = 480	6.3 yr	Bicalutamide = castration (hazard ratio = 1.20)	Bicalutamide = castration (hazard ratio = 1.05)
Boccardo et al. 1999 (84)	CAB	C/D; n = 220	38 mo	Bicalutamide: 25 mo CAB: 23 mo	Bicalutamide: 44 mo CAB: 45 mo
Chatelain et al. 1999 (85)	CAB	D2; n = 270	31 mo	NS	NS

CAB, combined androgen blockade; DES, diethystilboestrol; LH-RHa, luteinizing hormone-releasing hormone agonist; ND, not determined; NS, not significant; tds, three times daily.

6. TOLERABILITY

The side effects of NSAAs related to androgen withdrawal include breast pain, gynecomastia, and hot flushes. Breast symptoms occur more frequently during monotherapy, whereas hot flashes are more common during CAB *(84,85)*. Overall, there do not appear to be any clinically relevant differences between the three NSAAs regarding the incidence or severity of pharmacologic side effects. Importantly, sexual potency and libido are maintained in most patients during NSAA monotherapy *(67,82,83,89)*.

With respect to nonpharmacologic events, all three NSAAs slightly increase the incidence of nausea and vomiting, but there are no marked differences between the drugs. However, important differences in treatment-related diarrhea are seen. Diarrhea is most common and in some cases more severe with flutamide; for example, in the comparative trial within CAB, significantly more patients experienced diarrhea in the flutamide than the bicalutamide group (26 vs 12%; $p < 0.001$) and treatment withdrawal due to diarrhea also differed (6 and 0.5%, respectively) *(56)*. These figures are comparable with those quoted by other investigators *(44,73,76,89–91)*.

The incidence of diarrhea in bicalutamide monotherapy studies was only 2–5% *(82,83,92)*; frequencies of 5–20% have been cited for flutamide monotherapy *(81,89)*, and 2–4% for nilutamide monotherapy *(67,92,93)*.

Differences between the NSAAs are also apparent with respect to liver toxicity. Abnormal liver-function tests have been reported with all three NSAAs. The incidence of abnormalities varies widely, from 2–3% with nilutamide *(67,94,95)* and 4–62% with flutamide *(45,69,91,96–98)*. Many, but not all, cases may be at least partly due to underlying diseases and/or concomitant drug therapy. In the double-blind comparative study of flutamide and bicalutamide, the incidence of elevated transaminases was higher, but not significantly so, in the flutamide group *(56)*. Symptomatic and, in some cases, serious hepatotoxicity has also been reported for NSAAs. It has been estimated that the risk of severe, potentially fatal, hepatic failure with flutamide is 3/10000 patients *(99)*. Nilutamide hepatotoxicity is less well-documented, but can also have a fatal outcome *(100)*. A case of near-fatal fulminant hepatic failure in a patient on bicalutamide therapy (50 mg) has recently been published *(101)*, but it is uncertain whether this can be attributed to bicalutamide, as the symptoms developed after only two doses in a patient previously exposed to both cyproterone acetate and flutamide *(101)*.

Nilutamide is associated with several complications that have not been seen or have only rarely been reported with the other two NSAAs. The occurrence of interstitial pneumonitis and dyspnea without evidence of pulmonary infiltration during nilutamide therapy is a well-recognized complication *(92,103)*. The manufacturers of nilutamide have indicated that the overall incidence of interstitial pneumonitis is approx 1% *(103)*. Patients usually improve shortly after discontinuation of nilutamide, but complete resolution can take 6–12 mo. It has been suggested that oxidative stress secondary to the metabolism of nilutamide may cause both the pulmonary and hepatic toxicity associated with the drug, and simultaneous liver and lung toxicity has been reported in one patient *(104)*. Interstitial pneumonitis has not been reported with flutamide, but there has been one case in a patient receiving bicalutamide 200 mg *(105)*.

A significant proportion of patients receiving nilutamide (11–65%) experience delayed light/dark adaptation *(67,92–95,106–109)*. In an objective ophthalmologic study, the increase in adaptation time ranged from 20 s to 25 min, with a mean delay of 9 min *(106)*. Visual acuity is not impaired and no anatomic changes in the retina are apparent. Other unspecified visual side effects have also been linked with nilutamide *(92)*. A slight disulfiram-type reaction, with hot flashes and a rash has also been reported in 3–19% of patients receiving nilutamide as monotherapy or as a component of CAB *(67,92,94,95,107,108)*. No reports have suggested that either of these problems occur with flutamide or bicalutamide.

It should be noted that the reported incidence of adverse events is often higher during clinical trials, in which events are actively sought, than during routine clinical practice. In general, NSAA therapy is well-tolerated. A review of the CAB trials shows that between 7% and 18% of patients withdrew from the CAB group due to drug-related side effects. Most trials of NSAA monotherapy involved only small patient samples and, consequently, estimates of treatment withdrawals may be less accurate. In the large bicalutamide 150 mg monotherapy trials, less than 2% of patients withdrew due to adverse events.

7. FUTURE PERSPECTIVES

7.1. Neoadjuvant Therapy in Early Prostate Cancer

Approximately 50% of men with a clinical diagnosis of organ-confined disease have positive surgical margins, seminal-vesicle invasion, or extracapsular extension at radical prostatectomy, and are at risk of early biochemical relapse *(110)*. Neoadjuvant hormonal therapy is under investigation as one method of improving surgical outcome in these men. The histopathologic and PSA progression results from several controlled studies in which CAB was given for 3 mo preoperatively are now available (Table 4), but longer follow-up is needed to determine whether the advantages of neoadjuvant therapy with respect to reduction in tumor volume, surgically positive margins, and extracapsular penetration, translate into improved survival. The optimum duration of neoadjuvant therapy in this setting also remains to be defined; recent results presented by Gleave and colleagues *(119)* show that with an 8-mo course of neoadjuvant CAB, PSA levels continue to fall between 3 and 8 mo.

Neoadjuvant hormonal therapy has also been evaluated in patients undergoing radiotherapy. In a randomized study in 471 men with nonmetastatic (T2-4) dis-

Table 4
Results of Controlled Studies of 3 Mo Combined Androgen Blockade (Leuprolide/Goserelin Plus Flutamide) Before Radical Prostectomy in Early Prostate-cancer Patients

Study	Patient population (disease stage; no. of patients)	Decrease in tumor volume after neoadjuvant therapy	Rates of extracapsular penetration	Rates of positive surgical margins	Prostate-specific antigen progression during follow-up
Soloway et al 1995, 1997 (111,112)	T2b; n = 277	20%	CAB: 47% Controls: 78%	CAB: 18% Controls: 48%	NS at 2 yr
Cookson et al. 1997 (113)	T1, T2, T2/3; n = 141	38%	CAB: 26% Controls: 51%	CAB: 13% Controls: 36%	NS at median 35 mo
Fair et al. 1997 (110)	T1-2; n = 131	ND	CAB: 27% Controls: 44%	CAB: 17% Controls: 36%	NS at mean 28.6 mo
Schulman et al. 1997, Witjes et al. 1997 (114,115)	T2; n = 159	30%	CAB: 33% Controls: 66%	CAB: 14% Controls: 36%	NS at 3 yr
Labrie et al. 1994, 1997, Vaillancourt et al. 1996 (116–118)	B/C; n = 161	44%	CAB: 22% Controls: 51%	CAB: 8% Controls: 34%	ND

CAB, combined androgen blockade; ND, not determined; NS, not significant.

ease, neoadjuvant CAB (goserelin plus flutamide) given for 2 mo before and during radiotherapy significantly reduced local progression at 5 yr *(120)*. However, a significant difference in overall survival has yet to be determined. More recently, a Canadian group found significant advantages for neoadjuvant CAB in terms of PSA measurements over 3 yr of follow-up *(121,122)*. Continuing with CAB for 6 mo after radiotherapy conferred further early benefits. An additional advantage of CAB in this setting is a reduction in radiation-associated morbidity *(123)*.

7.2. Adjuvant Therapy in Early Prostate Cancer

The efficacy of adjuvant hormonal therapy in the setting of breast-cancer treatment *(124)* provides a rationale for a similar approach in early prostate cancer. Extensive clinical studies are currently underway using various modalities including NSAA monotherapy as adjuvant therapy. The largest of these studies (AstraZeneca trials 023, 024, and 025; data on file) aims to study the impact of bicalutamide monotherapy (150 mg/d) compared with placebo, on time to progression and survival in 8113 early prostate-cancer patients who have undergone radical prostatectomy or radiotherapy. Early results on time to recurrence from a smaller controlled trial of adjuvant flutamide involving 365 men with T3 disease appear promising *(125)*. Bicalutamide is also being assessed as a definitive approach for patients who are unsuitable for, or refuse, radical therapy.

7.3. Intermittent CAB

The concept of intermittent CAB is based on the hypothesis that intermittent androgen deprivation may prolong tumor sensitivity, thereby extending progression-free and/or ultimate survival *(126,127)*. This approach may also offer benefits in terms of quality of life, recovery of sexual potency, and drug costs. Intermittent CAB can be realized using reversible medical castration. Several investigators have recently reported their preliminary experience of intermittent CAB in small uncontrolled studies *(128–130)*. While their results suggesting equivalent survival and improved tolerability are encouraging, randomized controlled trials comparing intermittent with continuous CAB are needed to define fully the clinical advantages and risks of this approach.

7.4. New Combination Therapies

Another recent approach developed to try to extend the progression-free interval in advanced prostate cancer is the combination of CAB with chemotherapy. Pummer and colleagues *(131)* have evaluated CAB (orchiectomy and flutamide) combined with weekly epirubicin in a randomized controlled study in 145 previously untreated patients. At median follow-up of 81 mo, progression-free and overall survival increased by 6 and 8 mo, respectively ($p < 0.02$ and $p = 0.12$, respectively) in the epirubicin group. Quality of life was similar in the two groups.

Sequential androgen blockade is another innovative technique designed to mitigate the side effects of androgen suppression. This method of treatment uses a 5α-reductase inhibitor to suppress the conversion of testosterone to DHT in conjunction with an antiandrogen to antagonize the remaining androgens at the receptor level. Sequential androgen blockade should theoretically prevent the side effects of castration by maintaining high circulating testosterone levels, but prevent androgen-induced tumor growth. Pilot studies of finasteride combined with flutamide have been conducted *(132–135)*, and randomized trials are now underway.

Research into the mechanisms of tumor growth and refractoriness may lead to the development of further combination therapies for different stages of prostate cancer. For example, the antagonism of growth factors using suramin-like compounds may make endocrine blockade more complete *(136,137)*.

7.5. NSAAs as Second-Line Therapy

All current and investigative first-line treatments for advanced prostate cancer are palliative and research is therefore being directed at appropriate second-line therapies following relapse. Limited biochemical responses to both flutamide and bicalutamide have been observed following relapse after surgical or medical castration *(70,105,138–140)*. Interestingly, PSA responses to second-line high dose bicalutamide have also been seen in patients previously exposed to flutamide as part of CAB, both in those who did and did not demonstrate a response to flutamide withdrawal *(105,141)*. Bone-scan improvements were also seen in a small proportion of the patients who had an initial response to flutamide withdrawal. These findings demonstrate that only those tumors that continue to proliferate after trials of second-line hormonal manipulation should be defined as hormone-refractory *(142)*.

8. SUMMARY

NSAAs are currently most widely used as a component of CAB for advanced prostate cancer. The benefits of this approach have yet to be fully confirmed. Overall gains over castration alone are probably modest, and may be restricted to patients with few bone lesions. Within CAB, flutamide and bicalutamide are equally effective regarding overall survival outcome, but bicalutamide may be more advantageous in minimal disease. Recently it was suggested that prolonged NSAA therapy may result in prolonged survival when compared to short-term NSAA use as part of CAB therapy. Based on current data, antiandrogen-withdrawal therapy can be considered as a suitable option for patients who have progressed on CAB.

NSAA monotherapy offers palliative benefits in advanced disease, while enhancing certain quality of life domains compared with castration or CAB, specifically maintenance of sexual interest and potency. Bicalutamide has been more extensively studied as monotherapy than flutamide or nilutamide; survival with bicalutamide 150 mg monotherapy is equivalent to castration in M0 disease, whereas for certain M1 patients the quality of life gains may outweigh the slightly inferior survival.

Tolerability is an important consideration when choosing a NSAA. There are no clinically important differences between the NSAAs regarding pharmacologic side effects. However, these drugs differ with respect to the profile of nonpharmacologic toxicity. To date, bicalutamide appears to offer tolerability advantages over flutamide and nilutamide.

New therapeutic approaches that might reduce the mortality of patients with prostate cancer are being investigated. Research into the role of growth factors, oncogenes, tumor-suppressor genes, and inducers of apoptosis—together with ongoing/planned clinical studies of intermittent CAB and sequential androgen blockade in advanced disease, and neoadjuvant/adjuvant treatment for early prostate cancer—should provide a greater range of treatment options in the near future.

REFERENCES

1. Katchen B, Buxbaum S. Disposition of a new, nonsteroid, antiandrogen,α,α,α-trifluoro-2-methyl-4-nitro-m-propionotoluidide (flutamide), in men following a single oral 200mg dose. *J Clin Endocrinol Metab* 1975; 41:373–379.
2. Mukherjee A, Kirkovsky L, Yao XT, Yates RC, Miller DD, Dalton JT. Enantioselective binding of Casodex to the androgen receptor. *Xenobiotica* 1996; 26:117–122.
3. Huggins C, Stevens RE, Hodges CV. Studies in prostatic cancer, II. The effects of castration on advanced cancer of the prostate gland. *Arch Surg* 1941; 43:209–223.
4. Ayub M, Levell MJ. The effect of ketoconazole related imidazole drugs and antiandrogens on [3H]R1881 binding to the prostatic androgen receptor and [3H]5α-dihydrotestosterone and [3H]cortisol binding to plasma proteins. *J Steroid Biochem* 1989; 33:251–255.
5. Gaillard-Moguilewsky M. Pharmacology and antiandrogens and value of combining androgen suppression with antiandrogen therapy. *Urology* 1991; 37(Suppl):5–12.
6. Furr BJA, Tucker H. The preclinical development of bicalutamide: pharmacodynamics and mechanism of action. *Urology* 1996; 47(Suppl 1A):13–25.
7. Furr BJA, Valcaccia B, Curry B, Woodburn JR, Chesterson G, Tucker H. ICI 176, 334: a novel non-steroidal, peripherally selective antiandrogen. *J Endocrinol* 1987; 113:R7–R9.
8. Freeman SN, Mainwaring WIP, Furr BJA. A possible explanation for the peripheral selectivity of a novel non-steroidal pure antiandrogen, Casodex (ICI 176,334). *Br J Cancer* 1989; 60:664–668.
9. Marchetti B, Labrie F. Characteristics of flutamide action on prostatic and testicular functions in the rat. *J Steroid Biochem* 1988; 29:691–698.
10. Mahler C, Van Cangh P, Bouffioux C, Keuppens F, Coeck C, Ongena P, Denis L. Endocrine effects of Casodex. A new non-steroidal antiandrogen, in *Recent Advances in Urological Cancers* (Murphy G, Khoury S, eds). American Cancer Society, Atlanta, GA 1990:42–45.

11. Moguileswky M, Fiet J, Tournemine C, Raynaud JP. Pharmacology of an antiandrogen, anandron, used as adjuvant therapy in the treatment of prostate cancer. *J Steroid Biochem* 1986; 24:139–146.

12. Teutsch G, Goubet F, Baumann J, Bonfils A, Bouchoux F, Cerede E, et al. Non-steroidal antiandrogens: synthesis and biological profile of high-affinity ligands for the androgen receptor. *J Steroid Biochem* 1994; 48:111–119.

13. Winneker REC, Wagner MM, Batzold FH. Studies on the mechanism of action of WIN49596: a steroidal androgen receptor antagonist. *J Steroid Biochem* 1989; 33:1133–1138.

14. Luo S, Martel C, LeBlanc G, Candas B, Singh SM, Labrie C, Simard J, Belanger A, Labrie F. Relative potencies of flutamide and Casodex: preclinical studies. *Endocr-Rel Cancer* 1996; 3:229–241.

15. Kemppainen JA, Wilson EM. Agonist and antagonist activities of hydroxyflutamide and Casodex relate to androgen receptor stabilisation. *Urology* 1996; 48:157–163.

16. Furr BJA. Relative potencies of flutamide and Casodex. *Endocr-Rel Cancer* 1997; 4:197–202.

17. Kolvenbag GJCM, Furr BJA, Blackledge GRP. Receptor affinity and potency of non-steroidal antiandrogens: translation of preclinical findings into clinical activity. *Prostate Cancer Prostat Dis* 1998; 1:307–314.

18. Snyder BW, Winneker RC, Batzold FH. Endocrine profile of WIN 49596 in the rat: a novel androgen receptor antagonist. *J Steroid Biochem* 1989; 33:1127–1132.

19. Chandolia RK, Weinbauer GF, Behre HM, Nieschlag E. Evaluation of a peripherally selective antiandrogen (Casodex) as a tool for studying the relationship between testosterone and spermatogenesis in the rat. *J Steroid Biochem Mol Biol* 1991; 38:367–375.

20. Chandolia RK, Weinbauer GF, Simoni M, Behre HM, Nieschlag E. Comparative effects of chronic administration of the non-steroidal antiandrogens flutamide and Casodex on the reproductive system of the adult male rat. *Acta Endocrinol* 1991; 125:547–555.

21. Gromoll J, Weinbauer GF, Simoni M, Nieschlag E. Effects of antiandrogens and ethane dimethane sulphonate (EDS) on gene expression, free subunits, bioactivity and secretion of pituitary gonadotrophins in male rats. *Mol Cell Endocrinol* 1993; 91:119–125.

22. Darbre PD, King RJB. Progression to steroid autonomy in S115 mouse mammary tumor cells: role of DNA methylation. *J Cell Biol* 1984; 99:1410–1415.

23. Maucher A, von Angerer E. Antiproliferative activity of Casodex (ICI 176,334) in hormone-dependent tumors. *J Cancer Res Clin Oncol* 1993; 119:669–674.

24. Simard J, Singh SM, Labrie F. Comparison of in vitro effects of the pure antiandrogens OH-flutamide, Casodex, and nilutamide on androgen-sensitive parameters. *Urology* 1997; 49:580–589.

25. Wilding G, Chen M, Gelmann EP. Aberrant response in vitro of hormone-responsive prostate cancer cells to antiandrogens. *Prostate* 1989; 14:103–115.

26. Olea N, Sakabe K, Soto AM, Sonnenschein C. The proliferative effect of antiandrogens on the androgen-sensitive human prostate tumor cell line LNCaP. *Endocrinology* 1990; 126:1457–1463.

27. Schuurmans ALG, Bolt J, Veldscholte J, Mulder E. Simulatory effects of antiandrogens on LNCaP human prostate tumor cell growth. EGF-receptor level and acid phosphatase secretion. *J Steroid Biochem Mol Biol* 1990; 37:849–853.

28. Veldscholte J, Berevoets CA, Brinkman AO, Grootegoed JA, Mulder E. Antiandrogens and the mutated androgen receptor of LNCaP cells: differential effects on binding affinity, heat-shock protein interaction, and transcription activation. *Biochemistry* 1992; 31:2392–2399.

29. Culig Z, Hobisch A, Hittmair A, Cronauer MV, Radmayr C, Bartsch G, Klocker H. Androgen receptor gene mutations in prostate cancer. Implications for disease progression and therapy. *Drugs Aging* 1997; 10:50–58.

30. Fenton MA, Shuster TD, Fertig AM, Taplin ME, Kolvenbag G, Bubley GJ, Balk SP. Functional characterization of mutant androgen receptors from androgen-independent prostate cancer. *Clin Cancer Res* 1997; 3:1383–1388.

31. Joyce R, Fenton MA, Rode P, Constantine M, Gaynes L, Kolvenbag G, et al. High-dose bicalutamide for androgen-independent prostate cancer. *J Urol* 1998; 159:149–153.

32. Furr BJA. Casodex: preclinical studies. *Eur Urol* 1990; 18:2–9.

33. Aso Y, Akaza H, Kameyama S, Koyanagi T, Kumamoto Y, Funyu T. Clinical evaluation of flutamide, a pure antiandrogen, in prostatic cancer. Phase II dose-finding study. *Acta Urol Jpn* 1993; 39:391–403.

34. Denis L, Mahler C. Pharmacodynamics and pharmacokinetics of bicalutamide: defining an active dosing regimen. *Urology* 1996; 47(suppl 1A):26–28.

35. Blackledge GRP, Cockshott JD, Furr BJA. Casodex (bicalutamide): overview of a new antiandrogen developed for the treatment of prostate cancer. *Eur Urol* 1997; 31(Suppl 2):30–39.

36. Schellhammer P, Sharifi R, Block N, Soloway M, Venner P, Patterson AL, et al. A controlled trial of bicalutamide versus flutamide, each in combination with luteinizing hormone-releasing hormone analogue therapy, in patients with advanced prostate cancer. *Urology* 1995; 45:745–752.

37. Bales GT, Chodak GW. A controlled trial of bicalutamide versus castration in patients with advanced prostate cancer. *Urology* 1996; 47:38–43.

38. Schulz M, Schmeldt A, Donn F, Becker H. The pharmacokinetics of flutamide and its major metabolites after a single oral dose and during chronic treatment. *Eur J Clin Pharmacol* 1988; 34:633–636.

39. Pendyala L, Creaven PJ, Huben R, Tremblay D, Bertagna C. Pharmacokinetics of Anandron in patients with advanced carcinoma of the prostate. *Cancer Chemo Pharmacol* 1988; 22:69–76.

40. Cockshott ID, Cooper KJ, Sweetmore DS, Blacklock NJ, Denis L. The pharmacokinetics of Casodex in prostate cancer patients after single and during multiple dosing. *Eur Urol* 1990; 18 (Suppl 3):10–17.

41. McKillop D, Boyle GW, Cockshott ID, Jones DC, Phillips PJ, Yates RA. Metabolism and enantioselective pharmacokinetics of Casodex in man. *Xenobiotica* 1993; 23:1241–1253.

42. Kirby RS. Recent advances in the medical management of prostate cancer. *Br J Clin Pract* 1996; 50:88–93.

43. Bracci U, DiSilverio F. Role of cyproterone acetate in urology, in *Androgens and Antiandrogens* (Martini L, Motta M, eds). Raven Press, New York, 1977, pp 333–339.

44. Crawford ED, Eisenberger MA, McLeod DG, Spaulding JT, Benson R, Dorr FA, et al. A controlled trial of leuprolide with and without flutamide in prostatic carcinoma. *N Engl J Med* 1989; 321:419–424.

45. Denis LJ, de Moura CJL, Bono A, Sylvester R, Whelan P, Newling D, Depauw M. Goserelin acetate and flutamide versus bilateral orchidectomy: a phase III EORTC trial (30853). *Urology* 1993; 42:119–130.

46. Dijkman GA, Janknegt RA, de Reijke TM, Debrunye FMJ. Long-term efficacy and safety of nilutamide plus castration in advanced prostate cancer, and the significance of early prostate specific antigen normalization. *J Urol* 1997; 158:160–163.

47. Eisenberger M, Crawford ED, McLeod D, Loehrer P, Wilding G, Blumenstein B. A comparison of bilateral orchidectomy with or without flutamide in stage D2 prostate cancer (NCI INT-0105 SWOG/ECOG). *Proc Am Soc Clin Oncol* 1997; 16:2a (Abstr 3).

48. Prostate Cancer Trialists Collaborative Group. Maximum androgen blockade in advanced prostate cancer: an overview of 22 randomised trials with 3283 deaths in 5710 patients. *Lancet* 1995; 346:265–269.

49. Klotz LH, Newman T. Does maximal androgen blockade (MAB) improve survival? A critical appraisal of the evidence. *Can J Urol* 1996; 3:246–250.

50. Debruyne FM. Combined androgen blockade is the treatment of choice for patients with advanced prostate cancer: the argument for. *Eur Urol* 1996; 29 (suppl 2):34–36.

51. Caubet J-F, Tosteson TD, Dong EW, Naylon EM, Whiting GW, Ernstoff MS, Ross SD. Maximum androgen blockade in advanced prostate cancer: A meta-analysis of published randomized clinical trials using nonsteroidal antiandrogens. *Urology* 1997; 49:71–78.

52. Prostate Cancer Trialists Collaborative Group. Maximum androgen blockade in advanced prostate cancer: an overview of randomised trials. *Lancet* 2000; 355:1491–1498.

53. Labrie F, Dupont A, Cusan L, Gomez J-L, Diamond P. Major advantages of early administration of endocrine combination therapy in advanced prostate cancer. *Clin Invest Med* 1993; 16:493–498

54. Jörgensen T, Muller C, Kaalhus O, Danielson HE, Tveter KJ. Extent of disease based on initial bone scan: important prognostic predictor for patients with metastatic prostatic cancer. *Eur Urol* 1995; 28:40–46.

55. Sarosdy MF, Schellhammer PF, Johnson R, Carroll K, Kolvenbag GJCM. Does prolonged combined androgen blockade have survival benefits over short-term combined androgen blockade therapy? *Urology* 2000; 55:391–396.

56. Schellhammer P, Sharifi R, Block N, Soloway M, Venner P, Patterson AL, et al. Clinical benefits of bicalutamide (Casodex) versus flutamide (Eulexin) in combined androgen blockade for patients with advanced prostatic carcinoma: final report of a double-blind randomized, multicenter trial. *Urology* 1997; 50:330–336.

57. Soloway M, Schellhammer P, Sharifi R, Block N, Venner P, Patterson AL, et al. Differences between bicalutamide and flutamide, each in combination with LHRH analogs, in advanced prostate cancer patients: an exploratory analysis of extent of disease. *Prostate J* 2000; in press.

58. Scher HI, Kelly WK. The flutamide withdrawal syndrome: its impact on clinical trials in hormone-refractory prostatic cancer. *J Clin Oncol* 1993; 11:1566–1572.

59. Dupont A, Gomez J, Cusan L, Koutsilieris M, Labrie F. Response to flutamide withdrawal in advanced prostate cancer in progression under combination therapy. *J Urol* 1993; 150:908–913.

60. Sartor O, Cooper M, Weinberger M, Headlee D, Thibault A, Tompkins A, et al. Surprising activity of flutamide withdrawal, when combined with aminoglutethimide, in treatment of hormone-refractory prostate cancer. *J Natl Cancer Inst* 1994; 86:222–227.

61. Figg WD, Sartor O, Cooper MR, Thibault A, Bergan RC, Dawson N, et al. Prostate specific antigen decline following the discontinuation of flutamide in patients with stage D2 prostate cancer. *Am J Med* 1995; 98:412–414.

62. Herrada J, Hossan B, Amato R, Zukiwski A, von Esenbach A, Logothetis C. Characterization of patients with androgen independent prostate carcinoma whose serum prostate specific antigen decreased following flutamide withdrawal. *J Urol* 1996; 155:620–623.

63. Small EJ, Carroll PR. Prostate-specific antigen decline after Casodex withdrawal: evidence for an antiandrogen withdrawal syndrome. *Urology* 1994; 43:408–410.

64. Nieh PT. Withdrawal phenomenon with the antiandrogen Casodex. *J Urol* 1995; 153:1070–1073.

65. Huan SD, Gerridzen RG, Yau JC, Stewart DJ. Antiandrogen withdrawal syndrome with nilutamide. *Urology* 1997; 49:632–634.

66. Schellhammer P, Venner P, Haas G, Small EJ, Neih P, Seabaugh DR, et al. Prostate-specific antigen decreases after withdrawal of antiandrogen therapy with bicalutamide or flutamide in patients receiving combined androgen blockade. *J Urol* 1997; 157:1731–1735.

67. Decensi AU, Boccardo F, Guarneri D, Positano N, Paoletti C, Costantini M, et al. Monotherapy with nilutamide: a pure nonsteroidal antiandrogen, in untreated patients with metastatic carcinoma of the prostate. *J Urol* 1991; 146:377–381.

68. Jacobo E, Schmidt JD, Weinstein SH, Flocks RH. Comparison of flutamide (SCH-13521) and diethylstilbestrol in untreated advanced prostatic cancer. *Urology* 1976; 8:231–233.

69. Sogani PC, Vagaiwala MR, Whitmore WF. Experience with flutamide in patients with advanced prostatic cancer without prior endocrine therapy. *Cancer* 1984; 54:744–750.

70. Narayana AS, Loening SA, Culp DA. Flutamide in the treatment of metastatic carcinoma of the prostate. *Br J Urol* 1981; 53:152–153.

71. Keating MA, Griffin PP, Schiff SF. Flutamide in the treatment of advanced prostate cancer. *J Urol* 1986; 135:203a (Abstr 398).

72. Di Silverio F, Tenaglia R, Bizzarri M, Biggio A, Saragnano R. Experience with flutamide in advanced prostatic cancer patients refractory to previous endocrine therapy. *J Drug Dev* 1987; 1 (suppl 1):10–16.

73. Lundgren R. Flutamide as primary treatment for metastatic prostatic cancer. *Br J Urol* 1987; 59:156–158.

74. Prout GR, Keating MA, Griffin PP, Schiff SF. Long term experience with flutamide in patients with prostatic carcinoma. *Urology* 1989; 34:37–45.

75. Pavone-Macaluso M, Pavone C, Serretta Y, Daricello G. Antiandrogens alone or in combination for treatment of prostate cancer: the European experience. *Urology* 1989; 34:27–35.

76. Delaere KPJ, Van Thillo EL. Flutamide monotherapy as primary treatment in advanced prostatic carcinoma. *Semin Urol* 1991; 18:13–18.

77. Johansson JE, Andersson SO, Beckman KW, Lingardh G, Zador G. Clinical evaluation of flutamide and estramustine as initial treatment of metastatic carcinoma of prostate. *Urology* 1987; 24:55–59.

78. Lund F, Rasmussen F. Flutamide versus stilboestrol in the management of advanced prostatic cancer. *Br J Urol* 1988; 61:140–142.

79. Pavone-Macaluso M. Flutamide monotherapy versus combined androgen blockade in advanced prostate cancer. Interim report of an Italian multicenter, randomised study. SIU 23rd Congress, Sydney, Australia, September 1994 (Abstr 354).

80. Chang A, Yeap B, Davis T, Blum R, Hahn R, Khanna O, et al. Double blind randomized study of primary hormonal treatment of stage D2 prostate carcinoma: flutamide versus diethylstilbestrol. *J Clin Oncol* 1996; 14:2250–2257.

81. Boccon-Gibod L, Fournier G, Bottet P, Marechal JM, Guiter J, Rischman P, et al. Flutamide versus orchidectomy in the treatment of metastatic prostate carcinoma. *Eur Urol* 1997; 32:391–396.

82. Tyrrell CJ, Kaisary AV, Iversen P, Anderson JB, Baert L, Tammela T, et al. A randomised comparison of Casodex (bicalutamide) 150 mg monotherapy versus castration in the treatment of metastatic and locally advanced prostate cancer. *Eur Urol* 1998; 33:447–456.

83. Iversen P, Tyrrell CJ, Anderson JB, Baert L, Chamberlain M, Kaisary AV, et al. Comparison of Casodex (bicalutamide) 150 mg monotherapy with castration in previously untreated non-metastatic prostate cancer: mature survival results. *J Urol* 2000; 163 (Suppl):158 (Abs 704).

84. Boccardo F, Rubagotti A, Barichello M, Battaglia M, Carmignani, Comeri G, et al. Bicalutamide monotherapy versus flutamide plus goserelin in prostate cancer patients: results of an Italian prostate cancer project study. *J Clin Oncol* 1999; 17:2027–2038.

85. Chatelain C, Fourcader RO, Delchambre J. Bicalutamide (Casodex) versus combined androgen blockade (CAB): open French multicentre trial in patients with metastatic prostate cancer. *Br J Urol* 1997; 80 (Suppl 2):283 (Abstr 1111).

86. Kaisary AV, Tyrrell CJ, Beacock C, Lunglmayr G, Debruyne FA. Randomised comparison of monotherapy with Casodex 50 mg daily and castration in the treatment of metastatic prostate carcinoma. *Eur Urol* 1995; 28:215–222.

87. Chodak G, Sharifi R, Kasimis B, Block NL, Macramalla E, Kennealey GT. Single agent therapy with bicalutamide: a comparison with medical or surgical castration in the treatment of advanced prostate carcinoma. *Urology* 1995; 46:849–855.

88. Iversen P, Tveter K, Varenhorst E. Randomised study of Casodex 50 mg monotherapy vs orchidectomy in the treatment of metastatic prostate cancer. *Scand J Urol Nephrol* 1996; 30:93–98.

89. Oosterlinck W, Casselman J, Mattelaer J, van Velthoven R, Kurjatkin O, Schulman C. Tolerability and safety of flutamide in monotherapy, with orchiectomy or with LHRH-a in advanced prostate cancer patients. *Eur Urol* 1996; 30:458–463.

90. Boccardo F, Decensi A, Guarneri D, Rubagotti A, Oneto F, Martorana G, et al. Zoladex with or without flutamide in the treatment of locally advanced or metastatic prostate cancer: interim analysis of an outgoing PONCAP study. *Eur Urol* 1990; 18(Suppl 3):48–53.

91. Tyrrell CJ, Altwein JE, Klippel F, Varenhorst E, Lunglmayr G, Boccardo F, et al. A multicenter randomized trial comparing the luteinizing hormone-releasing hormone analogue goserelin acetate alone and with flutamide in the treatment of advanced prostate cancer. *J Urol* 1991; 146:1321–1326.

92. Chatelain C, Rousseau V, Cosaert J. French multicentre trial comparing Casodex (ICI 176,334) monotherapy with castration plus nilutamide in metastatic prostate cancer: a preliminary report. *Eur Urol* 1994; 26 (Supp 1):10–14.

93. Namer M, Toubol J, Caty A, Couette JE, Douchez J, Kerbrat P, Droz JP. A randomized double-blind study evaluating Anandron associated with orchiectomy in stage D prostate cancer. *J Steroid Biochem Mol Biol* 1990; 37:909–915.

94. Boccardo F, Decensi AU, Guarneri D, Martorana G, Fioretto L, Mini E, et al. Anandron (RU23908) in metastatic prostate cancer: preliminary results of a multicentric Italian study. *Cancer Detect Prev* 1991; 15:501–503.

95. Janknegt RA, Abbou CC, Bartoletti R, Bernstein-Hahn L, Bracken B, Brisset JM, et al. Orchiectomy and nilutamide or placebo as treatment of metastatic prostatic cancer in a multinational double-blind randomized trial. *J Urol* 1993; 149:77–83.

96. Boccardo F, Pace M, Rubagotti A, Guarneri D, Decensi A, Oneto F, et al. Goserelin acetate with or without flutamide in the treatment of patients with locally advanced or metastatic prostate cancer. *Eur J Cancer* 1993; 29A:1088–1093.

97. Iversen P, Rasmussen F, Klarskov P, Christensen IJ. Long-term results of Danish Prostatic Cancer Group Trial 86. *Cancer* 1993; 72(Suppl):3851–3854.

98. Rosenthal SA, Linstadt DE, Leibenhaut MH, Andras EJ, Brooks CP, Stickney DR, et al. Flutamide-associated liver toxicity during treatment with total androgen suppression and radiation therapy for prostate cancer. *Radiology* 1996; 199:451–455.

99. Wysowski DK, Fourcroy JL. Flutamide hepatotoxicity. *J Urol* 1996; 155:209–212.

100. Pescatore P, Hammel P, Durand F, Bertheau P, Bernuau J, Huc D, et al. Hepatite fulminante mortelle imputable au nilutamide (Anandron). *Gastroenterol Clin Biol* 1993; 17:499–501.

101. Dawson LA, Chow E, Morton G. Fulminant hepatic failure associated with bicalutamide. *Urology* 1997; 49:283–284.

102. Schellhammer PF. Fulminant hepatic failure associated with bicalutamide. *Urology* 1997; 50:827.

103. Pfizenmeyer P, Foucher P, Piard F, Coudert B, Braud ML, Gabez P, et al. Nilutamide pneumonitis: a report on 8 patients. *Thorax* 1992; 47:622–627.

104. Gomez J-L, Dupont A, Cuan L, Tremblay M, Tremblay M, Labrie F. Simultaneous liver and lung toxicity related to the nonsteroidal antiandrogen nilutamide (Anandron): a case report. *Am J Med* 1992; 92:563–566.

105. Scher HI, Liebertz C, Kelly WK, Mazumdar M, Brett C, Schwartz L, et al. Bicalutamide for advanced prostate cancer: the natural versus treated history of disease. *J Clin Oncol* 1997; 15:2928–2938.

106. Harnois C, Malenfant M, Dupont A, Labrie F. Ocular toxicity of Anandron in patients treated for prostatic cancer. *Br J Ophthalmol* 1986; 70:471–473.

107. Brisset JM, Bertagna C, Fiet J, de G ry A, Hucher M, Husson JM, et al. Total androgen blockade vs orchiectomy in stage D prostate cancer, in *Hormonal Manipulation of Cancer:*

Peptides, Growth Factors and New (Anti) Steroidal Agents (Klijn JGM, ed). Raven Press, New York, 1987, pp 19–30.

108. Beland G, Elhilali M, Fradet Y, Laroche B, Ramsey EW, Trachtenberg J, Venner PM, Tewari HD. Total androgen ablation: Canadian experience. *Urol Clin North Am* 1991; 18:75–82.

109. Crawford ED, Smith JA, Soloway MS, Lange PH, Lynch DF, Al-Juburi A, et al. Treatment of stage D2 prostate cancer with leuprolide and Anandron compared to leuprolide and placebo, in *Proceedings of the 3rd* International Symposium on Recent Advance in Urological Cancers: Diagnosis and Treatment (Murphy G, Khoury S, Chatelain C, Denis L, eds). Paris, SCI 1993, pp 61–63.

110. Fair WR, Cookson MS, Stroumbakis N, Cohen D, Aprikian AG, Wang Y, et al. The indications, rationale, and results of neoadjuvant androgen deprivation in the treatment of prostatic cancer: Memorial Sloan-Kettering Cancer Center results. *Urology* 1997; 49(Suppl 3A):46–55.

111. Soloway MS, Shairifi R, Wajsman Z, McLeod D, Wood DP, Puras-Baez A. Randomized prospective study comparing radical prostatectomy alone versus radical prostatectomy preceded by androgen blockade in clinical stage B2 (T2bNxM0) prostate cancer. *J Urol* 1995; 154:424–428.

112. Soloway MS, Shairifi R, Wajsman Z, McLeod D, Wood DP, Puras-Baez A. Radical prostectomy alone vs radical prostatectomy preceded by androgen blockade in cT2b prostate cancer – 24 month results. *Br J Urol* 1997; 80(suppl 2):259(Abs 1015).

113. Cookson MS, Sogani PC, Russo P, Sheinfeld J, Herr H, Dalbagni G, et al. Pathological staging and biochemical recurrence after neoadjuvant androgen deprivation therapy in combination with radical prostatectomy in clinically localized prostate cancer: results of a phase II study. *Br J Urol* 1997; 79:432–438.

114. Schulman CC, Debruyne FMJ, Forster G, van Cangh PJ, Witjes WPJ. Neoadjuvant combined androgen deprivation therapy in locally confined prostatic carcinoma. Three years of follow up of a European multicentric randomised study. *Br J Urol* 1997; 80(Suppl 2):259(Abs 1015).

115. Witjes WPJ, Schulman CC, Debruyne FMJ. Preliminary results of a prospective randomized study comparing radical prostatectomy versus radical prostatectomy associated with neoadjuvant hormonal combination therapy in $T_{2–3}N_0 M_0$ prostatic carcinoma. *Urology* 1997; 49(Suppl 3A):65–69.

116. Labrie F, Cusan L, Gomez J-L. Down-staging of early stage prostate cancer before radical prostatectomy: the first randomized trial of neoadjuvant combination therapy with flutamide and a luteinizing hormone-releasing hormone agonist. *Urology* 1994; 44:29–37.

117. Labrie F, Cusan L, Gomez J-L, Diamond P, Suburu R, Lemay M, et al. Neoadjuvant hormonal therapy: the Canadian experience. *Urology* 1997; 49(Suppl 3A):56–64.

118. Vaillancourt L, Tetu B, Fradet Y, Dupont A, Gomez J, Cusan L, et al. Effect of neoadjuvant endocrine therapy (combined androgen blockade) on normal prostate and prostatic carcinoma. *Am J Surg Pathol* 1996; 20:86–93.

119. Gleave M, Goldenberg SL, Jones E, Bruchovsky N, Sullivan L. Biochemical and pathological effects of 8 months of neoadjuvant hormonal therapy: an update on 125 consecutive patients. *Br J Urol* 1997; 80(Suppl 2):259(Abstr 1016).

120. Pilepich MV, Krall JM, Al-Sarraf M, John MJ, Scotte Doggett RL, Sause WT, et al. Androgen deprivation with radiation therapy compared with radiation therapy alone for locally advanced prostatic carcinoma: a randomized comparative trial of the Radiation Therapy Oncology Group. *Urology* 1995; 45:616–623.

121. Candas B, Gomes JL, Cusan L, Diamond P, Laverdiere J, Labrie F. Effects of neoadjuvant and adjuvant combined androgen blockade associated to radiation therapy on serum PSA. *Br J Urol* 1997; 80(Suppl 2):259 (Abstr 1017).

122. Laverdiere J, Gomez JL, Cusan L, Suburu ER, Diamond P, Lemay M, et al. Beneficial effect of combination hormonal therapy administered prior and following external beam

radiation therapy in localized prostate cancer. *Intl J Radiat Oncol Biol Phys* 1997; 37:247–252.

123. Zelefsky MJ, Harrison A. neoadjuvant androgen ablation prior to radiotherapy for prostate cancer: reducing the potential morbidity of therapy. *Urology* 1997; 49(Suppl 3A):38–45.

124. Early Breast Cancer Trialists Collaborative Group. Systemic treatment of early breast cancer by hormonal, cytotoxic or immune therapy. *Lancet* 1992; 339:1–14.

125. Wirth M, Frohmuller H, Marz F, Bolten M, Thieb M. Randomized multicenter trial on adjuvant flutamide therapy in locally advanced prostate cancer after radical surgery. *Br J Urol* 1997; 80(Suppl 2):263 (Abstr 1033).

126. Akakura K, Bruchovsky N, Goldenberg SL, Rennie PS, Buckley AR, Sullivan LD. Effects of intermittent androgen suppression on androgen-dependent tumors: apoptosis and serum prostate-specific antigen. *Cancer* 1993; 71:2782–2790.

127. Tunn UW. Intermittent endocrine therapy of prostate cancer. *Eur Urol* 1996; 30(suppl 1):22–25.

128. Goldenberg S1, Bruchovsky N, Gleave ME, Sullivan LD, Akakura K. Intermittent androgen suppression in the treatment of prostate cancer: a preliminary report. *Urology* 1995; 45:839–844.

129. Gleave M, Bruchovsky N, Goldenberg SL, Sullivan LD. Intermittent androgen suppression: rationale and clinical experience, in *Recent Advances in Prostate Cancer and BPH*. Proceedings of the 4th Congress on Progress and Controversies in Oncological Urology (PACIOU IV, Rotterdam, April 1996) (Schroeder FH, ed). 1997; 109–120.

130. Tunn UW. Clinical results of intermittent endocrine treatment in low-volume prostate cancer patients, in *Recent Advances in Prostate Cancer and BPH*. Proceedings of the 4th Congress on Progress and Controversies in Oncological Urology (PACIOU IV, Rotterdam, April 1996) (Schroeder FH, ed). 1997, pp 121–125.

131. Pummer K, Lehnert M, Stettner H, Hubmer G. Randomized comparison of total androgen blockade alone versus combined with weekly epirubicin in advanced prostate cancer. *Eur Urol* 1997; 32(Suppl 3):81–85.

132. Fleshner NE, Trachtenberg J. Combination finasteride and flutamide in advanced carcinoma of the prostate: effective therapy with minimal side effects. *J Urol* 1995; 154:1642–1646.

133. Fleshner NE, Fair WR. Anti-androgenic effects of combination finasteride plus flutamide in patients with prostatic carcinoma. *Br J Urol* 1996; 78:907–910.

134. Ornstein DK, Ran GS, Johnson B, Charlton ET, Andriole CL. Combined finasteride and flutamide therapy in men with advanced prostate cancer. *Urology* 1996; 46:901–905.

135. Brufsky A, Fontaine-Rothe P, Berlane K, Rieker P, Jiroutek M, Kaplan I, et al. Finasteride and flutamide as potency-sparing androgen-ablative therapy for advanced adenocarcinoma of the prostate. *Urology* 1997; 49:913–920.

136. Sklar GN, Eddy HA, Jacobs SC, Kyprianou N. Combined antitumour effect of suramin plus irradiation in human prostate cancer cells: the role of apoptosis. *J Urol* 1993; 150:1520–1532.

137. Dawson NA, Figg WD, Cooper MR, Sartor O, Bergan RC, Senderowicz AM, et al. Phase II trial of suramin, leuprolide and flutamide in previously untreated metastatic prostate cancer. *J Clin Oncol* 1997; 15:1470–1477.

138. MacFarlane JR, Tolley DA. Flutamide therapy for advanced prostatic cancer: a phase II study. *Br J Urol* 1985; 57:172–174.

139. Kucuk O, Blumenstein B, Moinpour C, Lew D, Coleman M, Eisenberger M, Crawford D. Phase II trial of Casodex in advanced prostate cancer (CaP) patients who failed conventional hormonal manipulation: a Southwest Oncology Group (SWOG) Study. *Proc Am Soc Clin Oncol* 1996; 15:245 (Abstr 618).

140. Datta SN, Thomas K, Matthews PN. Is prednisolone as good as flutamide in hormone refractory metastatic carcinoma of the prostate? *J Urol* 1997; 158:175–177.

17 LH-RH Agonist Role in Prostate Cancer Management

Amir V. Kaisary

CONTENTS

1. INTRODUCTION

In 1941, androgen sensitivity of adenocarcinoma of the prostate was demonstrated by Huggins and Hodges (1). The result was a considerable enthusiasm that androgen ablation by surgical orchidectomy or administration of estrogens would treat prostate cancer. Testosterone, a steroidal hormone produced by the testicular tissue, represents the vast majority of circulating androgen. It passes through the prostate-cell membrane, where it is converted to dihydrotestosterone (DHT) by the intracellular enzyme 5 alpha-reductase. DHT is believed to be the intracellular messenger responsible for stimulating the nucleus for protein synthesis after it binds to intracellular receptor (Fig. 1). Bilateral surgical orchidectomy leads to a decrease of the plasma testosterone level from 500 ng/100 mL to about 50 ng/100 mL in the majority of cases. The fall is very quick and ranges from 3–12 h, a mean of 8.6 h (2). Side effects of testosterone withdrawal include loss of libido, impotence, and hot flashes. Psychological aspects of castration became above all an important issue particularly with regards to the morale and quality of life of patients undergoing this form of therapy. Estrogen therapy, though previously utilized, fell out of favor in view of the cardiovascular and thrombo-embolic complications rates, which were as high as 25–30%. Hence was the search for alternatives of equivalent efficacy but without the prohibitive side effects.

From: *Hormone Therapy in Breast and Prostate Cancer*
Edited by: V. C. Jordan and B. J. A. Furr © Humana Press Inc., Totowa, NJ

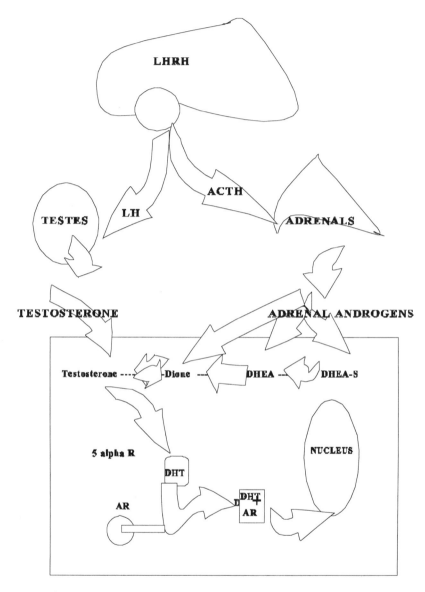

Fig. 1. Physiological control of prostate-gland cellular metabolism.

Leydig-cell production of testosterone is under the control of luteinizing hormone (LH) secreted by the anterior pituitary. However, the ultimate control of the entire cascade lies in the hypothalamus, where luteinizing hormone-releasing hormone (LH-RH) is released in a pulsatile fashion. LH-RH flows through the hypothalamic-pituitary portal venous system to reach the anterior

Glp - His - Trp - Ser - Tyr - Gly * - Leu - Arg - Pro - Gly * - NH₂

Fig. 2. Structure of the naturally occuring LH-RH. Replacement of the amino acids in positions 6 and 10 (*) is the bases of the pharmacologically produced analogues.

Table 1
LH-RH Agonists Available

Deca-peptyl SR	Triptorelin	4.2 mg	i.m./4 wk
Zoladex	Goserelin	3.6 mg	s.c./4 wk
Zoladex LA	Goserelin	10.8 mg	s.c./12 wk
Prostap SR	Leuprorelin	3.75 mg	s.c. or i.m./mo
Prostap 3	Leuprorelin	11.25 mg	s.c./3 mo

pituitary gland. Negative feedback inhibition by the circulating testosterone assures maintenance of natural levels. The naturally occurring LH-RH is a peptide where 10 amino acids are linked (Fig. 2).

In 1971, Schally and co-workers isolated and described the molecular structure of the naturally occurring decapeptide *(3)*. Amino acid substitutions at different positions lead to the production of some decapeptides with agonist and some with antagonist abilities. Several agonists were synthetised and are at present used therapeutically (Table 1). The synthetic analogues are approx 100 times more potent than the naturally occurring LH-RH *(4)*.

2. LH-RH AGONISTS FOR MEDICAL ORCHIDECTOMY

Several large clinical randomized studies were initiated comparing LH-RH agonists with surgical orchidectomy and estrogen therapy *(5,6)*. The results showed medical LH-RH agonist therapy to be as effective as surgical orchidectomy in terms of suppression of serum testosterone and its maintenance to within the surgically castrate range. No differences were shown in objective response rates, time to response, duration of response, and time to treatment failure (Table 2).

On initiation of LH-RH agonist therapy, an initial rise in LH with subsequent rise in testicular androgen production occurs. This rise could lead to serious effects in patients with large tumor burden, those with neurological signs of spinal-cord compression due to bone metastases and those with impending ureteric obstruction due to extensive local disease. Several reports recognized and confirmed this feature, which became subsequently known as the "flare phenomenon" *(7–12)*. Medical castration (LH-RH agonist therapy) gained favorable acceptance rapidly by patients. Lunglmayr and Girsch reported in 1987 their experience with 57 patients *(13)*. All patients were informed that both surgical and medical castration regimens were equally effective and identical in terms of side

Table 2
Objective Response Rates, Time to Responce, Duration of Response,
and Time to Treatment Failure *(5)*

Results	Zoladex 3.6 mg depot (148 pt)	Surgical orchi-dectomy (144 pt)	P_Value
Response %			
Complete and Partial	71	72	ns
Stable	18	22	ns
Progression	11	6	ns
Mean time to response (wk)	9.0	10.2	ns
Median duration of response (wk)	53.7	50.1	ns
Median time to treatment failure	26.9	40.3	ns

ns: Not a significant difference between medical and surgical castration.

effects. Forty-nine patients (86%)opted for LH-RH agonist medical castration. Their choice was mainly for cosmetic reasons (63%) and fear of surgery (35%). In 1990 the outcome of assessment of the treatment choice made by patients with advanced prostate cancer was reported by Soloway et al. *(14)*. The assessment was conducted via a questionnaire completed at home by 147 patients who had the chance to discuss it with their families. Overall, 115 patients (78%) selected LH-RH agonist therapy with the rest opting for surgical castration. Again, fear of surgery or the wish to avoid it was the main reason behind the choice made by those who opted for medical castration. Follow-up 3 mo after initiation of therapy showed that all those patients who received LH-RH agonist therapy but one indicated that they would have made the same choice again.

Patients who are offered castration as a treatment option, and their treating physicians, are usually keen to evaluate prospectively the outcome of treatment. As surgical and medical castration proved to be equivalent in objective response, time to treatment failure, and survival, further analysis of prognostic factors was conducted. In 292 patients reported, the relevant prognostic factors included: pre-treatment serum testosterone, performance status, alkaline phosphatase, and Gleason score (Table 3). Each factor was further analysed into subgroups and the results are shown in Fig. 3 *(15)*. LH-RH agonist therapy established its value in management of prostate cancer. Efforts were subsequently directed to achieve longer-acting depot formulations. Goserelin, which was initially evaluated as a daily s.c. injection, became later available as a four weekly s.c.depot injection (3.6 mg) and currently as a 12 weekly s.c.depot (10.8 mg). Other formulations available include: buserelin (initiation: s.c. injection 0.5 mg every 8 h for 7 d; maintainance: one application of nasal spray in each nostril 6 times daily), leuprorelin (3.75 mg s.c. or i.m. injection monthly and 11.25 mg s.c. 3 monthly)

Table 3
Prognostic Factors

◆ Performance status	$p < 0.0001$
◆ Alkaline phosphatase	$p < 0.0001$
◆ Tumor grade	$p = 0.0008$
◆ Serum testosterone	$p = 0.0039$

ns difference not significant.

Adapted with permission from ref. *(5)*.

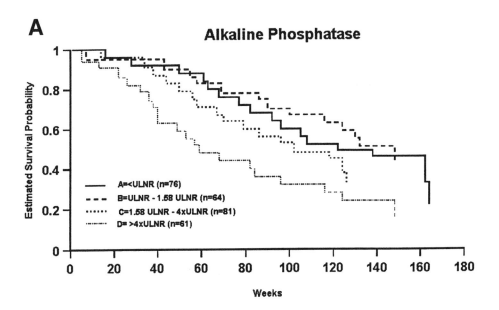

Fig. 3. Prognostic factors with regards to outcome in prostate-cancer patients undergoing castration.

and triptorelin (4.2 mg i.m. injection). Preliminary results of longer acting formulations, reaching up to 6 mo were recently reported *(16)*.

3. HISTOLOGICAL CHANGES IN RESPONSE TO LH-RH

Androgen blockade has effects on both the benign and malignant components.

3.1. LH-RH Effects on Benign Glands

There is a marked atrophy of the glands (Fig 4A). This is seen as a decrease in the overall lobular architecture as well as atrophy of individual acini. The removal of androgen support triggers off apoptosis and therefore degenerative

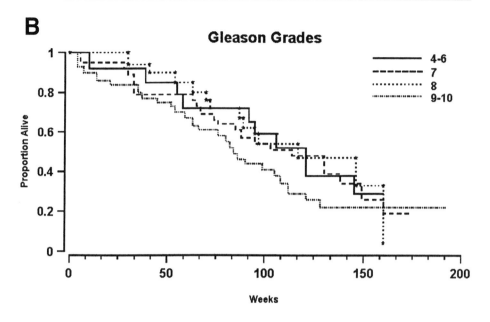

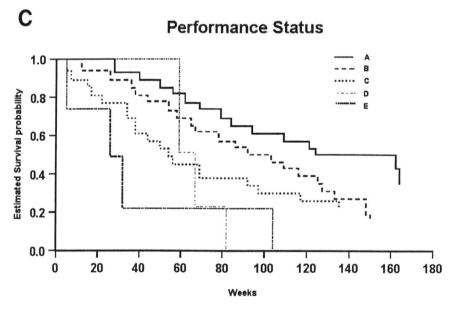

Fig. 3. *Continued.*

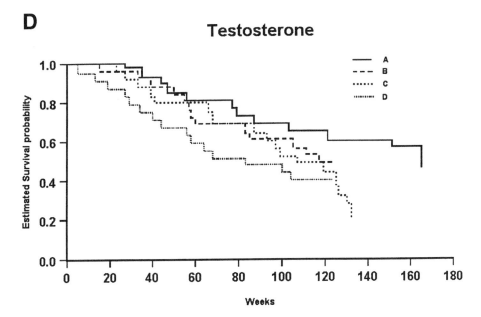

D

Testosterone

(Figure: line graph showing Estimated Survival probability (y-axis, 0.0 to 1.0) versus Weeks (x-axis, 0 to 180) for four curves A, B, C, D)

Fig. 3. *Continued.*

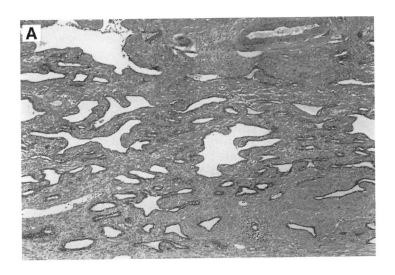

Fig. 4. Histological changes in response to LH-RH therapy. **(A)** Marked atrophy of benign glands in peripheral zone after LH-RH therapy. (H&E). **(B)** Prominence and mild hyperplasia of basal cells after LH-RH therapy. (Immunohistochemistry for high molecular weight cytokeratin LP34). **(C)** Areas of squamous metaplasia within benign prostatic glands after LH-RH therapy (H&E). **(D)** Carcinoma with marked clear cell change after LH-RH therapy. Note also the small nuclei without obvious nucleoli (H&E). **(E)** Early fibrosis and edema of stroma with small residual glands of carcinoma, after LH-RH therapy (H&E). Photographs courtesy of Dr. Michael Jarmulowicz, Senior Lecturer and Honorary Consultant in Histopathology, The Royal Free Medical School and NHS Trust.

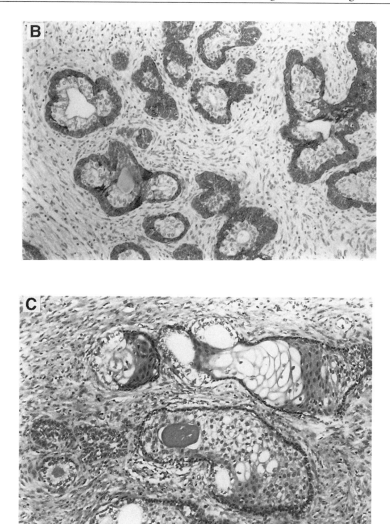

Fig. 4. *Continued.*

changes of cells are seen. In addition, there is condensation of the nucleoli, clearing of the cytoplasm, and often there is a vacuolar change at the luminal surface. The basal cells are not under androgen control and these become much more prominent, and often show basal-cell hyperplasia (Fig. 4B). The atrophy is most marked in the peripheral zone, with less pronounced changes being apparent in areas of nodular hyperplasia. Foci of squamous and transitional metaplasia are also common (Fig. 4C).

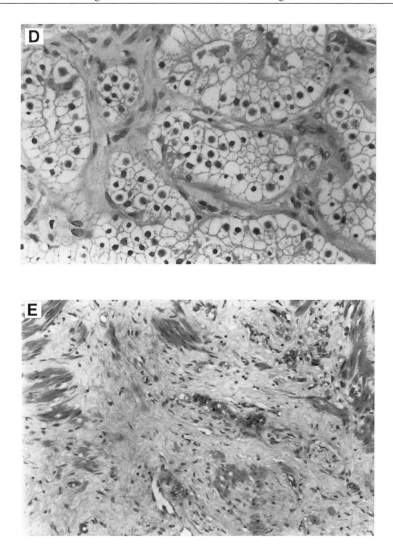

Fig. 4. *Continued.*

3.2. LHRH Effects on Malignant Tumors

The most dramatic effect on malignant glands is a decrease in the tumor-cell size with a corresponding nuclear condensation. The nuclear "atrophy" is also accompanied by a marked decrease in the prominence and size of nucleoli. The cytoplasmic clearing seen in the benign glands is very prominent in the malignant ones (Fig. 4D). The decrease in gland size, often with loss of obvious lumen, makes the glands appear further apart and often as solid nests. Such an architecture is given a higher Gleason score and explains the "upgrading" of tumors after LH-RH therapy. Although some have advocated a different set of criteria for Gleason-grading tumors after androgen blockade, the uncoupling of cytological and architectural appearances of the tumor is characteristic of androgen blockade and rarely causes confusion.

Although apoptosis is defined as programmed cell death without associated inflammation, there is often a lymphocytic infiltrate in areas of tumor. In the early stages there is stromal edema, which in later stages is replaced by fibrosis (Fig. 4E). In a neo-adjuvant (LH-RH agonist) radical prostatectomy, there is often quite marked variation of these changes across the specimen. This may reflect different responses of malignant clones to androgen blockade. Some may have escaped androgen control.

4. ADJUVANT/NEOADJUVANT HORMONE DEPRIVATION THERAPY

Despite the technological and clinical advances in early diagnosis and staging of prostate cancer, clinical understaging occurs in a significant number of patients, possibly in about 50% (17). This finding lead to an ongoing debate with regards to the choice between radical prostatectomy and radiation therapy in management of localized prostate cancer. As it has been recognized that a localized prostatic lesion can be reduced in size by hormonal deprivation (1), the place of pretreatment (neo-adjuvant) or simultaneous treatment (adjuvant) hormonal manipulation could enhance the outcome of the therapeutic modality offered.

4.1. Radiation Therapy

Radiation therapy aims at destroying malignant tissue while causing minimal damage to neighboring normal tissues. Androgen-ablation therapy leads to a reduction of the prostate volume allowing increased radiation dose to the prostate and seminal vesicles. The neighboring normal tissues, namely the bladder and rectum, thus receive less irradiation. Zelefsky and coworkers (18) reported a 25% decrease in the size of the prostate volume after 3 mo of neoadjuvant therapy. This in turn led to a decrease in the volume of the rectum receiving 95% of the prescribed dose from 36 to 30%. The bladder volume receiving 95% of the prescribed dose decreased from 53 to 35%. Comparable results were also reported by Forman et al. (19). In addition, in a randomized comparative trial of neoadjuvant hormone-ablation therapy and radiotherapy vs radiotherapy alone, Pilepich et al. (20) reported significant decrease in local progression (Table 4).

Bolla et al. (21) reported the results of a prospective randomized trial comparing external-beam irradiation alone with external-beam irradiation plus adjuvant treatment with goserelin in 415 patient with locally advanced prostate

Table 4
Androgen Deprivation with Radiation Therapy Compared to Radiation Alone for Locally Advanced Prostatic Carcinoma

Treatment modality	Local (%) progression (5 yr)	Distant metastases (%)	Progression free survival rate (%)
Neoadjuvant therapy + radiotherapy	46	34	36
Radiotherapy alone	71	41	15

Adapted with permission from ref. *(20)*.

Table 5
Improved Survival in Patients with Locally Advanced Prostate Cancer Treated with Radiotherapy and Goserelin

Treatment modality	Overall survival (5 yr)	Deaths	Disease-free survival	Disease pro-gression	5 Yr local control	Time to first treatment failure (yr)	5 Yr failure-free rate
Radiotherapy + Goserelin	79%	35[a]	85%	20 pt	97%	6.6	81%
Radiotherapy alone	62%	58[b]	48%	78 pt	77%	4.4	43%
p value	0.001		< 0.001		< 0.001	< 0.001	

[a] Six due to prostate cancer.

[b] 26 due to prostate cancer.

Adapted with permission from ref. *(21)*.

cancer. Patients in the combined treatment group received goserelin 3.6 mg subcutaneously starting on the first day of irradiation and continuing every 4 wk for 3 yr. The adjuvant treatment group showed improved local control and survival (Table 5).

4.2. Radical Prostatectomy

There is no clear-cut evidence that neoadjuvant therapy prior to radical prostatectomy improves the outcome of relapse compared with those having surgery alone. It is disputed in addition as to when to offer neoadjuvant therapy, in what form, and for how long. Partin et al. in 1997 *(22),* pointed out that 39% of T1c cancers, 52% with palpable abnormality (T2a or greater), 46% of those with a Gleason score of 6 or less and 36% in men with PSA value of 4.0 ng/mL or less, are already beyond the confines of the prostate. These findings

Table 6
Combination Therapies

I. Surgical castration and antiandrgens
    1. Orchidectomy + nilutamide
    2. Orchidectomy + flutamide
    3. Orchidectomy + cyprotrone acetate
    4. Orchidectomy + bicalutamide
II. Medical castration and antiandrogens
    1. Leuprolide + flutamide
    2. Goserelin + flutamide
    3. Busereline + cyprotrone acetate
    4. Goserelin + bicalutamide
III. Estrogens + antiandrogens

could be utilized as a pointer to choose patients for neoadjuvant therapy prior to radical prostatectomy in order to improve the organ-confined harvest. However, an increase in the organ-confined cancers neither necessarily implies an increased cure rate nor guarantees a cure. At present neoadjuvant hormonal therapy in prostate cancer is not a commonly accepted approach *(23)*. The clinical Phase III trials currently conducted have provided until now only preliminary data that do not support the adoption of such regimen as standard policy. It is only right to point out that discussing the various aspects by the treating clinician and individual patient could lead to a decision whether to use therapy prior to surgery or not.

5. COMBINED ANDROGEN BLOCKADE

For decades it has been known that the total available androgens in man include those secreted by the testis and adrenals. Following the observation that all prostate-cancer patients treated with castration eventually relapse, both orchidectomy and adrenalectomy were attempted by Huggins and Scott *(24)*. It was established that the concentration of DHT remained high within the prostate tissue after castration. Investigations of other means to control adrenal androgens stimulating effects were initially reported by Labrie et al. *(25)*. Widespread and enthusiastic studying of this therapeutic approach (Table 6) led to, and still causes, controversial views addressing its value.

The results of all studies addressing this approach have been inconclusive with regards to the value of this regimen. It seems that the greater survival advantage seen with combined androgen blockade is only in those patients with good prognostic profile. This includes minimal or lower tumor burden, good performance status, and perhaps well-differentiated histological grades of tumors. This approach in management has important economic and clinical consequences. Indeed it is far from over that all aspects of combined androgen blockade have been clearly verified and understood.

REFERENCES

1. Huggins C, Hodges CV. Studies on prostatic cancer. The effect of castration, of estrogen and of androgen injection on serum phosphatases in metastatic carcinoma of the prostate. *Cancer Res* 1941; 1:293–297.
2. Mackler MA, et al. The effect of orchidectomy and various doses of stilbestrol on plasma testosterone levels in patients with carcinoma of the prostate. *Invest Urol* 1972; 9:423–425.
3. Schally AV, Arimura A, Baba Y, et al. Isolation and properties of the FSH and LH-releasing hormone. *Biochem Biophys Res Commun* 1971; 43:393–399.
4. Dutta AS, Furr BJA, Giles MB, et al. Gonadotropin-releasing hormone receptors: Characterization, physiological regulation and relationship to reproductive function. *Biochem Biophys Res Commun* 1978; 81:382–390.
5. Kaisary AV, Tyrrell CJ, Peeling WB, Griffiths K. Comparison of LHRH analogue (Zoladex) with orchidectomy in patients with metastatic prostatic carcinoma. *Br J Urol* 1991; 67:502–508.
6. Vogelzang NJ, Chodak GW, Soloway MS, et al. Goserelin versus orchidectomy in the treatment of advanced prostate cancer: final results of a randomized trial. *Urology* 1995; 46:220–226.
7. Allen JM, O'Shea JP, Mashiter K, Williams G, Bloom SR. Advanced carcinoma of the prostate: treatment with a gonadotrophin releasing hormone agonist. *BMJ* 1983; 286:1607–1609.
8. Warner B, Worgul TJ, Drago J, et al. Effect of very high dose D-Leucine 6-gonadotropin releasing hormone proethyl-amide on the hypothalamic pituitary testicular axis in patients with prostate cancer. *J Clin Invest* 1983; 71:1842–1853.
9. Schroder FH, Lock TMTW, Chadha DR, et al. Metastatic cancer of the prostate managed with Buserelin versus Buserelin plus Cyproterone acetate. *J Urol* 1987; 137:912–918.
10. Kuhn JM, Billebaud T, Navratil H, et al. Prevention of the transient adverse effects of gonadotropin-releasing hormone analogue (buserelin) in metastatic prostatic carcinoma by administration of an antiandrogen (nilutamide). *N Engl J Med* 1989; 321:413–418.
11. Mahler C. Is disease flare a problem? *Cancer* 1993; 72(Suppl 12):3799–3802.
12. Faure N, Lemay A, Laroche B, et al. Preliminary results on the clinical efficacy and safety of androgen inhibition by an LHRH agonist alone or combined with an antiandrogen in the treatment of prostatic carcinoma *Prostate* 1983; 4:601–624.
13. Lunglmayr G, Girsch E. "Zoladex" – a new treatment for prostatic cancer, in (Chisholm GD, ed). International Congress and Symposium series, 125. Royal Society of Medicine Series, London 1987, pp 27–44.
14. Soloway MS, Cassileth BR, Vozelgang NJ, Schellhammer PS, Seidmon EJ, Kennealey GT. Patient's choice of treatment in stage D prostate cancer, in *Recent Advances in Urological Cancers Diagnosis and Treatment.* (Hendry, W. F., ed) Churchill-Livingstone, Paris 1990, pp 72–74.
15. Kaisary AV. 1991, unpublished data.
16. Kaisary AV, Bowsher WG, Gillatt DA, Anderson JB, Malone PR, Cesana M. Two 6-month sustained release depots of Avorelin, a new LHRH agonist: preliminary endocrinological and pharmacokinetic results in prostate cancer patients. *J Urol* 1999; 162:2019–2023.
17. Epstein J. Evaluation of radical prostatectomy capsular margins of resection: the significance of margins designated as negative, closely approaching and positive. *Am J Surg Pathol* 1990; 14:626–632.
18. Zelefsky MJ, Leibel SA, Kutcher GT, Harrison J, Happersett I, Fuks Z. Neoadjuvant hormones improve therapeutic ratio in patients with bulky carcinoma of the prostate treated with conformal radiation therapy. *Intl J Radiat Oncol Biol Phys* 1994; 29:755–761.

19. Forman JD, Kumar R, Hass G, Montie J, Porter AT, Mesina CF. Effect of neoadjuvant hormonal therapy on prostate size *Cancer Invest* 1995; 13:8–15.
20. Pilepich MV, Sause WT, Shipley WV, et al. Androgen deprivation with radiation therapy compared to radiation alone for locally advanced prostatic carcinoma: a randomised comparative trial of the Radiation Therapy Oncology Group. *Urology* 1995; 45:616–622.
21. Bolla M, Gonzales D, Wade P, Dubois JB, Mirimanoff RO, Storme G, et al. Improved survival in patients with locally advanced prostate cancer treated with radiotherapy and goserelin. *N Engl J Med* 1997; 337:295–300.
22. Partin AW, Kattan MW, Subong EN, Walsh PC, Wonjo KJ, Oesterling JE, et al. Combination of prostate-specific antigen, clinical stage, and Gleason score to predict pathological stage of localised prostate cancer. *JAMA* 1997; 277:1445–1451.
23. Abbass F, Scardino PT. Why neoandrogen deprivation prior to radical prostatectomy is unnecessary *Urol Clin North Am* 1996; 23:587–604.
24. Huggins C, Scott WW. Bilateral adrenalectomy in prostatic cancer; clinical features and urinary excretion of 17 – Ketosteroids and estrogen. *Ann Surg* 1945; 122:1031–1041.
25. Labrie F, Dupont A, Belanger A, et al. Combination therapy with flutamide and castration (LHRH agonist or orchidectomy) In advanced prostate cancer: a marked improvement in response and survival. *J Steroid Biochem* 1985; 23:833–842.

V PERSPECTIVE ON PROGRESS

18 Recent Progress in Breast Cancer Research

V. Craig Jordan and Barrington J. A. Furr

CONTENTS

1. INTRODUCTION

The goal of this final chapter is to highlight several important advances in basic and clinical research that may prove to be pivotal advances for the new millenium. Although it is not possible to be all-inclusive, we have selected advances that could be viewed as the most valuable for the control of hormone-dependent disease. We have developed our theme as advances in the clinic that exploit the strategic use of hormonal intervention followed by advances in laboratory research that provide an insight into the molecular mechanisms of antihormone action. We will consider advances in breast cancer as a model for future targeted therapies.

From: *Hormone Therapy in Breast and Prostate Cancer*
Edited by: V. C. Jordan and B. J. A. Furr © Humana Press Inc., Totowa, NJ

2. CHEMOPREVENTION OF BREAST CANCER

The National Surgical Adjuvant Breast and bowel Project (NSABP) P-1 study *(1)* was opened in 1992 with a primary endpoint of determining whether the use of tamoxifen for five years reduced the incidence of invasive breast carcinoma in high-risk women. Risk was calculated using the Gail model *(2)*, which includes age, age of menarche, parity and age at first live birth, number of first-degree relatives with breast cancer, number of breast biopsies, and a diagnosis of atypical hyperplasia. Prior to the NSABP P-1 trial, this model had been shown to predict risk accurately in two validation studies of women undergoing annual mammographic screening *(3,4)*. However, it is not a useful model for assessing risk in women with a strong family history of breast cancer suggestive of a genetic mutation, since it only includes first-degree relatives. The accuracy of the Gail model was examined using data from the 5969 white women in the placebo arm of the P-1 prevention trial *(5)*. After an average follow up of 48.4 mo, the ratio of expected to observed invasive cancers was 1.03 (95% CI 0.88–1.21) and 0.84 (95% CI 0.73–0.97) for both invasive and *in situ* cancers. In absolute numbers, the model predicted 159 invasive cancers and 155 occurred, indicating that the model is a clinically useful tool for counseling women about risk and identifying high-risk subjects for prevention interventions.

One of the most remarkable findings of the P-1 trial *(1)* is the consistent benefit of tamoxifen across all groups studied. A total of 368 invasive and noninvasive breast cancers occurred in the study participants, 124 in women on tamoxifen and 244 in those in the placebo group. Overall, a 49% reduction in the risk of invasive carcinoma was seen in the tamoxifen group (Fig. 1), a figure remarkably similar to the 47% reduction in contralateral breast cancer reported in the Overview Analysis *(6)*. A 50% reduction in noninvasive breast cancer (ductal carcinoma *in situ,* DCIS) was also observed in those receiving tamoxifen (Fig. 1), which is consistent with recent reports about the treatment of DCIS with tamoxifen *(7)*. Tamoxifen was found to be of benefit in all age groups, with relative risks ranging from 0.56 in women age 49 and younger, 0.49 for women age 50 to 59, and 0.45 for those age 60 and older. Although all women included in this study were defined as being at increased risk of breast cancer, a benefit was seen for all levels of risk within the study. Those at the lowest level of increased risk (≤ 2% over 5 yr) had a 63% reduction in breast-cancer risk, compared to 66% for those at the highest level of increased risk (≥ 5.01% over 5 yr). Women at risk on the basis of a family history of breast cancer, as well as those at risk due to other factors, were found to benefit from treatment. A particular benefit was observed in women at risk on the basis of lobular carcinoma *in situ* (LCIS) or atypical hyperplasia. In an updated analysis of this subgroup *(8)*, treatment with tamoxifen reduced risk by 65% in those with LCIS and 86% in those with atypical hyperplasia. In addition, the benefits

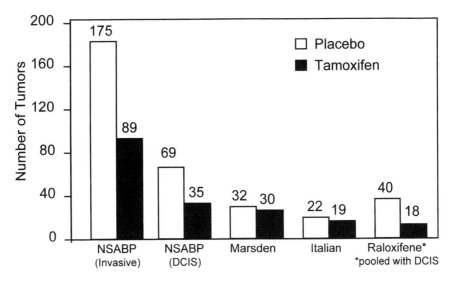

Fig. 1. A comparison of the studies to reduce the incidence of breast cancer. The NSABP P-1 trial is the only completed prospective clinical trial designed to test the value of an antiestrogen in preventing breast cancer in 13,388 high-risk women, selected on a validated mathematical risk model. The figure illustrates the effect of tamoxifen on both invasive and noninvasive (ductal carcinoma *in situ;* DCIS) breast cancer. By contrast, the Royal Marsden Study is a pilot project, and was stated to be a toxicity evaluation in 2,471 women at lower risk than the NSABP Study. These women were selected based on first-degree relatives with breast cancer. The Italian Study is from 3,984 normal-risk women, half of whom had already had an oophorectomy. Finally, the raloxifene result is estimated from published abstracts and is a secondary endpoint from 10,553 postmenopausal women around 70 yr of age who were participating in osteoporosis trials. The results for raloxifene are for both invasive and noninvasive breast cancer, but an effect of raloxifene on reducing DCIS alone has not been found because the events are too few.

of tamoxifen were consistent over time, with no evidence of diminution as the length of follow-up increased. Thus, the reduction in breast-cancer incidence was 55% in year two of the study, 49% in year four, and 55% in year six.

3. SECONDARY ENDPOINTS

The secondary aims of the NSABP study were to determine the effects of tamoxifen on the incidence of fractures of the hip, spine, and radius, and on the incidence of ischemic heart disease. Overall, 483 women in the placebo group and 472 in the tamoxifen group had fractures. Osteoporotic fractures occurred in 137 women on placebo and 111 on tamoxifen, a 19% reduction (RR 0.81; 95% CI 0.63–1.05). The greatest reduction was seen in hip fractures, where a 45% decrease was noted in women taking tamoxifen. Not surprisingly, the greatest reduction in fractures was seen in women age 50 or greater at study entry. Overall, these findings are consistent with the observations that tamoxifen increases bone density *(9)*. The lack of a statistically significant reduction in fracture incidence is most likely due to the fact that only 3995 of the 6681 women assigned to receive tamoxifen were age 50 or older, and only 1964 were age 60 or older. Thus, the number of women at significant risk for osteoporotic fracture receiving tamoxifen was relatively low.

No differences in the incidence of ischemic heart disease were observed. Overall, the annual rate of ischemic disease was 2.37 per 1000 in the placebo group and 2.73 per 1000 in the tamoxifen group. When myocardial infarction, fatal myocardial infarction, angina requiring angioplasty or surgery, and acute ischemic syndromes were considered individually, no differences between the placebo and tamoxifen groups were noted. However, unlike hormone-replacement therapy that is associated with an early increase in deaths from myocardial infarction before benefits are eventually observed, no early increase in the deaths are observed with tamoxifen *(10)*.

4. OTHER STUDIES OF TAMOXIFEN FOR PREVENTION

Although the results of the P-1 trial *(1)* were strongly positive and consistent with the laboratory data *(11)* and findings with contralateral breast cancer from the Overview *(6)*, the publication of two other studies that showed no decrease in breast-cancer incidence in women taking tamoxifen *(12,13)* raised significant questions regarding its efficacy. The Italian prevention trial *(13)* randomized 5408 of the planned 20,000 women aged 35–70 to tamoxifen 20 mg daily or placebo. There was no requirement for an increased level of breast-cancer risk to enter the study, and participants were required to have had a hysterectomy. Those women who had a premenopausal bilateral oophorectomy and hysterectomy (47% of participants) were actually at a reduced risk of breast-cancer development. The relatively low risk level of the participants in the study is evident from the breast-cancer incidence in the placebo arm of the study, 2.3 per 1,000 (compared to 6.7/1000 in the NSABP trial), and the small number of total cancers in the study, 41. In addition, although 5408 women were randomized, 1422 withdrew from the study and only 149 completed 5 yr of treatment. The failure of this study to demonstrate a benefit of tamoxifen is readily explained by its lack of statistical power due to small sample size, high dropout rate, and low level of baseline risk in the population studied. Nevertheless, those women who were taking estrogen-replacement therapy had a significant increase in breast cancer compared with those taking estrogen plus tamoxifen. This is a demonstration that tamoxifen can prevent estrogen-induced tumorigenesis.

The other report that failed to demonstrate a benefit for tamoxifen was from the Royal Marsden Hospital *(12)*. This study recruited 2484 women aged 30–70 who took tamoxifen 20 mg daily or placebo for up to 8 yr. Risk was primarily determined on the basis of a family history of breast cancer. Although the trial was initially described as a pilot study to evaluate toxicity *(14)*, it was subsequently analyzed for breast-cancer incidence. After a median follow-up of 70 mo, 70 breast cancers had occurred, with no difference in incidence between the tamoxifen and placebo arms. This study differed from the NSABP trial in that participants were younger and were allowed to use hormone-replacement therapy during the study. The authors reported that pedigree analysis of study participants was consistent with a high proportion of BRCA1 and two mutation carriers, leading them to hypothesize that the negative study results could indicate that tamoxifen chemoprevention is ineffective in this subgroup of women *(12)*. This explanation seems unlikely, since the breast-cancer incidence in the placebo arm of the study was only 5.5 per 1000, lower than that seen in the NSABP trial, and not suggestive of a study population enriched with carriers of a genetic mutation. Overall, the NSABP trial with its 46,858 women years of follow-up and 264 invasive malignancies is considerably more robust than the Royal Marsden and Italian studies, which together have only 103 malignant events as illustrated in Fig. 1. In addition, the NSABP trial is the only one of the three studies that was designed to be a definitive prevention trial, and the study results are completely consistent with data from the laboratory and the Overview Analysis. More recently, publication of the NSABP B 24 trial, in which women with DCIS were treated with excision and irradiation and randomized to tamoxifen 20 mg daily for 5 yr or placebo *(7)*, provides further confirmation of these results. The B 24 study demonstrates a 37% reduction in the risk of invasive and noninvasive breast cancer events in women taking tamoxifen. The somewhat smaller magnitude of benefit in this study in comparison to the prevention trial is consistent with the fact that DCIS lesions have progressed further along the pathway to the fully malignant phenotype than atypical hyperplasia or LCIS and would not be expected to be as responsive to a chemopreventive agent.

5. OTHER CONCERNS IN TAMOXIFEN PREVENTION

The use of tamoxifen for prevention has given rise to a number of concerns, many of which can be addressed with currently available data. The first of these is that since tamoxifen reduces the incidence of estrogen receptor (ER)-positive breast cancer, its use will increase the amount of poor prognosis, ER-negative breast cancer. Although the NSABP study confirms that tamoxifen reduces the annual rate of ER-positive breast cancer by 69%, it shows no difference in the incidence of ER-negative tumors *(1)*. In addition, there was no increase in the number of cancers with positive axillary nodes or those greater than 2.0 cm in size in the tamoxifen-treated group. Thus, although the *proportion* of ER-negative tumors will be higher in a population of women treated with tamoxifen, the *absolute number* will be unchanged.

The other major concern regarding tamoxifen is its toxicity. The most serious toxicities are an increased incidence of endometrial carcinoma and an increased risk of thrombotic vascular events. Although tamoxifen has been used to treat endometrial cancer, it is clear that the drug increases the incidence of the disease. In the P-1 trial, women taking tamoxifen had 2.5 times greater risk of developing endometrial carcinoma (95% CI 1.35–4.97) than those on placebo. The only significant increase in risk was in women age 50 and older. No excess of endometrial cancers was observed in younger women. Overall, the absolute increase in endometrial cancer was from 0.91 per 1000 women in the placebo group to 2.3 per 1000 in the tamoxifen group. All of the endometrial cancers in the tamoxifen group were Stage I. A review of the published literature on endometrial cancer associated with tamoxifen (15) confirms that these tumors do not differ in grade or stage from those occurring in the general population. Bernstein and co-authors (16) examined the relationship between tamoxifen use and known risk factors for endometrial cancer and found that both prior estrogen replacement and higher body-mass index were associated with a greater risk of endometrial cancer in tamoxifen-treated women. In the absence of these factors, the risk of endometrial cancers in women taking tamoxifen was quite low.

A recent epidemiology study in Holland has noted increases in endometrial cancer in postmenopausal patients treated with tamoxifen. However, unlike data derived from clinical trials, the authors claim an increase in poor grade disease associated with tamoxifen (17). The epidemiology study could be criticized because the database draws upon cases in the decade before the association between tamoxifen and endometrial cancer was well known. Today, gynecologic surveillance is an integral part of women's health and it would be unlikely that women who elected to use tamoxifen as a chemopreventive would not have annual gynecologic examinations.

Tamoxifen has also been noted to increase the incidence of thromboembolic events, although this increase in risk is seen only in women age 50 and older. In the prevention trial (1), significant increases in the risk of deep venous thrombosis (RR 1.71) and pulmonary embolism (RR 3.19) were seen in postmenopausal women. An excess of strokes was also seen, although this difference was not statistically significant. In addition to an increased risk of endometrial carcinoma and thromboembolic events, a marginally significant increase in cataract formation and an increase in cataract surgery were seen in tamoxifen-treated women. The rate of cataract development increased from 21.72 per 1000 in the placebo arm to 24.82 in the tamoxifen arm, and the use of cataract surgery increased from 3.0 to 4.72 per 1000 women.

While major toxicities of tamoxifen are rare, symptoms that may affect quality of life are more common. An analysis of 13,388 participants (82.6% of total accrual) in the P-1 trial was carried out to assess quality of life (18).

Significant increases in vasomotor and gynecologic symptoms such as vaginal discharge were noted in the tamoxifen group. Overall, no differences in scores on a depression scale or a short-form health-status survey were seen. This study also failed to confirm any increase in weight gain and depression, two problems anecdotally associated with tamoxifen therapy. A similar conclusion has recently been published (19) by analyzing the quality of life in the Marsden and ongoing International Breast Intervention Study.

6. FUTURE DIRECTIONS

The publication of the NSABP prevention trial was the culmination of three decades of laboratory and clinical investigation, and provides a valuable option for women at increased risk for breast cancer. However, many questions remain to be answered. These include the duration of benefit from a 5 yr course of tamoxifen for prevention. Clearly, the Overview Analysis indicates that benefit lasts for at least 5 yr after the drug is stopped, and 10 yr data will be available shortly. Does tamoxifen "imprint" the breast permanently? Is ongoing exposure to estrogen (i.e., menopausal status) a factor in determining the duration of benefit? What is the optimal time in a woman's life to give tamoxifen? Serious side effects are less frequent in younger women, but does this leave them at risk later in life when the baseline incidence of breast cancer is higher? Are we giving the optimal dose of tamoxifen or are we giving too much? The dose used in the chemoprevention trial (20 mg daily) was based on experience with the use of tamoxifen as a breast-cancer therapy, but could a much lower dose, say 10 mg 3 times a week, be just as effective in postmenopausal women? Pilot studies demonstrate that lower-dose treatment may be appropriate for future chemoprevention studies (20–23). Finally, are there more effective agents than tamoxifen? A decade ago, when selective ER modulation was first recognized (24–26), a paradigm shift occurred for drug development that has had important implications for breast-cancer prevention in postmenopausal women whose major breast-cancer risk factor is age. If tamoxifen, an anti-breast cancer drug, could maintain bone density and lower circulating levels of cholesterol, why not develop a drug to prevent osteoporosis that would prevent breast cancer as a beneficial side effect (27). The new strategy was simply stated:

> we have obtained valuable clinical information about this group of drugs that can be applied in other disease states. Research does not travel in straight lines and observations in one field of science often become major discoveries in another. Important clues have been garnered about the effects of tamoxifen on bone and lipids so it is possible that derivatives could find targeted applications to retard osteoporosis or atherosclerosis. The ubiquitous application of novel compounds to

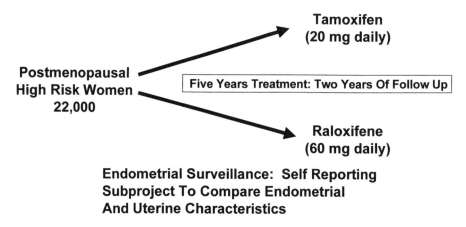

Fig. 2. The study of tamoxifen and raloxifene (STAR) is recruiting 22,000 high-risk post-menopausal women to be randomized to tamoxifen (20 mg/daily) or raloxifene (60 mg/daily). Risk is determined using the Gail Model. Recruitment is ongoing and should be completed by 2003. Results will be available 5 yr later.

prevent diseases associated with the progressive changes after menopause may, as a side effect, significantly retard the development of breast cancer. The target population would be postmenopausal women in general, thereby avoiding the requirement to select a high-risk group to prevent breast cancer *(27)*.

Raloxifene is the practical result of this strategy. Raloxifene is approved for the prevention of osteoporosis *(28),* but an evaluation of the incidence of breast cancer in study participants shows a decrease in women taking ralox-ifene compared with placebo (Fig. 1) *(29)*. However, breast-cancer incidence was a secondary endpoint of this study, and the breast cancer-risk status of the participants is unknown. The Study of Tamoxifen and Raloxifene (STAR) trial *(30)* (Fig. 2) will provide a definitive comparison of the risks and benefits of both drugs in a population of high-risk postmenopausal women. Raloxifene is not available for use in premenopausal women.

In the interim, tamoxifen is a viable option for breast-cancer-risk reduction in women at increased risk. Women must weigh the risks and benefits of tamoxifen chemoprevention against their personal level of breast-cancer risk and the alternatives of close observation or prophylactic mastectomy. A woman's overall health status is a critical component of this discussion. While all women who meet the risk criteria of the P-1 prevention trial will not choose to take tamoxifen, it is a particularly attractive option for women with LCIS or atypical hyperplasia, premenopausal women at increased risk, and post-menopausal women who have had a hysterectomy.

7. TREATMENT WITH ANTIHORMONES

Tamoxifen is the endocrine treatment of choice for all stages of ER-positive breast cancer *(6,31)*. However, we are now in a position to assess the overall impact of tamoxifen treatment through a continuing evaluation of the randomized clinical trials in the Oxford Overview Analysis. The recent analysis (September 2000) confirms the continuing effectiveness of tamoxifen as an adjuvant therapy in ER-positive, node-positive, and node-negative pre- and postmenopausal patients with breast cancer. Remarkably, tamoxifen continues to be effective for at least 10 yr after adjuvant therapy is stopped. This clinical observation naturally leads to the question of a mechanism for the long-term beneficial actions of tamoxifen. Some clues have recently been published from laboratory models. This new concept is addressed in the next section.

The success of tamoxifen has naturally lead to advances in therapeutics to avoid premature drug resistance. It is generally believed that drug resistance to tamoxifen occurs because of the intrinsic estrogen-like properties of the molecule. Tamoxifen-stimulated breast-cancer cells are selected for growth and, as a result, treatment fails.

A current strategy is to develop less estrogen-like modalities as first-line treatment. The pure antiestrogen Faslodex® has successfully been tested as a treatment for advanced breast cancer *(32,33)*, as has anastrozole *(34,35)* and the aromatase inhibitors anastrozole (Arimidex®), letrozole and exemestane are currently being evaluated against tamoxifen as an adjuvant therapy. A pivotal trial called Arimidex®, tamoxifen alone or in combination (ATAC) has randomized more than 9000 patients to receive 5 yr of tamoxifen, anastrazole, or the combination. Results will be available in late 2001. Since these treatment strategies, i.e., pure antiestrogens or aromatase inhibitors, do not have intrinsic estrogenic effects in the uterus, there will not be an increase in endometrial cancer as a side effect of therapy.

8. MODELS FOR DRUG RESISTANCE

There are still many gaps in our knowledge about drug resistance and new translational models are needed to explore the clinical issue of drug resistance to selective estrogen receptor modulators (SERMs) in patients. To this end, one of the authors (VCJ) has made a commitment to develop new models of SERM resistance to breast and endometrial cancer in vivo so that cross-resistance to tamoxifen can be evaluated for any new agent before valuable clinical resources are committed to national trials.

All current investigators of tamoxifen-stimulated breast-cancer growth are focused on the MCF-7 breast-cancer-cell line *(36),* but there is a requirement for diversity so that the multiplicity of drug-resistance pathways that are possible can be studied. About a quarter of breast cancers are mutated in the p53 gene so it would be reasonable to create a laboratory model to study the observation that patients with p53 mutations fail tamoxifen more rapidly *(37)*. Additionally, endometrial cancers that occur during long-term tamoxifen therapy are also mutant for p53 *(17)*. MCF-7 cells contain wild-type p53, and it is generally found that estrogen withdrawal produces a variety of cell lines that are estrogen independent for growth but retain ER and are still responsive to antiestrogens *(38–40)*. In contrast, the ER positive T47D breast cancer-cell line *(41)* is mutated for p53 and loses ER under conditions of estrogen withdrawal *(42)*. We chose to determine whether we could establish a new model of drug resistance to tamoxifen with the T47D cell line transplanted into athymic mice. Earlier studies had suggested that the cells were not only estrogen-responsive for growth but also required a pituitary factor for optimal growth *(43)*. Additionally, we hypothesized that tamoxifen would cause a rapid change from ER-positive to ER-negative *(42)*. We were incorrect, as transplantable estrogen-responsive tumors were rapidly converted to tamoxifen-stimulated tumors that retained the ER during high-dose (1.5 mg tamoxifen orally per day) tamoxifen treatment. The decrease in cell-cycle control through mutated p53 could potentially be the reason for the rapid failure of tamoxifen treatment both clinically and in the T47D model *(44)*. We are using the new model to classify novel SERMs *(45,46)*.

It is important to improve on tamoxifen because drugs that are clearly cross-resistant may be inappropriate for clinical use. We have already noted that unlike Faslodex® (ICI 182,780) which is not cross-resistant with tamoxifen in either model (or the tamoxifen-stimulated endometrial-cancer model *[47]*), other triphenylethylenes, toremifene or idoxifene, are cross-resistant *(45)*. The new SERMs related to raloxifene have mixed effects and display cross-resistance in some models but not others *(46)*.

The Overview Analysis *(6)* clearly demonstrated the beneficial effects of 5 yr of adjuvant tamoxifen treatment both for node-negative and node-positive patients. There is a significantly improved disease-free and overall survival in women treated with tamoxifen, and the beneficial effects are observed for up to 10 yr of follow-up. Based on these data, the question could be raised that if 5 yr of treatment is superior to shorter treatment periods, why stop tamoxifen at 5 yr, and why not propose the antiestrogen for a longer duration of treatment *(48)?* The NSABP *(49)* addressed this question by studying the effects of 5 vs more than 5 yr of tamoxifen treatment for breast cancer in ER-positive, lymph-node-negative patients. Using the data from the B-14 study, as well as recruiting other patients with the same criteria, the following important observations were made: 1) significantly better disease-free, distant disease-free, and overall survival at 10 yr was found in patients treated with tamoxifen for 5 yr compared to 5 yr of placebo; 2) tamoxifen therapy was associated with a 37% reduction in the incidence of contralateral breast cancer; and 3) advantages in disease-free and dis-

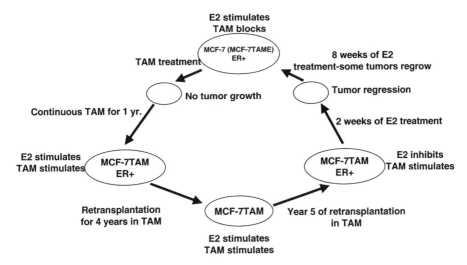

Fig. 3. Cyclical model of tumor sensitivity to TAM over a 5-yr period. MCF-7 breast tumors are ER-positive and respond to E_2, but TAM blocks this E_2-stimulated growth. After 1 yr of continuous TAM treatment, however, the tumors respond to both E_2 and TAM (MCF-7;TAM). After 4 yr of TAM treatment, the tumors are exclusively TAM-dependent, and 2 wk of E_2 treatment results in complete tumor regression. After 6–8 wk of E_2 treatment, some tumors will regrow, and these have reverted back to the original MCF-7 phenotype, with E_2 stimulating growth and TAM blocking this E_2-stimulated growth.

tant disease-free survival were found in patients who discontinued tamoxifen therapy at 5 yr compared to patients taking tamoxifen for 10 yr.

It is possible that tamoxifen-stimulated drug resistance occurs with more than 5 yr of adjuvant tamoxifen treatment, but the question could also be asked "Why does five years of tamoxifen confer a long-term survival advantage despite stopping tamoxifen?" A woman's endogenous estrogen would be expected to reactivate any residual ER-positive breast-cancer cells.

Until recently there was no model of long-term tamoxifen therapy. The MCF-7 models described previously *(50,51)* are representative of the development of drug resistance during the treatment of advanced breast cancer with tamoxifen. On average, tamoxifen therapy is effective for approximately 1 yr. To address this deficiency, we serially transplanted MCF-7 tamoxifen-stimulated tumors into tamoxifen-treated mice for up to 5 yr *(52)*.

Based on extensive laboratory studies on the actions of E_2 and tamoxifen on tumor-growth regulation, we propose the following sequential stages of hormone sensitivity in breast cancer that appear to follow a 5-yr cycle (Fig. 3): 1) tamoxifen acts as an antiestrogen by blocking tumor growth; 2) tamoxifen-stimulated tumors occur, and these tumors can grow with either tamoxifen or

E_2; 3) eventually only tamoxifen stimulates tumor growth, but E_2 causes a dramatic regression of tumor size; 4) E_2 subsequently stimulates the regrowth of some tumors, but tamoxifen blocks E_2 stimulated growth. In our study, only physiological doses (premenopausal levels) of estrogen were used to prevent tumor growth, to induce tumor regression, or to stimulate tumor growth. We suggest that the repeated transplantation of these tumors into tamoxifen-treated animals has resulted in the selection of a MCF-7 tumor that is now supersensitive to the cytotoxic effects of estrogen.

Overall, this new model system of changing hormonal sensitivity in breast cancer can be applied to provide an insight into the long-term control of breast cancer relapse following 5 yr of adjuvant tamoxifen. We suggest that if the micrometastases around a woman's body become supersensitized to the actions of estrogen by tamoxifen, then a women's own estrogen may provoke an antitumor effect after 5 yr of tamoxifen treatment (52). The conclusions would also imply that patients could benefit from tamoxifen rechallange following recurrence several years after their adjuvant therapy. Clearly, these conclusions should be tested in clinical trials.

9. A SELECTION OF SERMS

The successful development of tamoxifen as a breast-cancer preventive, and the introduction of raloxifene to prevent osteoporosis, has encouraged the investigation of "new" molecules that may have unforeseen advantages. Droloxifene, 3-hydroxytamoxifen, and idoxifene (Fig. 4) are similar molecules to tamoxifen that potentially have multiple applications as SERMs. Droloxifene is active as an estrogen-like agent in rat bone (53), but has activity in the clinic (54) as a breast-cancer drug. Similarly, idoxifene is active in rat bone (55) and is an antitumor agent in models of breast cancer (56).

The compounds listed in Fig. 5 (with the exception of ICI 182,780) can potentially be applied either as breast-cancer therapies or as agents for osteoporosis or both. The drugs GW 5638 (Fig. 4) and CP 336,156 (Fig. 5) are both particularly interesting because they maintain bone density in animals (57,58) and could find an application as preventives for osteoporosis but with the potential to prevent breast cancer (59) because of their structural similarity to tamoxifen and nafoxidine, respectively. Furthermore, the new SERM LY 353385 (60) is designed to be more bioavailable than raloxifene, which is only 2% (61) so that a more sustained blood level can be maintained. The compound is in clinical trial for breast cancer (62). However, the new drug EM-652 currently being developed by Schering-Plough is a surprise. The compound has been evaluated rigorously in animal models and is classified as an orally active pure antiestrogen because the molecule silences both AF1 and AF2 in ERα (63). The formula of the drug is drawn in the publications to show a structural similarity to the pure antiestrogen ICI 182, 780 (64).

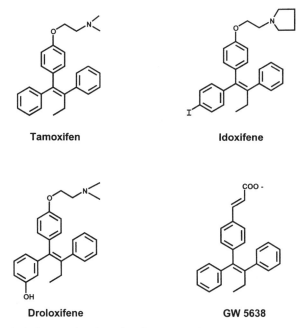

Tamoxifen

Idoxifene

Droloxifene

GW 5638

Fig. 4. Triphenylethylene molecules related to tamoxifen that have been evaluated as selective ER modulators in bone and breast. Neither compound is being pursued for further clinical development.

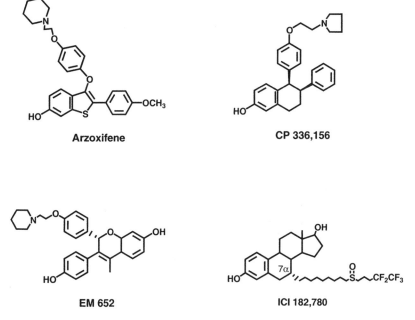

Arzoxifene

CP 336,156

EM 652

ICI 182,780

Fig. 5. Nonsteroidal compounds under active laboratory and clinical evaluation as selective estrogen receptor modulators. The steroidal compound ICI 182,780 (Faslodex®) being evaluated as a pure antiestrogen for breast-cancer treatment.

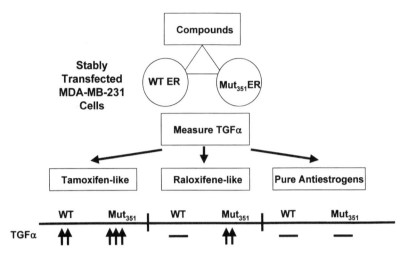

Fig. 6. Antiestrogens can be classified by their interaction with the ER. Tamoxifen analogs with a similar side chain are promiscuous and readily activate the TGF-α gene in MDA-MB-231 cells stably transfected with cDNAs for ER. Raloxifene analogs have increased estrogenicity with a mutated ER (Asp351Tyr) because this changes the protein conformation to increase activating functions. Pure antiestrogens are not affected by the ER mutation at 351.

We have developed an assay system in vitro that can distinguish between tamoxifen-like compounds, raloxifene-like compounds, and pure antiestrogens (Fig. 6). The assay depends on the differential regulation of the transforming growth factor-α (TGF-α) via wild-type and Asp351Tyr mutant ER *(65–67)*. EM-652 is reclassified as a raloxifene-like compound *(68)* and not a pure antiestrogen. The compound EM-652 may not have use as a second-line drug after tamoxifen failure, but there is potential to prevent coronary heart disease and/or osteoporosis if toxicity in preliminary studies proves acceptable. EM-652 has recently been shown to preserve bone density in rats *(69)*, thus validating the laboratory-assay system. Since new SERMs can now be rapidly classified based on functional assays, only selected agents need to be crystallized to confirm the biologic data. This approach to drug discovery will make clinical testing of compounds more predictable in the future.

10. A MOLECULAR MECHANISM OF SERM ACTION

Over the past five years, new models to describe the interaction of raloxifene and tamoxifen have been developed through a combination of X-ray crystallography and structure-function relationships of the ER. It is not possible to crystallize the whole ER for technical reasons, but a shortened ligand-binding domain has been crystallized with estradiol, diethylstilbestrol

(DES) raloxifene, and 4-hydroxytamoxifen *(70,71)*. Similarly, the ligand-binding domain of ERβ crystallized with raloxifene *(72)* and the pure antiestrogen ICI 164,384 *(73)* have been reported. The findings advance earlier structure function studies that proposed that estrogens are locked within the ligand-binding domain to cause activation of the ER complex, but the side chain of antiestrogens wedges the ligand-binding domain open so the ER is not fully activated *(74,75)*.

X-ray crystallography demonstrated that estrogens are bounded within the hydrophobic ligand-binding domain and helix 12 folds across the top of the pocket sealing the estrogen inside. The correct positioning of helix 12 now permits coactivator binding so that estrogen-responsive genes can be transcribed *(70,71)* (*see* Chapter 3). In contrast, raloxifene does not permit the locking of the ligand within the hydrophobic pocket and helix 12 is repositioned in the site on the surface of the ER normally occupied by a coactivator. 4-Hydroxytamoxifen produces a similar repositioning of helix 12, but there are subtle differences in the structures of the ER complex *(71)* that can explain the differences in the estrogen-like properties of tamoxifen when compared to raloxifene. X-ray crystallography revealed an intimate connection between the antiestrogenic side chain of raloxifene and amino acid 351 aspartate in the ligand-binding domain of ER *(70)*. However, the side chain of 4-hydroxytamoxifen is not as close to aspartate 351 *(71)* (Fig. 7). We propose that the remaining negative charge that surrounds the surface amino acid aspartate in the 4-hydroxytamoxifen: ER complex is the key to the estrogen-like actions of the complex. This, we reason, could form the basis for a novel binding site for coactivators and explain the promiscuous estrogen-like effects of 4-hydroxytamoxifen compared to raloxifene. However, it had previously been suggested that the estrogen-like actions of 4-hydroxytamoxifen was because activating functions (AF1) at the far end of the ER from the ligand-binding domain was constitutive and unaffected by ligands *(76)*. We have addressed these issues through a study of structure-function relationships of mutated ERs at target genes based on an initial observation of a naturally mutated ER discovered in a tamoxifen-stimulated tumor *(77)*.

A single-point mutation in the cDNA for ER was detected in a MCF-7 tamoxifen-stimulated tumor line using single-stranded conformational polymorphism *(78)*. This resulted in a D351Y change in the amino acid sequence. However, the mutation was outside the traditional AF2 region of the ligand binding domain, and studies using techniques of transient transfection and artificial reporter genes show very little changes in intrinsic activity for tamoxifen and raloxifene ER complexes when compared with estradiol *(79)*. In contrast, the structure-function relationship of wild-type and mutant ERs using stable transfection of cDNAs was evaluated in the ER-negative breast-cancer-cell line MDA-MB-231 *(80)*. The rationale for the use of MDA-MB-231 cells was

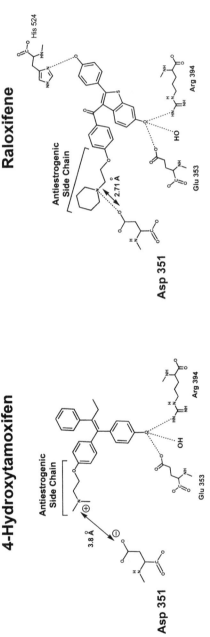

Fig. 7. Diagram based on the crystal structure of the ER LBD complexed with either E_2, 4-OHT or Ral. The amino acids that interact with the lig- and have been identified, and bond lengths, when important, have been noted. The significant difference between E_2 and the antiestrogens is the interaction with aspartate 351. However, the antiestrogenic side chain of Ral appears to be closer than is possible for the side chain for 4-OHT. We propose that this is an important difference between 4-OHT and Ral complexes that could result in an increased E_2-like action of the 4-OHT:ER complex.

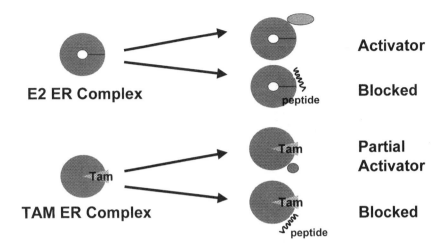

Fig. 8. A diagrammatic representation of the hypothesis *(82)* that coactivators bind to the estradiol ER complex at a different place than the tamoxifen ER complex to initiate gene transduction. These data were generated using random phage-display technology with peptides to block coactivator action. Different peptides were discovered that blocked coactivators for the different complexes.

that they would be replete with transcription factors relevant to breast cancer. Additionally, it was found that the complex promoter for TGF-α could be activated by ER *(81)* so this was selected as the gene target *in situ.*

We found that there was a profound difference between tamoxifen and raloxifene ER complexes in the stable transfectants with wild type ER. Tamoxifen was a complete estrogen at the TGF-α gene *(65),* whereas raloxifene was an antiestrogen *(66).* Most importantly, the D351Y transfected cells converted raloxifene from an antiestrogen to an estrogen *(66).* We conclude that aspartate at amino acid 351 was extremely important for the expression of antiestrogenic and estrogenic actions of raloxifene because a mutation to tyrosine changes the relationship of the ligand side chain and the protein *(67).* The interactions of the piperidine ring that shields the charge at the small aspartate is no longer possible when tyrosine is substituted so coactivators can now activate the D351Y: ER raloxifene complex to transcribe TGF-α. The hypothesis was consolidated with further information about the 4-hydroxytamoxifen: ER complex. Norris and coworkers *(82)* used a phage-display assay to identify different coactivator binding sites on the estradiol and 4-hydroxytamoxifen: ER complex (Fig. 8). It was reasoned that the 4-hydroxytamoxifen: ER complex could have a binding site for coactivators that included aspartate 351. If the binding of coactivators at the novel site, (which we have named AF2b), is dependent on a correctly positioned negative charge for LXXLL binding, then removal of the charge or displacement of the charge should result in loss of estrogen-like properties for the 4-hydroxytamoxifen ER complex. Addressing the first point, a D351G cDNA stable transfectant was prepared in MDA-MB-231 and it was found that 4-hydroxytamoxifen loses estrogen-like properties but retains antiestrogenic properties *(83)*. Most importantly, these data demonstrate that it is possible to silence the "constitutive activity" of AF1 in the 4-hydroxytamoxifen: ER complex by an allosteric interaction at the ligand-binding domain. To the second point, a novel derivative of tamoxifen called GW 7604 was examined. Unlike all other SERMs, GW 7604 and the pro-drug GW 5638 (Fig. 4) have an antiestrogenic side chain that contains a carboxylic acid rather than a tertiary nitrogen atom. The pro-drug has virtually no uterotropic activity in the rat but is estrogen-like in the bone *(57,84)* and is classified as a novel SERM with actions on the ER like a pure antiestrogen *(85)*. Computer-assisted ligand docking showed *(86)* that GW 7604, the presumed active metabolite of GW 5638, dramatically repels AA 351 aspartate, and this is correlated with a loss of estrogen-like properties at the TGF-α gene. In broad terms, we reclassified GW 7604 as a raloxifene-like drug because D351Y ER weakly reactivates the TGF-α gene *(86)*.

In summary, the previous models of estrogen and antiestrogen action *(70,74,75,87)* have recently been advanced to describe a complex interaction between putative coactivators for the ER complex that could control SERM actions. The site for coactivator binding on the E_2 ER complex (AF2) is distinct from the site on the 4-hydroxytamoxifen: ER complex (AF2b) *(83,86)*. Norris and coworkers originally proposed a new coactivator site on the ER, which they call AF2a *(88)*. However, the site is probably more complex than originally thought as it must involve helix 12 and a correctly positioned and charged amino acid at the surface site 351 that then acts synergistically *(89)* with AF1. This new SERM site AF2b could be a target for further drug discovery, but only if there is selective specificity at the target site that would avoid general toxicity. Indeed, it has recently been shown that the intrinsic estrogenicity of the complex can easily be modulated through alterations in the charge of the amino acid in position 351 *(89)*.

11. FINAL THOUGHTS

We were encouraged to edit this book by the proven success of endocrine therapy for breast and prostate cancer. Thirty years ago, none of the targeted therapeutic agents routinely used today was available to the physician. We offer this volume as proof of principle that targets in cancer can be discovered and that drugs with selective toxicity to the tumor and not the host can be developed. This is not a new idea, but it is one that was almost forgotten during the past 40 years of testing cytotoxic chemotherapy. The concept of destroying a parasite with chemotherapy was demonstrated just when Professor Paul

Ehrlich successfully tested his 606th compound salvarsan to cure syphilis nearly 100 years ago *(90)*.

The key to rational drug discovery in cancer is either the application of a novel chemopreventive strategy *(91,92)* or the identification of an appropriate target in the tumor. The use of the proposed SERM strategy *(27)* to develop a molecule to prevent osteoporosis but to reduce the risk of breast cancer is a further idea that has been exploited with some success. Raloxifene is available to prevent osteoporosis *(28,93)*, but with a reduction in breast-cancer incidence *(29,94)* compared with the elevated risk observed with hormone-replacement therapy. The wide-spread use of SERMs, i.e., tamoxifen and raloxifene, will potentially reduce the incidence of breast cancer, but these agents will also shift the primary endocrine treatment of breast cancer away from tamoxifen towards aromatase inhibition or the use of a pure antiestrogen such as Faslodex. Additionally, patients who receive SERMs for prevention will admittedly have reduced incidence of breast cancer, but an increased proportion of endocrine-refractory breast cancer. New targets are currently being developed to address this treatment issue specifically. Tumor-specific tyrosine kinase inhibitors such as Irressa are proving successful in a wide range of cancers.

However, future targets are required for effective chemoprevention and treatment in breast and prostate cancer. The completion of the Human Genome Project to sequence each chromosome and the application of gene array technology *(95)* will allow the description of novel pathways to modulate cell replication and apoptosis. These molecular targets will extend the proven principles illustrated in this volume.

REFERENCES

1. Fisher B, Costantino JP, Wickerham DL, Redmond CK, Kavanah M, Cronin WM, et al. Tamoxifen for prevention of breast cancer: report of the National Surgical Adjuvant Breast and Bowel Project P-1 Study. *J Natl Cancer Inst* 1998; 90:1371–1388.
2. Gail MH, Brinton LA, Byar DP, Corle DK, Green SB, Schairer C, Mulvihill JJ. Projecting individualized probabilities of developing breast cancer for white females who are being examined annually. *J Natl Cancer Inst* 1989; 81:1879–1886.
3. Spiegelman D, Colditz GA, Hunter D, Hertzmark E. Validation of the Gail et al. model for predicting individual breast cancer risk. *J Natl Cancer Inst* 1994; 86:600–607.
4. Bondy ML, Lustbader ED, Halabi S, Ross E, Vogel VG. Validation of a breast cancer risk assessment model in women with a positive family history. *J Natl Cancer Inst* 1994; 86:620–625.
5. Costantino JP, Gail MH, Pee D, Anderson S, Redmond CK, Benichou J, Wieand HS. Validation studies for models projecting the risk of invasive and total breast cancer incidence. *J Natl Cancer Inst* 1999; 91:1541–1548.
6. EBCTCG Tamoxifen for early breast cancer: an overview of the randomised trials. *Lancet* 1998; 351:1451–1467.

7. Fisher B, Dignam J, Wolmark N, Wickerham DL, Fisher ER, Mamounas E, et al. Tamoxifen in treatment of intraductal breast cancer: National Surgical Adjuvant Breast and Bowel Project B-24 randomised controlled trial. *Lancet* 1999; 353:1993–2000.

8. Wickerham DL, Costantino J, Fisher B, Kavanah M, Wolmark N. Average annual rates of invasive and noninvasive breast cancer by history of LCIS and atypical hyperplasia for participants in the BCPT, in *Proceedings of the American Society for Clinical Oncology,* 1999, pp 87a (#327).

9. Love RR, Mazess RB, Barden HS, Epstein S, Newcomb PA, Jordan VC, et al. Effects of tamoxifen on bone mineral density in postmenopausal women with breast cancer. *N Engl J Med* 1992; 326:852–856.

10. Reis SE, Constantino JP, Wickerham DL, Tan-Chiu E, Wang J, Kavanah M. Cardiovascular effects of tamoxifen in women with and without heart disease: breast cancer prevention trial. National Surgical Adjuvant Breast and Bowel Project Breast Cancer Prevention Trial Investigators. *J Natl Cancer Inst* 2001; Jan 3;93:16–21.

11. Jordan VC. Effect of tamoxifen (ICI 46,474) on initiation and growth of DMBA-induced rat mammary carcinomata. *Eur J Cancer* 1976; 12:419–424.

12. Powles T, Eeles R, Ashley S, Easton D, Chang J, Dowsett M, et al. Interim analysis of the incidence of breast cancer in the Royal Marsden Hospital tamoxifen randomised chemoprevention trial. *Lancet* 1998; 352:98–101.

13. Veronesi U, Maisonneuve P, Costa A, Sacchini V, Maltoni C, Robertson C, et al. Prevention of breast cancer with tamoxifen: preliminary findings from the Italian randomised trial among hysterectomised women. Italian Tamoxifen Prevention Study. *Lancet* 1998; 352:93–97.

14. Powles TJ, Hardy JR, Ashley SE, Farrington GM, Cosgrove D, Davey JB, et al. A pilot trial to evaluate the acute toxicity and feasibility of tamoxifen for prevention of breast cancer. *Br J Cancer* 1989; 60:126–131.

15. Assikis VJ, Jordan VC. Gynecologic effects of tamoxifen and the association with endometrial carcinoma. *Intl J Gynaecol Obstet* 1995; 49:241–257.

16. Bernstein L, Deapen D, Cerhan JR, Schwartz SM, Liff J, McGann-Maloney E, et al. Tamoxifen therapy for breast cancer and endometrial cancer risk. *J Natl Cancer Inst* 1999; 91:1654–1662.

17. Bergman L, Beelen ML, Gallee MP, Hollema H, Benraadt J, van Leeuwen FE. Risk and prognosis of endometrial cancer after tamoxifen for breast cancer. Comprehensive Cancer Centres' ALERT Group. Assessment of Liver and Endometrial cancer Risk following Tamoxifen. *Lancet* 2000; 356:881–887.

18. Day R, Ganz PA, Costantino JP, Cronin WM, Wickerham DL, Fisher B. Health-related quality of life and tamoxifen in breast cancer prevention: A report from the National Surgical Adjuvant Breast and Bowel Project P-1 study. *J Clin Oncol* 1999; 17:2659–2669.

19. Fallowfield L, Fleissig A, Edwards R, West A, Powles TJ, Howell A, Cuzick J. Tamoxifen for the prevention of breast cancer: psychological impact on women participating in two randomized controlled trials. *J Clin Oncol* 2001; 19:1885–1892.

20. Decensi A, Robertson C, Rotmensz N, Severi G, Maisonneuve P, Sacchini V, et al. Effect of tamoxifen and transdermal hormone replacement therapy on cardiovascular risk factors in a prevention trial. Italian Chemoprevention Group. *Br J Cancer* 1998; 78:572–578.

21. Decensi A, Bonanni B, Guerrieri-Gonzaga A, Gandini S, Robertson C, Johansson H, et al. Biologic activity of tamoxifen at low doses in healthy women. *J Natl Cancer Inst* 1998; 90:1461–1467.

22. Decensi A, Gandini S, Guerrieri-Gonzaga A, Johansson H, Manetti L, Bonanni B, et al. Effect of blood tamoxifen concentrations on surrogate biomarkers in a trial of dose reduction in healthy women. *J Clin Oncol* 1999; 17:2633–2638.

23. Costa A, Bonanni B, Manetti L, Guerrieri Gonzaga A, Torrisi R, Decensi A. Prevention of breast cancer: focus on chemoprevention. *Recent Results Cancer Res* 1998; 152:11–21.

24. Gottardis MM, Jordan VC. Antitumor actions of keoxifene and tamoxifen in the N-nitro-somethylurea-induced rat mammary carcinoma model. *Cancer Res* 1987; 47:4020–4024.

25. Jordan VC, Robinson SP. Species-specific pharmacology of antiestrogens: role of metabolism. *Fed Proc* 1987; 46:1870–1874.

26. Jordan VC, Phelps E, Lindgren JU. Effects of anti-estrogens on bone in castrated and intact female rats. *Breast Cancer Res Treat* 1987; 10:31–35.

27. Lerner LJ, Jordan VC. Development of antiestrogens and their use in breast cancer: Eighth Cain memorial award lecture. *Cancer Res* 1990; 50:4177–4189.

28. Delmas PD, Bjarnason NH, Mitlak BH, Ravoux AC, Shah AS, Huster WJ, et al. Effects of raloxifene on bone mineral density, serum cholesterol concentrations, and uterine endometrium in postmenopausal women. *N Engl J Med* 1997; 337:1641–1647.

29. Cummings SR, Eckert S, Krueger KA, Grady D, Powles TJ, Cauley JA, et al. The effect of raloxifene on risk of breast cancer in postmenopausal women: results from the MORE randomized trial. Multiple Outcomes of Raloxifene Evaluation. *JAMA* 1999; 281:2189–2197.

30. Jordan VC, Morrow M. Tamoxifen, raloxifene, and the prevention of breast cancer. *Endocr Rev* 1999; 20:253–278.

31. Osborne CK. Tamoxifen in the treatment of breast cancer. *N Engl J Med* 1998; 339:1609–1618.

32. Howell A, Robertson JFR, Quaresma Albano J, et al. Comparison of the efficacy of Fulvestrant (Faslodex) with Anastrozole (Arimidex) in post menopausal women with advanced breast cancer. *Breast Cancer Res Treat* 2000; 64:27 (Abstr 6).

33. Osborne CK, on behalf of the North American Faslodex Investigator Group. A double blind randomized trial comparing the efficacy and tolerability of Faslodex (Fulvestrant) with Arimidex (Anastrozole) in postmenopausal women with advanced breast cancer. *Breast Cancer Res Treat* 2000; 64:27(Abstr 7).

34. Bonneterre J, Thurlimann B, Robertson JF, Krzakowski M, Mauriac L, Koralewski P, et al. Anastrozole versus tamoxifen as first-line therapy for advanced breast cancer in 668 postmenopausal women: results of the tamoxifen or arimidex randomized group efficacy and tolerability study. *J Clin Oncol* 2000; 18(22):3748–3757.

35. Nabholtz JM, Buzdar A, Pollark M, Harwin W, Burton G, et al. Anastrozole is superior to tamoxifen as first-line therapy for advanced breast cancer in postmenopausal women: results of a North American multicenter randomized trial. Arimidex study group. *J Clin Oncol* 2000; 18(22):3758–3767.

36. Levenson AS, Jordan VC. MCF-7: the first hormone-responsive breast cancer cell line. *Cancer Res* 1997; 57:3071–3078.

37. Berns EM, Foekens JA, Vossen R, Look MP, Devilee P, Henzen-Logmans SC, et al. Complete sequencing of TP53 predicts poor response to systemic therapy of advanced breast cancer. *Cancer Res* 2000; 60:2155–2162.

38. Welshons WV, Jordan VC. Adaptation of estrogen-dependent MCF-7 cells to low estrogen (phenol red-free) culture. *Eur J Cancer Clin Oncol* 1987; 23:1935–1939.

39. Katzenellenbogen BS, Kendra KL, Norman MJ, Berthois Y. Proliferation, hormonal responsiveness, and estrogen receptor content of MCF-7 human breast cancer cells grown in the short-term and long-term absence of estrogens. *Cancer Res* 1987; 47:4355–4360.

40. Pink JJ, Jiang SY, Fritsch M, Jordan VC. An estrogen-independent MCF-7 breast cancer cell line which contains a novel 80-kilodalton estrogen receptor-related protein. *Cancer Res* 1995; 55:2583–2590.

41. Keydar I, Chen L, Karby S, Weiss FR, Delarea J, Radu M, et al. Establishment and characterization of a cell line of human breast carcinoma origin. *Eur J Cancer* 1979; 15:659–670.

42. Pink JJ, Bilimoria MM, Assikis J, Jordan VC. Irreversible loss of the estrogen receptor in T47D breast cancer cells following prolonged estrogen deprivation [published erratum appears in *Br J Cancer* 1997; 75:1557]. *Br J Cancer* 1996; 74:1227–1236.

43. Dembinski TC, Leung CK, Shiu RP. Evidence for a novel pituitary factor that potentiates the mitogenic effect of estrogen in human breast cancer cells. *Cancer Res* 1985; 45:3083–3089.

44. MacGregor Schafer J, Lee E-S, O'Regan RM, Yao K, Jordan VC. Rapid development of tamoxifen stimulated mutant p53 breast tumors (T47D) in athymic mice. *Clin Cancer Res* 2000; 6:4373–4380.

45. Lee E-S, MacGregor Schafer J, Yao K, England G, O'Regan RM, De los Reyes A, Jordan VC. Cross resistance of triphenylethylene-type antiestrogen but not ICI 182,780 in tamoxifen-stimulated breast tumors grown in athymic mice. *Clin Cancer Res* 2000; 6:4893–4899.

46. MacGregor Schafer J, Lee E-S, Dardes RC, Bentrem DJ, O'Regan RM, De los Reyes A, Jordan VC. Analysis of cross-resistance of the selective estrogen receptor modulators arzoxifene (LY353381) and LY117018 in tamoxifen-stimulated breast cancer xenografts. *Clin Cancer Res* 2001; in press.

47. O'Regan RM, Cisneros A, England GM, MacGregor JI, Muenzner HD, Assikis VJ, et al. Effects of the antiestrogens tamoxifen, toremifene, and ICI 182,780 on endometrial cancer growth. *J Natl Cancer Inst* 1998; 90:1552–1558.

48. Bilimoria MM, Assikis VJ, Jordan VC. Should adjuvant tamoxifen therapy be stopped at 5 years? *Cancer J Sci Am* 1996; 2:140.

49. Fisher B, Dignam J, Bryant J, DeCillis A, Wickerham DL, Wolmark N, et al. Five versus more than five years of tamoxifen therapy for breast cancer patients with negative lymph nodes and estrogen receptor-positive tumors. *J Natl Cancer Inst* 1996; 88:1529–1542.

50. Osborne CK, Coronado EB, Robinson JP. Human breast cancer in the athymic nude mouse: cytostatic effects of long-term antiestrogen therapy. *Eur J Cancer Clin Oncol* 1987; 23:1189–1196.

51. Gottardis MM, Jordan VC. Development of tamoxifen-stimulated growth of MCF-7 tumors in athymic mice after long-term antiestrogen administration. *Cancer Res* 1988; 48:5183–5187.

52. Yao K, Lee ES, Bentrem DJ, England G, Schafer JI, O'Regan RM, Jordan VC. Antitumor action of physiological estradiol on tamoxifen-stimulated breast tumors grown in athymic mice. *Clin Cancer Res* 2000; 6:2028–2036.

53. Ke HZ, Simmons HA, Pirie CM, Crawford DT, Thompson DD. Droloxifene, a new estrogen antagonist/agonist, prevents bone loss in ovariectomized rats. *Endocrinology* 1995; 136:2435–2441.

54. Rauschning W, Pritchard KI. Droloxifene, a new antiestrogen: its role in metastatic breast cancer. *Breast Cancer Res Treat* 1994; 31:83–94.

55. Nuttal ME, Bradbeer JN, Stroup GB, Nadeau DP, Hoffman SJ, Zhao H, et al. Idoxifene: a novel selective estrogen receptor modulator prevents bone loss and lowers choleterol levels in ovariectomized rats and decreases uterine weight in intact rats. *Endocrinology* 1998; 139:5224–5234.

56. Johnston SR, Boeddinghaus IM, Riddler S, Haynes BP, Hardcastle IR, Rowlands M, et al. Idoxifene antagonizes estradiol-dependent MCF-7 breast cancer xenograft growth through sustained induction of apoptosis. *Cancer Res* 1999; 59:3646–3651.

57. Willson TM, Norris JD, Wagner BL, Asplin I, Baer P, Brown HR, et al. Dissection of the molecular mechanism of action of GW5638, a novel estrogen receptor ligand, provides insights into the role of estrogen receptor in bone. *Endocrinology* 1997; 138:3901–3911.

58. Ke HZ, Paralkar VM, Grasser WA, Crawford DT, Qi H, Simmons HA, et al. Effects of CP-336,156, a new, nonsteroidal estrogen agonist/antagonist, on bone, serum cholesterol, uterus and body composition in rat models. *Endocrinology* 1998; 139:2068–2076.

59. Connor CE, Norris JD, Broadwater G, Willson TM, Gottardis MM, Dewhirst MW, McDonnell DP. Circumventing tamoxifen resistance in breast cancers using antiestrogens that induce unique conformational changes in the estrogen receptor. *Cancer Res* 2001; 61:2917–2922.

60. Sato M, Turner CH, Wang T, Adrian MD, Rowley E, Bryant, HU. LY353381.HCl: a novel raloxifene analog with improved SERM potency and efficacy in vivo. *J Pharmacol Exp Ther* 1998; 287:1–7.

61. Snyder KR, Sparano N, Malinowski JM. Raloxifene hydrochloride. *Am J Health Syst Pharm* 2000; 57:1669–1678.

62. Munster PN, Buzdar A, Dhingra K, Enas N, Ni, L, Major M, et al. Phase I study of a third-generation selective estrogen receptor modulator, LY353381.HCl, in metastatic breast cancer. *J Clin Oncol* 2001; 19, No. 7:2002–2009.

63. Labrie F, Labrie C, Belanger A, Simard J, Gauthier S, Luu-The V, et al. EM-652 (SCH 57068), a third generation SERM acting as pure antiestrogen in the mammary gland and endometrium. *J Steroid Biochem Mol Biol* 1999; 69:51–84.

64. Gauthier S, Caron B, Cloutier J, Dory YL, Favre A, Larouche D, et al. (S)-(+)-4-[7-(2,2-dimethyl-1-oxopropoxy)-4-methyl-2-[4-[2-(1-piperidinyl)-ethoxy]phenyl]-2H-1-benzopyran-3-yl]-phenyl2,2-dimethylpropanoate (EM-800): a highly potent, specific, and orally active nonsteroidal antiestrogen. *J Med Chem* 1997; 40:2117–2122.

65. Levenson, AS, Tonetti DA, Jordan VC. The estrogen-like effect of 4-hydroxytamoxifen on induction of transforming growth factor alpha mRNA in MDA-MB-231 breast cancer cells stably expressing the estrogen receptor. *Br J Cancer* 1998; 77:1812–1819.

66. Levenson, AS, Catherino WH, Jordan VC. Estrogenic activity is increased for an antiestrogen by a natural mutation of the estrogen receptor. *J Steroid Biochem Mol Biol* 1997; 60:261–268.

67. Levenson, AS. Jordan VC. The key to the antiestrogenic mechanism of raloxifene is amino acid 351 (aspartate) in the estrogen receptor. *Cancer Res* 1998; 58:1872–1875.

68. MacGregor Schafer J, Liu H, Tonetti DA, Jordan VC. The interaction of raloxifene and the active metabolite of the antiestrogen EM-800 (SC 5705) with the human estrogen receptor. *Cancer Res* 1999; 59:4308–4313.

69. Martel C, Picard S, Richard V, Belanger A, Labrie C, Labrie F Prevention of bone loss by EM-800 and raloxifene in the ovariectomized rat. *J Steroid Biochem Mol Biol* 2000; 74:45–56.

70. Brzozowski AM, Pike AC, Dauter Z, Hubbard RE, Bonn T, Engstrom O, et al. Molecular basis of agonism and antagonism in the estrogen receptor. *Nature* 1997; 389:753–758.

71. Shiau AK, Barstad D, Loria PM, Cheng L, Kushner PJ, Agard DA, Greene GL. The structural basis of estrogen receptor/coactivator recognition and the antagonism of this interaction by tamoxifen. *Cell* 1998; 95:927–937.

72. Pike AC, Brzozowski AM, Hubbard RE, Bonn T, Thorsell AG, Engstrom O, et al. Structure of the ligand-binding domain of estrogen receptor beta in the presence of a partial agonist and a full antagonist. *EMBO J* 1999; 18:4608–4618.

73. Pike AC, Brzozowski AM, Walton J, Hubbard RE, Thorsell A, Li Y, et al. Structural insights into the mode of action of a pure antiestrogen. *Structure* 2001; 9(2):145–153.

74. Lieberman ME, Gorski J, Jordan VC. An estrogen receptor model to describe the regulation of prolactin synthesis by antiestrogens in vitro. *J Biol Chem* 1983; 258:4741–4745.

75. Tate AC, Greene GL, DeSombre ER, Jensen EV, Jordan VC. Differences between estrogen- and antiestrogen-estrogen receptor complexes from human breast tumors identified with an antibody raised against the estrogen receptor. *Cancer Res* 1984; 44:1012–1018.

76. Berry M, Metzger D Chambon P. Role of the two activating domains of the estrogen receptor in the cell-type and promoter-context dependent agonistic activity of the anti- estrogen 4-hydroxytamoxifen. *EMBO J* 1990; 9:2811–2818.

77. Wolf DM, Jordan VC. Characterization of tamoxifen stimulated MCF-7 tumor variants grown in athymic mice. *Breast Cancer Res Treat* 1994; 31:117–127.

78. Wolf DM, Jordan VC. The estrogen receptor from a tamoxifen stimulated MCF-7 tumor variant contains a point mutation in the ligand binding domain. *Breast Cancer Res Treat* 1994; 31:129–138.

79. Anghel SI, Perly V, Melancon G, Barsalou A, Chagnon S, Rosenauer A, et al. Aspartate 351 of estrogen receptor alpha is not crucial for the antagonist activity of antiestrogens. *J Biol Chem* 2000; 275:20867–20872.

80. Jiang SY, Jordan VC. Growth regulation of estrogen receptor-negative breast cancer cells transfected with complementary DNAs for estrogen receptor. *J Natl Cancer Inst* 1992; 84:580–591.

81. Jeng MH, Jiang SY, Jordan VC. Paradoxical regulation of estrogen-dependent growth factor gene expression in estrogen receptor (ER)-negative human breast cancer cells stably expressing ER. *Cancer Lett* 1994; 82:123–128.

82. Norris JD, Paige LA, Christensen DJ, Chang CY, Huacani MR, Fan D, et al. Peptide antagonists of the human estrogen receptor. *Science* 1999; 285:744–746.

83. MacGregor Schafer J, Liu H, Bentrem DJ, Zapf JW, Jordan VC. Allosteric silencing of activating function 1 in the 4-hydroxytamoxifen estrogen receptor complex is induced by substituting glycine for aspartate at amino acid 351. *Cancer Res* 2000; 60:5097–5105.

84. Willson TM, Henke BR, Momtahen TM, Charifson PS, Batchelor KW, Lubahn DB, et al. 3-[4-(1,2-Diphenylbut-1-enyl)phenyl]acrylic acid: a non-steroidal estrogen with functional selectivity for bone over uterus in rats. *J Med Chem* 1994; 37:1550–1552.

85. Wijayaratne AL, Nagel SC, Paige LA, Christensen DJ, Norris JD, Fowlkes DM, McDonnell DP. Comparative analyses of mechanistic differences among antiestrogens. *Endocrinology* 1999; 140:5828–5840.

86. Bentrem DJ, Dardes RC, Liu H, MacGregor-Schafer JI, Zapf JW, Jordan VC. Molecular mechanism of action at estrogen receptor alpha of a new clinically relevant antiestrogen (GW7604) related to tamoxifen. *Endocrinology* 2001; 142:838–846.

87. McDonnell DP, Clemm DL, Hermann T, Goldman ME, Pike JW. Analysis of estrogen receptor function in vitro reveals three distinct classes of antiestrogens. *Mol Endocrinol* 1995; 9:659–669.

88. Norris JD, Fan D, Kerner SA, McDonnell DP. Identification of a third autonomous activation domain within the human estrogen receptor. *Mol Endocrinol* 1997; 11:747–754.

89. Liu H, Lee ES, De Los Reyes A, Zapf JW, Jordan VC. Silencing and reactivation of the estrogen receptor modulator (SERM)-ER alpha complex. *Cancer Res,* 2001; 61:3632–3639.

90. Baumler E. *Paul Ehrlich, Scientist for Life.* Holmes & Meier, New York, 1984, p 288.

91. Sporn MB. Approaches to prevention of epithelial cancer during the preneoplastic period. *Cancer Res* 1976; 36:2699–2702.

92. Sporn MB, Dunlop NM, Newton DL, Smith JM. Prevention of chemical carcinogenesis by vitamin A and its synthetic analogs (retinoids). *Fed Proc* 1976; 35:1332–1338.

93. Ettinger B, Black DM, Mitlak BH, Knickerbocker RK, Nickelsen T, Genant H K, et al. Reduction of vertebral fracture risk in postmenopausal women with osteoporosis treated with raloxifene: results from a 3-year randomized clinical trial. Multiple Outcomes of Raloxifene Evaluation (MORE) Investigators. *JAMA* 1999; 282:637–645.

94. Cauley JA, Norton L, Lippman ME, Eckert S, Krueger KA, Purdie DW, et al. Continued breast cancer risk reduction in postmenopausal women treated with raloxifene: 4-year results from the MORE trial. *Breast Cancer Res Treat* 2001; 65(2):125–134.

95. Perou CM, Sorlie T, Eisen MB, van de Rijn M, Jeffrey SS, Rees CA, et al. Molecular portraits of human breast tumours. *Nature* 2000; 406:747–752.

Index

409